HEALTH AND SAFETY FOR TOXICITY TESTING

HEALTH AND SAFETY FOR TOXICITY TESTING

Edited by

Douglas B. Walters
Head, Chemical Health and Safety Section/
   Program Resources Branch
National Institute of Environmental Health Sciences (USDHHS)
Research Triangle Park, North Carolina

C.W. Jameson
Head, Chemistry Section/
   Program Resources Branch
National Institute of Environmental Health Sciences (USDHHS)
Research Triangle Park, North Carolina

BUTTERWORTH PUBLISHERS
Boston • London
Sidney • Wellington • Durban • Toronto

An Ann Arbor Science Book

Ann Arbor Science is an imprint of Butterworth Publishers.

Library of Congress Cataloging in Publication Data
Main entry under title:

Health and safety for toxicity testing.

   Bibliography: p.
   Includes index.
   1. Toxicity testing—Safety measures.   2. Chemical laboratories—
Safety measures.   I. Walters, Douglas B.   II. Jameson, C.W.
[DNLM 1. Laboratories—Standards—Congresses.   2. Accidents,
Occupational—Prevention and control—Congresses.
3. Toxicology—Standards—Congresses.   4. Environmental
pollution—Prevention and control—Congresses. WA465 H4337 1982]
RA119.H43   1984   615.9'07   83-20846
ISBN 0-250-40546-6

Butterworth Publishers
80 Montvale Avenue
Stoneham, MA 02180

10 9 8 7 6 5 4 3 2 1

Printed in the United States of America

To Eugene T. Walters, Sr.,
whose love and devotion helped foster the belief:

*You are never given a wish without also being given the power to make it true.
You may have to work for it, however.*

Richard Bach, *Illusions* 1977

CONTENTS

The Editors   ix

The Contributors   xi

Preface   xiii

I. **DESIGN AND FACILITIES**   1

1. Chemical Health and Safety Concerns for Toxicity Testing
    in the National Toxicology Program
    Douglas B. Walters   3

2. Chemical Containment Design Criteria for Toxicity Testing
    Facilities
    Douglas B. Walters, R. Scott Stricoff, and James M. Harless   33

3. Components in the Design of a Hazardous Chemicals Handling
    Facility
    James M. Harless   45

4. Health and Safety in the Design of Toxicity Testing
    Laboratories
    R. Scott Stricoff, E. Robinson Hoyle, and Douglas B. Walters   73

5. Barrier Laboratory Facilities: A Fire Control Manager's
    Perspective
    Robert G. Nemchin   91

6. Hazard Containment in an Inhalation Toxicology Laboratory
    W.B. Reid, J.R. Klok, and B.K.J. Leong   111

7. Human Factors Considerations in the Handling of Toxic
    Chemicals
    Eileen J. Phelan, Carla M. Snyder, and Douglas B. Walters   121

II. **ESTABLISHMENT OF A SAFETY PROGRAM**   135

8. Preparation of Chemical-Specific Health and Safety
    Documents
    *Andrew T. Prokopetz, Douglas B. Walters, William S.
    Baillargeon, Elizabeth M. Prescott, and R. Scott Stricoff*   137

9. The Requirements and Pitfalls of Laboratory Worker Medical Surveillance
   G. Stewart Young   159

10. Safety Training Programs for Toxicity Testing Laboratories
    J. David Sakura   183

11. A Respirator Protection Program for Toxicology Laboratories
    Joseph A. Coco   193

III. SAFETY MONITORING AND MANAGEMENT   211

12. Practical Aspects of Packaging and Shipping Test Chemicals for Research
    Richard L. Trammell, Lawrence H. Keith, Douglas B. Walters, and Andrew T. Prokopetz   213

13. Bulk Chemical Management for Chronic Toxicity Studies
    Steven W. Graves, E.J. Woodhouse, K.M. Stelting, and C. W. Jameson   221

14. Safety Problems in a Chemical Testing Program
    Henry Mahar, and Richard E. Shaff   241

15. Laboratory Hood Performance in Toxicity Testing Laboratories
    E. Robinson Hoyle, R. Scott Stricoff, and Douglas B. Walters   255

16. Industrial Hygiene Monitoring of Chemical Contaminants at Bioassay Laboratories
    J.J. Beres   275

IV. WASTE MANAGEMENT   281

17. A Risk Assessment Program for Toxicology Laboratory Waste Disposal
    Robert G. Nemchin and Joseph A. Coco   283

18. Chemical-Contaminated Waste Management: Disposal Concerns, Regulations and Surplus Chemicals
    Neil B. Jurinski   299

19. Incinerator Design and Operation for Chemical Waste Disposal
    Maurice W. Hunt   309

INDEX   335

THE EDITORS

DOUGLAS B. WALTERS

Douglas B. Walters is head of the Chemical Health and Safety Section for the Program Resources Branch at the National Institute of Environmental Health Sciences (USDHHS) in Research Triangle Park, North Carolina. He is the former chief of the safety office and the former technical programs manager of the Laboratory of Environmental Chemistry at National Institute of Environmental Health Sciences. His Ph.D. was earned at the University of Georgia concentrating on the analytical chemistry of metal-complex interactions using NMR spectroscopy and organophosphorus synthesis. Until 1977 he was an active researcher with the USDA's Tobacco and Health Program specializing in the fractionation, characterization, and bioassay of cigarette smoke.

Since joining National Institute of Environmental Health Sciences, he has been involved in diverse projects which apply chemistry principles to a broad range of environmental health and safety concerns. Included in these areas are the design of high-hazard chemistry laboratories, establishment of a chemical repository with associated analytical and synthetic support, implementation of a comprehensive health and safety program, and foundation of health and safety guidelines and requirements for various types of toxicology studies. Dr. Walters' work covers a range of areas of interest including: design of specialty equipment and facilities for chemical containment; application of human factors engineering to chemical health and safety; chemical control and management of environmental quality, health and safety in multidisciplinary operations; and use and application of chemical health and safety information. He has organized, developed, and implemented internationally recognized programs in chemical health and safety for the National Toxicology Program which utilize interdisciplinary knowledge of chemistry, industrial hygiene, and toxicology as applied to problems of environmental concern.

Dr. Walters is the current chairman and past secretary of the Division of Chemical Health and Safety of the American Chemical Society (ACS). He is the past chairman of the Northeast Georgia Section of the ACS and was appointed by the National ACS headquarters from 1973 to 1978 as ACS science advisor to U.S. Senator Herman Talmadge and U.S. Congressmen Robert G. Stephens and Doug Barnard, all of Georgia. He has lectured throughout the United States and is the author or coauthor of numerous publications, including 17 book chapters.

Dr. Walters has edited the unique two-volume set *Safe Handling of Chemical Carcinogens, Mutagens, Teratogens and Highly Toxic Substances,* and serves on the editorial board of the *International Journal of Chemical Health and Safety* and the *Handbook of Environmental Chemistry: Chemical Waste* volume.

C.W. JAMESON

C.W. Jameson, a research chemist at the National Institute of Environmental Health Sciences (USDHHS) in Research Triangle Park, North Carolina, is the Acting Chief for the Program Resources Branch and is also head of the Chemistry Section of that branch. He received his Ph.D. from the University of Maryland, specializing in the synthesis and photochemistry of aliphatic amides and imides and the interaction of nuclear magnetic resonance shift reagents with substrates in solution. He has been an active participant in the National Institutes of Health's Carcinogenesis Testing Program since 1976.

Since joining the National Institute of Environmental Health Sciences, he has assumed responsibility for the chemistry aspects of the testing and research programs of the Toxicology Research and Testing Program. In addition, Dr. Jameson has served as program leader for chemistry in the Department of Health and Human Service's National Toxicology Program since its inception. In this position, he has developed chemistry standards for toxicity studies that have been widely accepted as an integral part of many toxicology testing programs.

Dr. Jameson is currently an active member of the Division of Analytical Chemistry of the American Chemical Society, serving as a member of the division's Committee on Regulatory Affairs. He has lectured throughout the United States and is the author or coauthor of numerous publications.

THE CONTRIBUTORS

William S. Baillargeon
Radian Corporation
Austin, Texas

J.J. Beres
IBM
Manassas, Virginia

Joseph A. Coco
Office of Occupational Safety and
    Health
Litton Bionetics, Inc.
Kensington, Maryland

Steven W. Graves
Midwest Research Institute
Kansas City, Missouri

James M. Harless
Radian Corporation
Austin, Texas

E. Robinson Hoyle
Arthur D. Little, Inc.
Acorn Park
Cambridge, Massachusetts

Maurice W. Hunt
Rollins Environmental Services (NJ)
    Inc.
Bridgeport, New Jersey

C.W. Jameson
National Toxicology Program
Research Triangle Park,
    North Carolina

Neil B. Jurinski
NuChemCo, Inc.
Burke, Virginia

Lawrence H. Keith
Radian Corporation
Austin, Texas

J.R. Klok
Client Engineering, Pharmaceutical
    Research and Development
The Upjohn Company
Kalamazoo, Michigan

B.K.J. Leong
Industrial Toxicology Laboratory
The Upjohn Company
Kalamazoo, Michigan

Harry Mahar
Division of Safety
National Institutes of Health
Public Health Service
U.S. Department of Health and
    Human Services
Bethesda, Maryland

Robert G. Nemchin
Office of Occupational Safety and
    Health
Litton Bionetics, Inc.
Kensington, Maryland

E.J. Phelan
Westinghouse Electric Corporation
Baltimore, Maryland

Andrew T. Prokopetz
National Toxicology Program
Research Triangle Park,
   North Carolina

Elizabeth M. Prescott
Arthur D. Little, Inc.
Acorn Park
Cambridge, Massachusetts

W.B. Reid
Facility Planning and Environmental
   Regulatory Affairs
The Upjohn Company
Kalamazoo, Michigan

J. David Sakura
Arthur D. Little, Inc.
Acorn Park
Cambridge, Massachusetts

Richard E. Shaff
Division of Safety
National Institutes of Health
Public Health Service
U.S. Department of Health and
   Human Services
Bethesda, Maryland

K.M. Stelting
Midwest Research Institute
Kansas City, Missouri

R. Scott Stricoff
Arthur D. Little, Inc.
Acorn Park
Cambridge, Massachusetts

Richard L. Trammell
Radian Corporation
Austin, Texas

Douglas B. Walters
National Toxicology Program
Research Triangle Park,
   North Carolina

E.J. Woodhouse
Midwest Research Institute
Kansas City, Missouri

G. Stewart Young
Arthur D. Little, Inc.
Acorn Park
Cambridge, Massachusetts

PREFACE

Toxicological characterization of environmental chemicals often involves potentially hazardous materials from both the acute and chronic standpoint. Such a toxicity testing program must protect both the worker and the environment, conform to guidelines and regulations, and help ensure the integrity of the study. Control of almost all health and safety concerns in this context center on an in-depth knowledge of the chemical-physical properties of the test chemicals. In addition, successful administration of such a program necessitates interdisciplinary knowledge and cooperation with fields such as industrial hygiene, engineering, toxicology, occupational medicine, information retrieval, biology, regulatory activities, and management. Input from chemical health and safety for such toxicology studies begins with the initial experimental design to ensure special requirements are met and to provide chemical-specific health and safety guidelines. Involvement continues through initial laboratory design evaluation, site visits, program reviews, report monitoring, recommended changes in procedures, facilities' design, as well as response to emergency situations and concern with eventual waste disposal and record archiving. Included in such a program is maintenance of a program-specific, state-of-the-art, chemical health and safety effort which encompasses: industrial hygiene surveys; chemical monitoring; periodic review of training needs; and formulation of standards, guidelines, and safety plans.

The origin of this book lies with the formulation of the National Toxicology Program (NTP) which was established by the secretary of the Department of Health, Education and Welfare (now DHHS) in November 1978. This program joined the toxicology testing efforts of the National Institutes of Health's National Institute of Environmental Health Sciences and National Cancer Institute; the Food and Drug Administration's National Center for Toxicological Research; and the Center for Disease Control's National Institute for Occupational Safety and Health. The goals of this program are to consolidate the departments' activities in toxicological testing of chemicals of public concern and to develop and validate new and better test methods. This department-wide effort provides scientifically tested information about potentially toxic chemicals to regulatory and research agencies.

The need for such a program evolved from increasing scientific, regulatory, and public concerns over the human health effects of environmental chemicals. Many increases in human diseases can be related to chemical exposure. Thus, decreasing and controlling such exposure should prevent many human diseases and disorders.

This book is an outgrowth of my earlier two-volume work *Safe Handling of Chemical Carcinogens, Mutagens, Teratogens and Highly Toxic Substances.* Much of what was presented at that time provided the foundation for the establishment of chemical health and safety efforts of the National Toxicology Program. The focus of this work is intended to reflect the broad knowledge and experience which has been gained since the formation of the National Toxicology Program. Chapters are included to describe chemical health and safety concerns on many aspects of *in vivo* toxicology testing. This includes information on chronic rodent bioassays using various methods of dose administration such as dosed feed, dosed water, gavage, skin painting, and inhalation. In addition, chemical containment control procedures for *in vitro* studies such as *Salmonella* microsome testing, *Drosophila* mutagenesis, cytogenetics, and other short-term tests are included.

The book is divided into four parts which focus on the progressive stages of chemical health and safety development in a toxicology testing program. Part I describes specific concerns, requirements, principles, and concepts for the design of facilities in which toxicology testing of environmental chemicals will be conducted. The novel source, path, receiver concept is presented in conjunction with chemical containment principles and the combined use of engineering controls, operational practices, and personal protection. Included are the often neglected areas of fire control in a barrier facility and human factors considerations in handling chemicals.

Part II describes some of the requirements for establishment of a safety program for toxicity testing laboratories. Included are chapters on the preparation of chemical-specific health and safety documents, training programs geared to professionals and highly trained workers, and requirements for a respirator protection program. Particularly unique is the chapter on requirements and pitfalls of medical surveillance programs for laboratory workers.

Once the toxicology testing program is established and operational, it becomes necessary to monitor and manage the program to ensure its effectiveness. Part III concerns problems encountered in day-to-day operations of such a program. Topics covered include practical aspects of packaging and shipping test chemicals for toxicology research, bulk chemical management, laboratory hood performance criteria, and industrial hygiene monitoring of chemical contaminants.

Part IV presents a new risk assessment approach for management of laboratory waste followed by in-depth discussions on waste management concerning actual disposal, regulations, and handling of surplus test chemicals. Finally a full description of proper incinerator design for disposal of hazardous chemicals is presented.

Contributors include authorities in the field who represent an extensive cross section of knowledge in the many aspects of chemical health and safety. Many disciplines are involved, illustrating the difficulties of a field which encompasses a diversity of expertise.

The chapters in this book, with the exception of 6 and 10, are adaptations of presentations from the symposium, "Chemistry and Safety for Toxicity Testing of Environmental Chemicals," which was presented at the 183rd national American Chemical Society meeting in Las Vegas, Nevada, in March 1982. Chapter 6 has been reprinted with permission from Basil Leong, the Upjohn Company, and Ann Arbor Science from Leong, Basil, K.J. Ed. *Inhalation Toxicology and Technology* (Ann Arbor, MI: Ann Arbor Science, 1981) pp. 1–10, and is included since it represents an excellent discussion of hazardous chemical containment in inhalation toxicity testing laboratories. Chapter 10 has been included to complete Part II and is an excellent discussion of training requirements and presents several thought-provoking ideas.

I said in my first books three years ago, "A work of this nature would have been very difficult to write a few years ago because of the scant knowledge available and the lack of concern toward safe chemistry." Current trends still indicate changes which are increasing our knowledge in this area, but we still have a long way to go. For example, four years ago the ACS Division of Chemical Health and Safety had approximately 350 members; today's membership now tops 1,300.

The interdisciplinary nature of chemical health and safety illustrates the need for all practitioners in the field to continually strive to bridge the communication gap which often exists between disciplines. In so doing, the quest for knowledge and order becomes a rapidly moving progression. We become continually motivated by the insight gained from other disciplines which can then be applied as new concepts to our own fields of expertise. I hope this book will stimulate further interest, growth, and research in this exciting area.

I wish to thank Andrew T. Prokopetz and Scott Stricoff for their valuable advice, suggestions, and constructive criticism throughout the many steps involved in this undertaking. The assistance and patience of Mr. Prokopetz in editing and Mrs. Jerry Gray in clerical support are very gratefully acknowledged.

Douglas B. Walters

PART I

Design and Facilities

CHAPTER 1

Chemical Health and Safety Concerns for Toxicity Testing in the National Toxicology Program

Douglas B. Walters
National Toxicology Program, National Institute of
Environmental Health Sciences, Post Office Box 12233,
Research Triangle Park, North Carolina 27709

INTRODUCTION

The activities in a toxicological testing program for environmental chemicals are broad and involve research and testing of wide ranges of potentially hazardous materials from both the chronic and acute standpoint. The purposes of health and safety efforts are to:

- protect the worker
- safeguard the environment
- comply with regulations and guidelines
- help ensure the integrity of the study

It is the responsibility of health and safety to guard both the worker and the environment against excessive exposure to the test materials, their metabolites, and their degradation products. This can be accomplished, in part, by setting standards and establishing guidelines and recommendations to help ensure that pertinent federal, state, and local regulations are followed. Monitoring and tracking, both chemically and managerially, are then used to help evaluate the effectiveness of compliance with regulations and to respond in the event of an emergency. It should be emphasized that the safety purposes listed above must be accomplished without compromising the integrity of the toxicity studies and should not impact negatively on the efficiency or effectiveness with which the testing of chemicals is performed. Exercise of considerable creativity and cleverness is often necessary to institute acceptable engineering controls; to change, relocate, or redesign equipment and facilities; and to modify established, but faulty, operating procedures. Occasionally comfort, as well as appearance, must also be considered with respect to use of personnel protection.

Finally, the importance of communication with and input from the employee cannot be overstressed. Perhaps the old cliché could better be stated: The happy worker is not only productive but also safer.

A chemical health and safety effort is needed in a toxicology testing program to help institute uniform effective industrial hygiene practices across the entire program and to account for particular safety needs of individual as well as highly specialized toxicology disciplines and their accompanying support programs (e.g., chemistry, laboratory animal medicine, pathology). Frequently special safety requirements are needed because of a particular chemical's properties or the unique needs of the specific toxicology experiment. The effectiveness of a health and safety program depends, as usual, on its support from management, branch chiefs, and section heads and the dedication of the health and safety staff and their interaction with these leaders.

A well-run chemical health and safety program for toxicology testing studies includes knowledge from the following list of disciplines to maximize effectiveness.

- chemistry (physical, analytical, organic)
- industrial hygiene
- safety specialties (fire, etc.)
- engineering (mechanical, industrial, chemical)
- toxicology
- biology
- occupational medicine
- information retrieval
- regulations
- management

The most important personnel requirement in such a program is a strong background in chemistry, since almost all health and safety concerns in such toxicology studies relate directly or indirectly to the individual test chemicals and their physical-chemical properties. Particularly important, therefore, is a good understanding of physical, analytical, and organic chemistry. In addition, sound knowledge and experience are necessary in other areas to permit the recognition, evaluation, and control of hazards usually encountered. It is important to emphasize that the role of safety personnel should not be to act as monitors or police officers, but should stress interaction as a coworker in a helpful and advisory capacity. Generally speaking, if newly instituted safety procedures require substantially more time or effort or are uncomfortable they must be reevaluated. Such reevaluation will require more time and in-depth knowledge of the problem area by the safety personnel. In addition, significant creativity and originality are essential. It should only be the rare exception for safety procedures to impact negatively on the efficiency of a study.

Conceivably it could be argued that once a safety program is implemented it should, to a large extent, run itself. It must be stressed, however, that safety must be as viable and dynamic as its accompanying toxicology program to be effective. New regulations are always promulgated; changes are constantly occurring in regulations; toxicology programs and accompanying support disciplines grow, alter, are eliminated and new ones formed—all of which require changes in the focus of safety. Improvements and innovations must be supported by state-of-the-art safety research to accompany similarly developing toxicology and to meet special toxicology and chemical needs. In addition, as funds for toxicology testing often become tighter due to inflation and other economic factors, the screening program may select fewer chemicals. Since these selections are subjected to more vigorous scrutinizing, their potential health and safety risks are often higher. Lastly, it is usually the unanticipated which causes the greatest problems.

Safety in a toxicology testing program is complex because of the many scientific disciplines it serves, the many tasks it performs, and the fact that any type of chemical can be tested. Hence, the relevance of a chemical health and safety effort is directly related to the primary mission of the testing program. Just as chemicals are tested to help protect the public health, it is important that the program protect the worker and the environment from any hazards involved in testing these chemicals.

NATIONAL TOXICOLOGY PROGRAM

Structure

Figure 1-1 illustrates programs requiring health and safety input, including *in vivo* and *in vitro* toxicology studies as well as support programs. It is helpful at this point to briefly explain the structure of the National Toxicology Program (NTP). Chemicals are selected for testing by the NTP Board of Scientific Counselors' [1,2,3] Subcommittee for Chemical Nomination and Selection. This subcommittee is composed of representatives from the Consumer Product Safety Commission (CPSC), Envi-

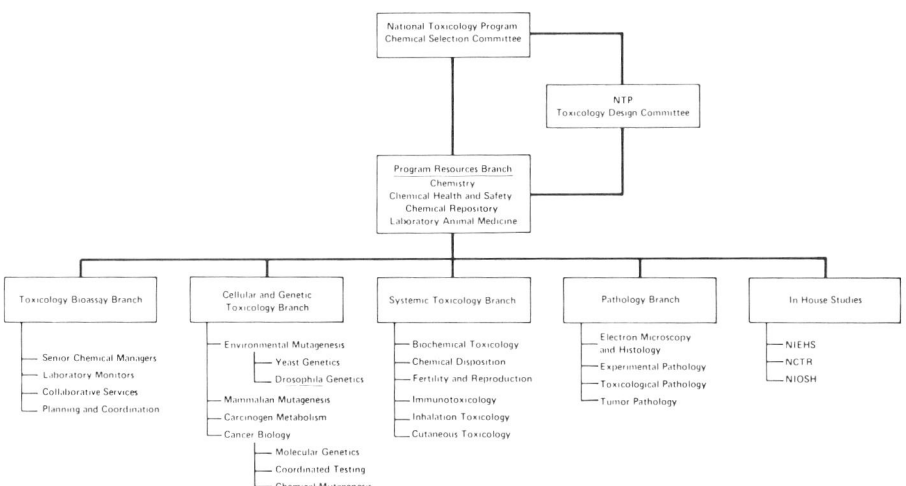

Figure 1-1.   National Toxicology Program Organizational Structure.

ronmental Protection Agency (EPA), Food and Drug Administration (FDA), Occupational Safety and Health Administration (OSHA), National Cancer Institute (NCI), National Institute of Environmental Health Sciences (NIEHS), National Institute for Occupational Safety and Health (NIOSH), National Center for Toxicological Research (NCTR), and National Toxicology Program (NTP).

To help achieve the goals of the NTP, discipline leaders (i.e., chemical health and safety, chemistry, laboratory animal care, toxicology, and pathology) also function as chemical managers for at least one chemical under test in the program. After a chemical has been selected for toxicology bioassay testing a chemical manager is assigned to ensure that the chemical receives a complete scientific evaluation. The chemical manager follows the progress of the chemical through each of the various testing phases and has the responsibilities listed in Table 1–1. The chemical manager also maintains liaison with the organization (government, public, industry) which nominated the chemical and with the industry that manufactures or uses the chemical. The major purpose for having discipline leaders function in this capacity is to help ensure that a comprehensive familiarity with all aspects of the NTP is achieved.

Before going to the *Program Resources Branch*, chemicals selected for *in vivo* toxicological bioassay studies go to the Toxicology Design Committee where the chemical manager prepares a protocol after doing a complete literature search. These chemicals are next located, procured, and analyzed for purity and stability, in the neat form as well as in the dose vehicle [4,5], at the NTP analytical resources contract laboratory under the Program Resources Branch. In addition animals are obtained for the study, and detailed Chemical-Specific Health and Safety Guidelines are prepared [6]. Chemicals selected for *in vitro* testing as well as most chemicals selected for systemic toxicology and in-house studies go directly to the NTP chemical repository managed by the Program Resources Branch since the protocols are either less complicated or are clearly research endeavors. Analysis, in most instances, is not required until completion of the studies. While a complete description of each of the major testing areas in the NTP is not appropriate for this chapter, and is given elsewhere [1,2], a brief synopsis of each field is helpful in understanding the interaction of chemical health and safety in these areas.

Table 1–1. Responsibilities of Chemical Manager

1. Know and understand the relevant scientific literature.
2. Present draft protocols to the Toxicology Design Committee to ensure that testing is developed to measure relevant endpoints.
3. Keep up to date on the experiment's progress and maintain current awareness.
4. Provide liaison with groups doing special studies on the chemical.
5. Assist in data evaluation.
6. Draft the technical bioassay reports.
7. Be available to present test results at the Technical Reports Review Subcommittee meetings.
8. Prepare the final technical report and journal manuscripts.
9. Respond to request for information on that chemical after obtaining clearance from the agency which regulates the chemical.

Carcinogenesis and toxicological bioassays have been changed under the NTP from the standard acute, two-week repeated dose, subchronic, and chronic two-year carcinogenesis bioassay to include broadened toxicologic characterization of chemicals. Information is now collected relating to target organ effects and includes detailed studies of functional, biochemical, and structural aspects of test compounds.

The *cellular and genetic toxicology* efforts use short-term test systems to evaluate genetic activity and to increase understanding of mechanisms of interaction. Emphasis is presently placed on tests that measure mutagenicity and aneuploidy in microbial cells, as well as mutagenicity, cytogenetic damage, and transformation in mammalian cells. The eventual goal is use of short-term tests to predict carcinogenicity and mutagenicity and reduce the need for *in vivo* assays and to assist in setting testing priorities for long-term bioassays.

Systemic toxicology includes testing for biochemistry, chemical disposition, fertility and reproductive disorders, immunotoxicology, and neurobehavioral and inhalation toxicology.

Finally the *chemical pathology* branch conducts research and testing as well as provides support to other areas of the NTP in the fields of electron microscopy and histology, experimental pathology, toxicological pathology, and tumor pathology.

In-house studies are conducted at the National Center for Toxicological Research; the National Institute of Environmental Health Sciences; and the National Institute for Occupational Safety and Health in all branch areas of NTP toxicology testing concern.

Most of the NTP work is performed at approximately 50 different toxicology contract laboratories, the majority of which are in the United States with a few in Western Europe. In addition, in-house studies are conducted to help maintain state-of-the-art excellence and to ensure that NTP project officers in charge of individual contracts remain active in laboratory research and are aware of the latest developments in their fields. Interagency agreements are also in effect for some of the work carried out in cooperation with the Departments of Defense and Energy and for studies done at many of the national laboratories (e.g., Oak Ridge).

HEALTH AND SAFETY FUNCTIONS

Table 1–2 summarizes some of the major functions of the NTP Chemical Health and Safety Office. Input from chemical health and safety for NTP studies begins with the initial experimental design to ensure special requirements are met and to provide chemical-specific health and safety guidelines. Involvement continues through initial laboratory evaluation, follow-up site visits, program reviews, report monitoring, recommended changes in procedures, facilities design, etc., as well as response to emergency situations and concern with eventual waste disposal and record archiving. Included is maintenance of a program-specific, state-of-the-art chemical health and safety research effort; chemical monitoring and industrial hygiene surveys; periodic review of training needs; and formulation of standards, guidelines, and safety plans. Chemical health and safety coverage also includes the receipt, storage, shipment, and

Table 1-2. NTP Chemical Health and Safety Functions

Establish guidelines, standards, and requirements for work practices.
Conduct site visits and assess adequacy of contractor laboratories.
Monitor and track for compliance with regulations.
Perform industrial hygiene surveys and conduct chemical monitoring.
Participate in program reviews.
Recommend changes in procedures and facilities design.
Conduct state-of-the-art research.
Provide expertise and serve as an information resource.
Provide chemical specific guidelines, safety and handling documents, and emergency procedures documents.
Respond to emergency situations.
Provide specific training needs for personnel.
Oversee waste management.
Provide repository services for NTP test chemicals.
Establish an archive for test chemicals.

---

handling of test chemicals by the Chemical Repository. In addition, the NTP Chemical Health and Safety Office advises and serves as a resource for in-house efforts.

Figure 1–2 illustrates the support the NTP Office of Chemical Health and Safety receives for some of these functions from contractors and in-house NIEHS health and safety personnel. A contract for health and safety support services has been awarded to A.D. Little, Inc., Cambridge, Massachusetts, to provide assistance in many of the functions listed in Table 1–2. Examples of some of this support is the subject in Chapters 4, 8, and 15.

Chemical Repository

The Chemical Repository also falls under the auspices of the NTP Office of Chemical Health and Safety and is serviced by contract with the Radian Corporation, Austin, Texas. The Chemical Repository provides a centralized management system for test and control chemicals and has been fully described elsewhere [3,6,7,8]. Major activities include locating and acquiring chemicals and their safe storage, handling, packaging, and shipping as well as the preparation of chemical safety data sheets for all test chemicals. Because of the involvement of health and safety and the unique nature of the repository facility, it is felt that managerially the Office of Health and Safety functions best as a focal point for this operation.

A close working relationship between the NTP and NIEHS Offices of Health and Safety is advantageous to help accomplish many of the program's goals. The NTP office serves as a resource for health and safety information, which is often unique or difficult to obtain for test chemicals and chemicals structurally similar to them. In addition, it provides advice and expertise on special health and safety concerns regarding chemistry and toxicology in general. Participation in relevant meetings and committees as well as screening of in-house NTP safety protocols for

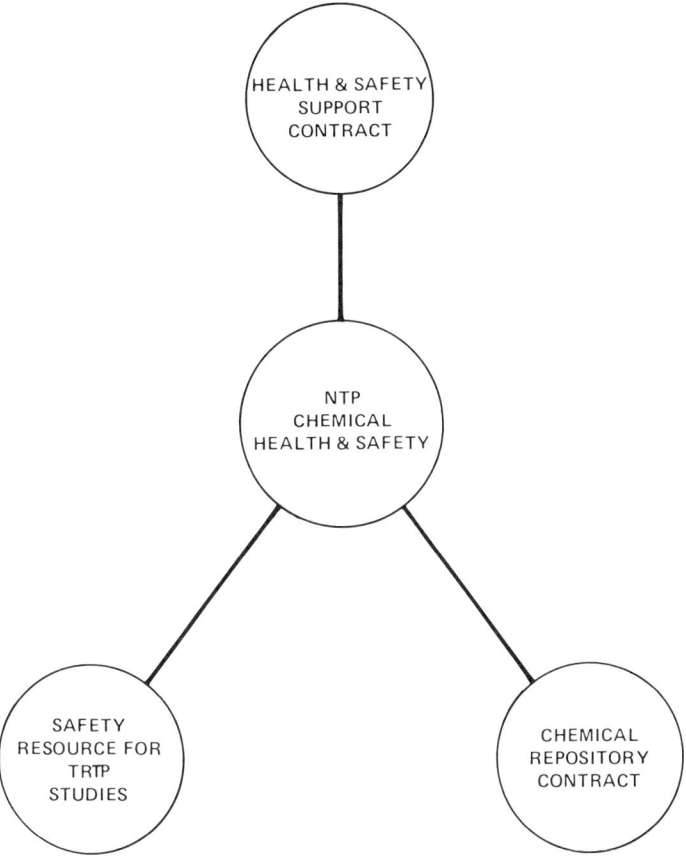

Figure 1-2.   NTP Chemical Health and Safety Functional Structure.

accuracy and completeness before submission to the NIEHS Health and Safety Office are additional responsibilities. The NIEHS office assists the NTP by providing complementary health and safety expertise and information, particularly in the areas of epidemiology and biohazard safety. In addition the NIEHS office arranges for institution of a medical surveillance program and distribution of safety glasses and respirators to all NIEHS-based NTP employees. The NIEHS office is responsible for the approval of safety protocols for all NIEHS in-house NTP studies and has responsibility for monitoring the health and safety aspects of these studies.

HEALTH AND SAFETY REQUIREMENTS

The NTP health and safety functions begin with the formulation of health and safety guidelines, standards, and minimum requirements for work performance and equipment. In the NTP, minimum requirements have been written for studies performed in the cellular and genetic toxicology, toxicology bioassay, and pathology branches. Similar documents are in the process of being written for the systemic toxicology effort. These documents are reprinted in Appendixes A, B, and C of this chapter. These minimum requirements were written by the NTP Office of Chemical Health and Safety and the contractor for health and safety support services, A.D. Little. Attached to the actual minimum requirements (but, for brevity, not reprinted here) are two appendixes. The first is a detailed description of the recommended methodology for evaluation of laboratory hoods and local exhaust systems, as applied to toxicology testing laboratories (see Chapter 15). The second is a brief description of a recommended respiratory protective equipment program. In order to effect the orderly transition necessary to implement these requirements, they were instituted first as guidelines for existing contracts and then made minimum requirements for newly awarded contracts. In-house work is the responsibility of the parent organizations and is covered by their respective health and safety programs [6,9].

Pathology and cellular and genetic toxicology work is usually performed in one, two, or three rooms at most. In almost all instances small quantities of test chemicals are used for short duration (hours or days). This ranges from milligram to gram quantities in the cellular and genetic toxicology labs to only trace contamination present in the animals themselves in pathology laboratories. Pathology laboratories have the added concern of large amounts of hazardous solvents such as formaldehyde and xylenes. In both instances safety officers are appointed but are rarely trained safety professionals (i.e., possess formal health and safety or industrial hygiene course work). The small quantities of hazardous agents used are generally highly localized to specific areas (e.g., hoods) in the work rooms.

The contract bioassay laboratories use large amounts of material in many rooms, and the work practices (e.g., dosed-feed preparation) often make chemical contamination more difficult to contain. The bioassay studies often take place over several years and require interaction of several disciplines (toxicology, chemistry, animal laboratory medicine, pathology) and require an on-site formally trained health and safety officer. Additional comparisons of the work practices and design criteria for these areas of work with respect to health and safety are presented in Chapter 2.

The main point to be made is that the minimum requirements for each major area of toxicology research in the NTP are formulated to meet the needs of that particular program. The health and safety requirements are written to provide safe working conditions without significantly slowing down or making the performance of the work inconvenient. This requires in-depth knowledge by the safety officer of the program as well as considerable creativity.

One purpose of formulating such guidelines and requirements is to ensure compliance with applicable regulations such as OSHA [10, 11], EPA [12], Department of Transportation (DOT) [13], FDA [14], Nuclear Regulatory Commission (NRC) [15], in addition to various guidelines [16,17,18]. In all instances, NTP health and safety minimum requirements meet and usually exceed existing regulations. The relationship of various regulations, guidelines, and practices is shown in Figure 1-3.

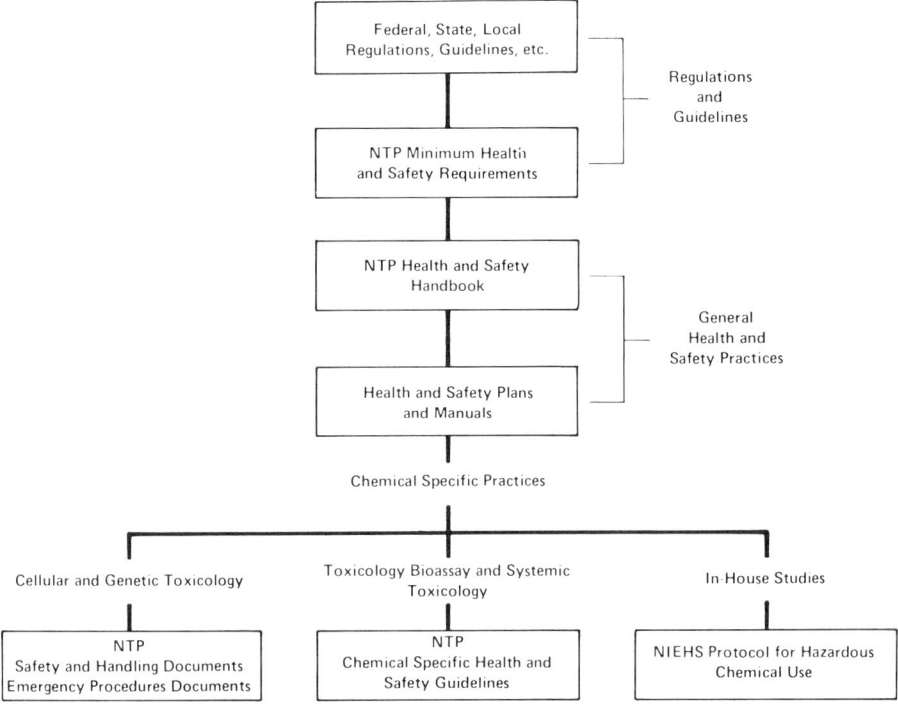

Figure 1–3.   NTP Health and Safety Requirements, Guidelines, and Practices.

The minimum requirements are used contractually to ensure that bidders meet the various regulations and qualify for immediate participation in the NTP effort in the event they are awarded a contract.

Health and Safety Handbook

Writing is in progress on an NTP health and safety handbook. The purpose of this document will be twofold: (1) it will set NTP health and safety policy, and (2) it will serve as a resource for the writers of laboratory-specific health and safety plans or manuals. Hence, the handbook will serve as a guide for the revision of present NTP contractor health and safety plans in order to achieve uniform policy and procedures. The handbook will include background and descriptive information and present opinions on which NTP policy and decisions are based. The NTP suggestions of equipment and procedures will be based on good industrial hygiene practices and conform to the needs of NTP work practices. The handbook will not be a mundane document which does not permit deviation, but will form an NTP choice tailored to the needs of its program. It will be emphasized that other choices and options are available which may be better suited to programs differing from the NTP.

Table 1-3.   Safety Plan for Bioassay Laboratories

Functions as a safety manual.
Contains pertinent standard operating procedures (SOPs).
Addresses all phases of testing program.
Conforms to local, state, and federal regulations.
Includes operating procedures on:

Waste disposal	Dose preparation
Traffic patterns	Accident and emergency response
Training	Medical surveillance
Respirator program	Use of radiolabeled materials
Ventilation maintenance	Spill cleanup
Storage and transportation	

Safety Plans

The health and safety plans or manuals of the individual contractors, including those for in-house studies [9], set down specific policy and work practices for individual locations and generally do not allow for deviations or offer options for compliance to requirements. Table 1-3 lists the contents of a typical safety plan for a bioassay laboratory. Safety plans are necessary for each contractor since facilities are used for other studies in addition to those of the NTP and because none of the facilities were built or designed specifically for NTP work. In addition, geography and climate sometimes dictate differences unique to particular facilities. Just as the minimum requirements provide a way to ensure uniform, general compliance with regulations, the health and safety plans provide a method for evaluation of particular policies and procedures.

Health and Safety Documents

Chemical-specific practices are described by the NTP in three different ways before a study is started. The documents which describe these practices have been fully described elsewhere and will merely be summarized here (see Chapter 8).

Cellular and genetic toxicology studies are often undertaken using blind, coded samples whose identities are not divulged to the testing laboratory. To help ensure safe conditions two documents are shipped with each specially sealed chemical [3, 19]. The first is a Safety and Handling Document (SHD) which provides adequate information to work safely with the material (i.e., protective clothing and equipment required, ventilation needed, pertinent properties such as solubility, volatility) but does not identify the chemical. Second, in a specially sealed envelope, is the Emergency Procedures Document (EPD) which is to be opened in the event of an emergency or situation involving potential exposure. The EPD breaks the code, identifies the material, and provides information on first aid, spill cleanup, and properties. These documents are supported by written standard operating procedures (SOPs) which are developed by contractor laboratories to conform to the particular studies they are conducting. The SOPs are site specific to meet the unique needs of each facility and are in accordance with company policies.

Chemical-specific Health and Safety Guidelines are written for all chemicals tested in the toxicology bioassay and systemic toxicology programs. Chemicals are tested in these programs as knowns, hence a single comprehensive document, complete with references, is written, bearing in mind that the particular study may continue for up to five years and may require occasional updates. Once again these documents are used in conjunction with written SOPs from the testing contractor.

In-house studies take place at NIEHS only after a protocol for hazardous chemical use has been written, peer reviewed, and approved by the NIEHS Office of Health and Safety. These protocols may be written with the assistance of the NTP Health and Safety Office but are the responsibility of and approved by the NIEHS office.

Contractor Monitoring

The evaluation of toxicology testing laboratories which participate in the NTP can involve up to six steps:

- qualifications to participate in program
- bid proposal evaluation
- pre- or postaward site visit
- evaluation of special procedures
- safety plan review
- annual program review

In the large-scale toxicology bioassay program, evaluations begin with the review of eligibility in accordance with the minimum requirements discussed above, to determine which laboratories qualify under the master agreement to participate in the program. This evaluation is performed by nongovernment experts in the various disciplines used in these studies.

The next phase of evaluations takes place during the review by NTP staff of bid packages submitted in response to requests for proposals for NTP studies. If recent changes (e.g., in facilities or staff) have occurred at a laboratory, it may be necessary to conduct a preaward site visit to confirm qualifications. If the study involves special techniques or chemical hazards, a postaward site visit may be required. In addition during the initial award period, safety plans and specific SOPs are reviewed and suggestions for updates and changes are made, where necessary.

Finally, annual program reviews are performed to review the performance of the contractor laboratory. The review includes an in-depth examination of the technical aspects of the specific toxicology study as well as support functions such as health and safety and chemistry. Shortly before such reviews occur detailed health and safety surveys are conducted at the contract laboratory. These reviews include an evaluation of the items listed in Table 1–4. Such site visits are intended to assist both the NTP and contract laboratories in protecting the health and safety of the testing personnel, while maintaining the scientific integrity of the study. The surveys include an initial briefing by the site visit team, the principal investigator, safety officer, and other appropriate personnel to discuss health and safety procedures, facilities, SOPs and protocols employed in handling test chemicals from receipt through dose preparation and administration, to final disposal of surplus chemical and contaminated waste. A review of health and safety documentation such as training materials and injury and illness records also takes place.

In addition the site visit team and laboratory personnel walk through laboratories reviewing the facility safety features (ventilation, eyewashes, safety showers, etc.) and operating practices of personnel. This includes (but is not limited to) monitoring of hood face velocities with smoke tubes and velometers and donning of protective equipment to enter regulated or restricted areas. Chemical monitoring may be included for specific test chemicals (where NIOSH-approved methods exist) as well as for formaldehyde. Particular attention is paid to areas of high risk where the neat chemical is used such as the receipt, chemical storage, dose preparation, and test administration rooms as well as the use of proper transport and packaging proce-

Table 1–4.   Health and Safety Baseline Survey

General background information
  Staff
  Policies and guidelines
  Training
  Medical surveillance
  OSHA reporting (accident/injuries)
  Emergency procedures, spill control
  Labeling and signs
  Contractor chemical monitoring programs
  Waste management
  Annotated floor plans
Toxicology operations
  Test chemical receipt
  Chemical/sample transport
  Chemical storage
  Diet, sample, dose preparation
  Test chemical administration
  Analytical chemistry
  Histopathology
  Clinical chemistry
  Waste disposal
  Ventilation
  Measurements
  Chemical monitoring (formaldehyde and specific chemicals) performed
    during site visit
  Photographs

dures. Areas of concern are indicated and discussed with the laboratory personnel during the walk through.

A debriefing meeting is held for discussion of health and safety items that require further explanation. Typically, bioassay health and safety surveys require one to two days, whereas cellular and genetic toxicology laboratory reviews can be completed in a single day. Written reports which list attention items are communicated to the laboratory and the NTP project officer in charge. Direct communication as well as monthly reports are used to follow up on the correction of the deficiencies.

Information presented in the monthly reports is as follows:

- action item response
- accident/incident reports
- personnel changes
- training programs offered
- floor plan with air flow direction
- room air changes (quarterly basis)
- temperature excursions (above 80° F)
- miscellaneous items of concern

In addition to response to attention items, floor plans showing air flow directionality are presented every month; quarterly reports contain complete information on monitoring of hood velocities, other ventilation systems, as well as the number of animal room air changes. Information on accidents and incidents is presented to help ascertain where special or additional training may be necessary and sometimes may reflect changes in personnel. Lastly, the temperature of the rooms where protective clothing is worn is monitored to ensure excursions above 80° F do not occur which could lead to heat stress. All monthly reports for each laboratory are reviewed at least once a year. In this manner trends are sometimes observed in particular rooms, areas, or hoods which may have ventilation problems; particular times of the year may be noted when higher than normal accident rates occur; and areas of improvement for training programs may be realized (e.g., high number of animal bites, and high incidence of back strain resulting from not relubricating cage rack wheels after washing cages).

When serious problems are noted, the following special responses may be required:

- special or follow-up site visits
- industrial hygiene surveys which may include chemical monitoring
- modification of operating procedures
- redesign of areas and/or equipment
- approval and/or input on renovations
- interaction with appropriate personnel

A follow-up site visit by the project officer assigned to that laboratory may be all that is necessary to ensure changes were made. If the problem is more serious or cannot be clearly defined at the time of the baseline survey a follow-up industrial hygiene survey which may include chemical monitoring may be required. While a more complete description of chemical monitoring concerns in toxicology laboratories is presented in Chapter 16, a summary of the principal aspects for attention is given in Table 1–5. Generally, chemical monitoring must always be chemical specific, wherever possible using NIOSH-approved methods [20]. Since many of the NTP test chemicals are research chemicals, approved monitoring methods do not always exist and must be developed to conform to program requirements. It is important to interface the chemical monitoring with a complete view of the industrial hygiene aspects of the work. This interface usually involves a combination of personal and area monitoring and determination (where applicable) of eight-hour threshold limit values (TLVs), short-term exposure limits (STEL), as well as ceiling limits. The monitoring should be related to the facility and the operations performed there, concentrating on areas of high risk—for example, where the neat chemical is used. Data and results must then be interpreted and corrective action taken, bearing in mind that containment of the chemical contamination and worker protection should be accomplished using a hierarchical approach. Reliance should be placed first on engineering controls, then on operational and administrative controls (e.g., order and use only the amount of chemical needed), and last on protective equipment. This is a basic application of the concept of control at the source, then path, and finally the receiver (employee) (see Chapters 2 and 7).

Other problems that may occur at testing laboratories that require special responses or site visits are modifications to operating procedures, redesign of work

Table 1–5.   Chemical Monitoring Concerns

Chemical specific
Interface with industrial hygiene aspects
Relate to test facility and operations
  Study dosage
  Route of administration
  Areas monitored
    Storage
    Analysis
    Dose preparation
    Administration
    Cage handling
    Waste handling
    Support services
  Personnel and area monitoring
  Worker protection
    Engineering controls
    Operational practices
    Protective equipment
    Administrative controls
Interpret and relate data and results

Table 1-6.   Miscellaneous Health and Safety Duties

Track health and safety status at approximately 50 contract NTP laboratories.
Archive records.
Provide health and safety services to NTP technical staff.
Provide respirators.
Provide safety glasses.
Provide medical surveillance.
Review in-house safety protocols.
Interact with in-house safety officer.
Serve on safety-related committees and work groups.
Monitor for return of intact emergency procedures documents from cellular and genetic toxicology labs.

areas and/or equipment, and renovations to facilities. In all cases interaction with appropriate personnel, such as the corporate safety officer, NTP laboratory project officer, and affected personnel is important.

Miscellaneous duties of the NTP Office of Chemical Health and Safety are shown in Table 1-6. These duties include the tracking and monitoring of the ongoing status of the approximately 50 NTP contract laboratories and the archiving of pertinent records. In addition the NTP section works through the NIEHS Health and Safety Office to provide NTP staff based at NIEHS with safety glasses, respirators, and cartridge changes as well as coverage for medical surveillance. Similarly personnel stationed at other NTP sites work through health and safety offices at those locations to obtain these services. In addition, the NTP office reviews and inputs into the safety protocols for in-house studies before they are submitted to the NIEHS Office of Health and Safety for approval and interacts with appropriate health and safety committees and groups and takes part in related meetings. Finally, the Emergency Procedures Documents from the NTP Chemical Repository are monitored to ensure that they are returned from the testing laboratories unopened, which indicates the studies' integrity has not been compromised.

HEALTH AND SAFETY RESEARCH AREAS

As stated earlier, it is essential that research in chemical health and safety be carried out to keep pace with state-of-the-art developments in toxicological studies and to solve problems as soon as they become apparent. In part, the laboratory problems which necessitate research for solutions often arise from the health and safety section's function in serving as a resource for relevant information and expertise and providing advice. Insight is also gained from actual visits and surveys of laboratories and from response to emergency situations. Special health and safety research projects currently under way in the NTP include:

- incinerator evaluation
- special chemical and industrial hygiene monitoring

- human factors evaluation
- medical surveillance/biological monitoring investigation
- glove permeabilities
- determination of flash points

The evaluation of the efficacy of the incinerator used to dispose of large amounts of neat bulk chemicals from the bioassay program, and on-site incinerators used for special studies (e.g., Polybrominated Biphenyl, PBB) have been performed integrating chemical monitoring and industrial hygiene to determine the extent of observed problems. Periodically, marker chemicals (e.g., sodium fluorescein or radiolabeled chemicals) have been used as indicators to study the possible spread of contamination resulting from particular work practices or to verify containment by properly functioning engineering controls. Human factors evaluations are often considered an integral part of the complete NTP health and safety picture when analyzing potential problems, changing work practices, or redesigning equipment. Human factors have had major emphasis in the design of tissue trimming and necropsy work stations, evaluation of the health and safety of the specially designed, high-containment Hazardous Material Laboratory used by the Radian Corporation for the chemical repository, analysis of accident and incident reports, and examination of special work practices such as weighing of hazardous materials for dose preparation. Additional projects include study of the interrelationship of medical surveillance and biological monitoring (see Chapter 9). As a result of this study it does not appear that biological monitoring is generally feasible for studies involving research chemicals. Glove permeabilities are being determined for homologous series of test chemicals to derive a useful relationship based on structure-activity in order to predict and recommend specific glove types for research chemicals whose characteristics are not fully known. Finally, flash points are determined for many compounds to assist in classifying them according to DOT regulations when such information is not available on research materials.

CONCLUSION

The purpose of health and safety in a toxicology testing program is to safeguard employees and the environment against exposure to any test chemicals. This necessitates continued interaction from initial chemical selection and study design to final waste disposal. Proper fulfillment of this responsibility can best occur when safety personnel have complete familiarity with all aspects of toxicology testing and have a strong foundation in chemistry. Similar expertise in other specialty fields, such as biohazards, engineering, and epidemiology, is necessary if the program emphasis is in these directions. Safety effectiveness is greatly enhanced by application of an understanding of human factors and applied work psychology. This aspect of safety is best accomplished by assuming the role of coworker to assist and participate in the study rather than interactions which may lead to confrontations and be interpreted in an adversary manner. It should be remembered that the institution of inconvenient, uncomfortable or time-consuming constraints should be discouraged unless absolutely necessary. Alternate solutions that are effective and efficient, however, often require more time and ingenuity by safety professionals.

Application of the fundamentals of industrial hygiene to observe and recognize, evaluate and identify, and to then eliminate problems necessitates initiation of industrial hygiene research to effect long-term solutions. Safety can only be as strong as management's commitment to the program. The function of the safety office to aid in attaining the toxicological program goals depends largely on the safety professional.

REFERENCES

1. "National Toxicology Program, Annual Plan," DHHS Report NTP-81-94 (1982).
2. Moore, J.A., J.E. Huff, L. Hart, and D.B. Walters. "Overview of the National Toxicology Program," in *Environmental Health Chemistry*, J.D. McKinney, Ed. (Ann Arbor, MI: Ann Arbor Science, 1981), pp. 555–574.
3. Walters, D.B., L.H. Keith, and J.M. Harless. "Chemical Selection and Handling Aspects of the National Toxicology Program," in *Environmental Health Chemistry*, J.D. McKinney, Ed. (Ann Arbor, MI: Ann Arbor Science, 1981), pp. 575–592.
4. Jameson, C. W. "Analytical Chemistry Requirements for Toxicity Testing of Environmental Chemicals," in *Chemistry for Toxicity Testing*, C.W. Jameson and D.B. Walters, Eds. (Ann Arbor, MI: Ann Arbor Science, 1983).
5. Jameson, C.W., G.O. Kuhn, and J.J. Rollheiser. "Stability Determinations of Chemical/Vehicle Mixtures," in *Chemistry for Toxicity Testing*, C.W. Jameson and D.B. Walters, Eds. (Ann Arbor, MI: Ann Arbor Science, 1983).
6. Walters, D.B., J.D. McKinney, A. Norstrom, and N. DeWitt. "Control of Potential Carcinogenic, Mutagenic and Toxic Chemicals via a Protocol Review Concept and a Chemistry Containment Laboratory," in *Safe Handling of Chemical Carcinogens, Mutagens, Teratogens and Highly Toxic Substances, Vol. 1*, D.B. Walters, Ed. (Ann Arbor, MI: Ann Arbor Science, 1980), pp. 3–30.
7. Harless, J.M., K.E. Baxter, L.H. Keith, and D.B. Walters. "Design and Operation of a Hazardous Materials Laboratory," in *Safe Handling of Chemical Carcinogens, Mutagens, Teratogens and Highly Toxic Substances, Vol. 1*, D.B. Walters, Ed. (Ann Arbor, MI: Ann Arbor Science, 1980), pp. 79–100.
8. Keith, L.H., J.M. Harless, and D.B. Walters. "Analysis and Storage of Hazardous Environmental Chemicals for Toxicological Testing," in *Environmental Health Chemistry*, J.D. McKinney, Ed. (Ann Arbor, MI: Ann Arbor Science, 1981), pp. 593–621.
9. Walters, D.B., Ed. "NIEHS Safety and Health Manual," DHHS NIH–79–1848 (1979).
10. *Code of Federal Regulations*, Title 29, Part 1910, "Occupational Safety and Health Standards for General Industry," April 1981.
11. *Code of Federal Regulations*, Title 29, Part 1990, "Identification, Classification and Regulation of Potential Occupational Carcinogens," Occupational Safety and Health Administration, *Federal Register*, January 1980.
12. *Code of Federal Regulations*, Title 40, "Hazardous Waste and Consolidated Permit Regulations," Environmental Protection Agency, *Federal Register*, May 19, 1980.
13. *United States Code*, Title 49, 1801 *et. seq.* 88 Statute 2156, P.L 93–633, "Hazardous Materials Transportation Act."

14.   "Nonclinical Laboratory Studies, Good Laboratory Practice Regulations" DHHS, FDA, Title 21, *Federal Register*, December 22, 1978, Part II.

15.   *Code of Federal Regulations*, Title 10, "Standards for Protection Against Radiation," United States Nuclear Regulatory Commission.

16.   "National Cancer Institutes Safety Standards for Research Involving Chemical Carcinogens," DHEW (NIH) 77–900 (1975).

17.   "National Institutes of Health (NIH) Guidelines for the Laboratory Use of Chemical Carcinogens," DHHS NIH–81–2385.

18.   Montesano, R., H. Bartsch, E. Boyland, G. Della Porta, L. Fishbein, R.A. Griesemer, A.B. Swan, and L. Tomatis, Eds. *Handling Chemical Carcinogens in the Laboratory: Problems of Safety, No. 33* (Lyon, France: International Agency for Research on Cancer, 1979).

19.   Ward, W. T., C.H. Williams, Jr., C.D. Wolbach, L.H. Keith, and D.B. Walters. "Transportation of Materials from Radian Corporations Hazardous Materials Laboratory," in *Safe Handling of Chemical Carcinogens, Mutagens, Teratogens and Highly Toxic Substances, Vol. 1*, D.B. Walters, Ed. (Ann Arbor, MI: Ann Arbor Science, 1980), pp. 101–127.

20.   Taylor, David, Ed. *NIOSH Manual of Analytical Methods, Second Edition, Vols. 1–6*, DHEW (NIOSH) Publication Numbers 77–157–A, B, C, 78–175, 79–141, 80–125.

APPENDIX A

National Toxicology Program Health and Safety Minimum Requirements for Bioassay Laboratories*

1. HEALTH AND SAFETY OFFICER

A qualified health and safety officer will be designated to monitor worker health and safety conditions during all phases of the work. The health and safety officer should be administratively responsible to someone other than the Principal Investigator (P.I.) and the P.I.'s subordinates, and will have the authority to bring to the attention of higher management and the NTP Project Officer and Safety Office unsafe conditions.

The following qualifications for the health and safety officer are used as evaluation factors:

a. Graduate of an institution of higher education with at least a Bachelor's degree, majoring in chemistry, biology, chemical engineering or a closely related field.

b. At least two years experience (part-time) in occupational health and safety *along with* completion of courses in general occupational health and hazard control indicating the acquisition of successively greater levels of knowledge regarding industrial hygiene. Training should have been completed within the last 18 months, and should be refreshed with additional training at an interval not exceeding 18 months. The health and safety officer may have other responsibilities within the offeror's organization; however, the amount of time devoted explicitly to health and safety is to be commensurate with the scale of the offerer's operations. (A Master's degree in industrial hygiene, or a Bachelor's degree in industrial hygiene with one year of experience, is an acceptable substitute for this experience requirement.)

c. Documented experience in working with the requirements of local, state, and federal statutes relating to occupational health and safety, environmental protection and monitoring.

---

*Reprinted by permission of the NTP Office of Chemical Health and Safety and the contractor for health and safety support services, Arthur D. Little, Inc., Cambridge, Massachusetts.

d.   Ability to deal effectively with the scientific and managerial staffs in responsibly implementing the health and safety program (including the identification of problem areas and the execution of corrective actions) required.

2. PROTECTIVE EQUIPMENT

Personnel who may be exposed to test compounds or dosed animals will use appropriate protective clothing and equipment where the chemical-specific health and safety guidelines prepared by the NTP indicate the need for protective clothing. A complete set of clean protective clothing and equipment will be provided to anyone entering the animal test and dose formulation areas at the laboratory (minimally, a disposable laboratory suit, e.g., Tyvek; safety glasses or goggles; two pairs of gloves; boots or disposable shoe covers or sneaker shoes; and head covering). Such clothing will be worn by anyone entering the facility. Protective clothing is not to be worn outside the bioassay work areas. Disposable items will be discarded as hazardous waste after each use. Other items should be stored in covered containers until washed. If washing is done by laboratory personnel, they will wear gloves and disposable suits while handling contaminated items. If washing is done by an outside service, they will be notified that they are handling items with potential chemical contamination. Specific details of the protective clothing program shall be provided by the offeror in the proposal.

3. RESPIRATORS

NIOSH-approved respirators of the type designated in each compound's Health and Safety package will be worn by personnel working in those areas in which compounds or dosed animals are present (unless the chemical-specific package indicates that no respirator is needed). A respirator program which meets the requirements of OSHA regulation 29 CFR 1910.134 will be implemented, and a copy of the program will be submitted as an attachment to the proposer's offer for evaluation by NTP. The respirator program will specifically indicate who is responsible for each program element. Simply paraphrasing the OSHA regulation is not adequate.

4. OCCUPATIONAL MEDICAL SURVEILLANCE

Medical examinations will be performed at the time personnel are assigned to the program or will be working with test compounds or animals, and before they are exposed to potentially hazardous chemicals. Follow-up medical examinations will be performed at least annually and upon termination of an individual's participation in the project. (Pre-employment physicals are not a program charge.) The scope of the medical examination will be specified in the laboratory's Health and Safety Plan.

Cardiac and pulmonary function tests are advised (i.e., non-stress EKG and vital capacity) for persons wearing respirators.

A record will be kept of any incident resulting in minor or major personal injury (including animal bites) or probable personnel exposure to test chemicals. Those records will include a full description of the incident, the chemical involved, the medical attention required, any remedial actions taken, and planned follow-up if pertinent. Copies of such incident reports will be included in the Monthly Progress Report submitted by the laboratory. Follow-up actions taken to prevent recurrence of accidents will be reported in subsequent monthly progress reports. In addition, occupational injury and illnesses will be recorded and reported according to the OSHA recording system.

5.   BARRIER SYSTEMS AND ACCESS RESTRICTION

The "barrier systems" are incorporated into bioassay laboratories to protect the integrity of experiments and to maximize safe work conditions. To fulfill this objective, the facility's barrier system will meet the following criteria:

a.   The dose preparation area will be isolated from general traffic. This may be accomplished by locating the dose preparation area within the animal facility barrier system, or by establishing a separate barrier for dose preparation. If the latter approach is used, all areas into which laboratory workers may bring used protective equipment (including gloves, shoes, head covers, and clothing), respirators, and/or containers of dosed feed or water will be considered to be behind the barrier. Also, any hallways used by workers for reaching the shower facility will be considered to be behind the barrier.

b.   Within the animal facility, no entry from an animal room to the clean corridor is permitted. This requirement applies to the clean hallway(s) serving rooms used for NTP test work; therefore, entry from non-NTP animal rooms to the clean hallway is not acceptable.

c.   Within the shower facility, the "clean" and "dirty" areas should be physically separated by the shower or by another physical barrier. The facility design and procedures will be arranged so that it is not necessary to cross over to the clean side prior to showering, or to the dirty side after showering (e.g., to store or retrieve items such as shoes, towels, respirators, etc.).

6.   HEALTH AND SAFETY PLAN

Except where otherwise indicated in the chemical-specific health and safety package, each test agent will be considered a potential toxigenic agent. Accordingly, all necessary precautions will be taken to protect personnel and the environment against possible exposure to the compounds under test. A Health and Safety Plan that addresses the particular control options that the laboratory intends to follow to minimize the potential risk of personnel exposure to, or environmental release of, the material under test will be submitted with the proposal. No laboratory will participate in the bioassay program without a health and safety plan in effect which has been approved by the NTP. An updated health and safety plan will be submitted every two years to the NTP for review and approval. In addition, the NTP will be informed of any updates to the health and safety plans during the course of the contract. The scope of each Health and Safety Plan should include pertinent chemical, physical, and biological hazards present. Standard operating procedures as outlined in Section 9 of these minimum requirements will be included in the Health and Safety Plan. All phases of the testing program will be addressed in the Plan, from the acquisition of test material, to the storage or ultimate disposal of contaminated waste. The Plan should address (but need not be limited to) housekeeping, eating and smoking areas, signs and labels, emergency procedures, chemical storage, personal protective equipment, respirator programs, waste disposal, and training. All work shall conform to the applicable local, state, and federal statutes relating to occupational health and safety, transportation and handling, and environmental protection.

The NTP may inspect the laboratory facility to assure that the health and safety plan is being implemented.

7. ENGINEERING CONTROLS

All dose preparation and all gavage and inhalation administration will be performed in hoods or other vented enclosures. The proposer should fully describe the facilities which will be used for such operations.

Each laboratory will have a hood inspection program providing periodic checks of hood air flow velocities and general ventilation systems. At a minimum, the following inspections are required:

- Laboratory hoods and all other local exhaust ventilation enclosures (e.g., mixer enclosures, vented necropsy and histology work stations, dumping stations) should have their proper operation verified by measurement of airflow at least quarterly during long-term studies. For studies of 90 days or less duration, each hood or other vented enclosure will be verified within 45 days prior to the beginning of the study. Face velocities of laboratory hoods and of necropsy and tissue trimming work stations will be 100 feet per minute ($\pm$ 20) as recommended by the American Conference of Governmental Industrial Hygienists for the control of chemical vapors.
- Relative pressures of laboratory areas will be checked monthly with smoke tubes to verify that air flows from relatively clean to relatively dirty areas.
- Confirmation of at least 10 air changes per hour in animal rooms will be verified at least twice yearly.

Records of these ventilation system checks will be maintained by the health and safety officer. The records will indicate for each hood, room, and area, at a minimum, when air flow was tested, what was found, who conducted the test, and what test equipment was used.

Documentation (e.g., schematic diagram) will be provided indicating the relative location of external air intakes and exhausts for both local and general ventilation systems, as well as the direction of prevailing winds. Also, a detailed description (with illustrations) of controls employed in the dose preparation area will be provided.

Chemicals will not be handled in hoods which exhaust less than 70% of their airflow. Recirculation of air from local exhaust systems into occupied spaces will not be permitted. Effluent exhaust vapor from analytical instruments (e.g., gas chromatographs) will be vented outside of the building.

Test chemicals and solvents will not be stored in unvented areas.

Air exhausted from dose preparation areas will be passed through HEPA filters. If volatile chemicals are handled, charcoal filters will also be used.

8.   WASTE DISPOSAL

Surplus bulk chemical will be shipped to the NTP Chemical Repository for disposal by the NTP, and will be packaged in accordance with NTP and DOT requirements.

All potentially contaminated material (carcasses, bedding, labware, etc.) will be incinerated in a manner consistent with federal (EPA) and local regulations, or disposed of in a licensed hazardous waste landfill. The laboratory will indicate whether it plans to fulfill this requirement with its own incinerator or by use of a licensed waste disposal firm. If the laboratory's incinerator is to be used, specifications and operating procedures will be provided to NTP for evaluation. If a contract disposer is to be used, information on the firm's licensure will be provided.

9.   STANDARD OPERATING PROCEDURES

The laboratory will be required to have written standard operating procedures for at least the following activities:

a.   Waste Disposal
b.   Entry and Exit from the Bioassay Area (including traffic patterns of dose prep facility and animal handling and testing room)
c.   Spill Clean-up, Accident and Emergency Response
d.   Employee Training
e.   Respirator Protection and Fit
f.   Ventilation System Maintenance
g.   Storage and Transportation of Test Materials
h.   Use of Radio-labelled Materials (if applicable)
i.   Dose Preparation
j.   Medical Surveillance
k.   Cleaning of exposed pipes and light fixtures

10. WORKER EXPOSURE SAMPLING

When the test chemical has a Threshold Limit Value of 10 ppm or less, or 0.1 mg/m^3 or less, or the chemical-specific health and safety guideline requires chemical monitoring, the laboratory performing the work will be required to sample worker exposures. This sampling will be performed at least once during initial dose preparation and once during initial dose administration and at the midpoint of the study. Exposure sampling will be performed when both test chemical and controls are handled. Samples should be collected using the method indicated in the Health and Safety package for that specific chemical.

11. FORMALDEHYDE CONTROL

Histology, necropsy, and tissue trimming operations will be conducted in a manner which employs engineering controls to ensure that exposures to formaldehyde are kept below 1 ppm.

12. MISCELLANEOUS

The offeror's proposal will describe the location (preferably with schematic diagram) of fire control equipment and plumbed eyewash stations and emergency showers.

Animal rooms and dose preparation rooms will be constructed of wall, floor, and ceiling materials which form chemical-tight surfaces. Animal room doors should include windows to permit observation of workers within each room.

Emergency power generator systems will be described, including information on maintenance and testing programs.

Chemical storage facilities will be described.

Within the barrier facility, walls, floors, and ceilings will be sealed around all incoming and outgoing pipes, conduits, and other utilities.

Where not superseded by this document, guidelines provided by "NIH Guidelines for the Laboratory Use of Chemical Carcinogens" (NIH Publication 81-2385, May 1981), will be followed.

Other pertinent personnel, operational and administrative practices and engineering controls necessary for the containment and safe handling of potential chemical carcinogens will be explained in the offeror's proposal.

The procedures used for decontamination of Toxicology Data Management System (TDMS) terminals should be consistent with spill clean up provisions in the chemical-specific health and safety packages. Terminals should be disconnected from electrical power source before decontamination, and care should be taken to ensure that any solvents used to do not damage the plastic of the TDMS terminal.

HEALTH AND SAFETY MINIMUM REQUIREMENTS
FOR INHALATION STUDIES

The NTP Health and Safety Minimum Requirements for Bioassay laboratories will be followed with the following additions and changes:

1. The test atmosphere generation apparatus will be contained in a vented enclosure. All connections in the piping and/or ducting between the test atmosphere generator and the exhaust air filters will be either threaded; welded; or enclosed and vented.
2. At least one sampling port connected to the test chemical concentration monitoring system will be located in each animal room involved in the study. Daily maximum concentration detected at that sampling port will be reported in the health and safety section of the Monthly Report.
3. When a test chemical is flammable, sampling of test chemical concentration will be done in the chamber air supply line, in the chamber, and in the chamber exhaust line. The sampling apparatus will be connected so as to sound an alarm if the concentration at any point exceeds 50% of the lower explosive limit. This alarm will be designed to be heard in the study room, the adjacent corridor(s), and at least one remote, normally occupied location within the facility.

   If the dose level is to exceed 50% of the lower flammable limit, the following provisions will be made:
   a. All electrical fixtures in the study room will be explosion-proof, conforming to the National Electrical Code.
   b. All equipment through which test chemical flows will be electrically grounded and bonded.
   c. The study room will have explosion venting or an explosion suppression system.
4. At least two NIOSH-approved, 30-minute positive pressure self-contained breathing apparatus will be available for use if emergency entry into a study room following a leak is required. These units will be maintained and inspected as recommended by the manufacturer.
5. The personal protection requirements specified in the NTP Health and Safety Minimum Requirements for Bioassay Laboratories will apply except as follows:
   a. When animals are within a closed chamber and the ambient sampling port indicates that the study room is not contaminated, personnel entering the study room need not wear respirators and disposable overgarments. However, when the chamber is opened and/or when animals are outside of the chamber, the normal requirements for entering dose administration rooms apply.
   b. When the test chemical is a particulate (dust, mist, or aerosol), necropsy personnel will wear the same respiratory and protective equipment required of animal-handling staff in the dose administration area. Necropsy will be performed in a vented enclosure.

APPENDIX B

National Toxicology Program Health and Safety Minimum Requirements for Cellular and Genetic Toxicology Laboratories*

The following precautions will be taken by laboratories which handle test chemicals from the NTP Repository at Radian. These requirements, taken together, are intended to help assure safe conditions at NTP Cellular and Genetic Toxicology laboratories. They will be treated as a group and not taken out of context.

1. An isolated laboratory separate from other laboratory facilities will be provided for unpacking, storing, weighing, and diluting of test chemical and/or positive controls.
2. The above isolated laboratory will be a limited access area and have its air supply under negative pressure with respect to connecting laboratories and hallways.
3. A record will be kept of all personnel entering/exiting any limited access area(s).
4. Weighing of the test chemical and/or positive controls will be performed on an analytical balance with a sensitivity of 0.1 mg. This balance will be placed at all times in an effective laboratory hood or a vented enclosure. Protocols for testing will be designed to use the minimum possible quantities of "neat" chemical in preparing test solutions.
5. An effective laboratory hood for weighing, diluting and administering of test chemicals and/or positive controls will provide sufficient contaminant capture velocities, as evaluated by a combination of velometer and smoke tube tests. Hoods used for weighing, diluting and administering of test chemicals will be vented to the outside. Biological safety cabinets used for dilution or administration of toxic chemicals will recirculate no more than 30% of their air (i.e., Class II Type A hoods will not be used). Laboratory hoods will be routinely monitored as described in Appendix I. [Not reprinted here.]
6. Plastic-backed absorbent matting will be secured inside of any hood wherever the test chemicals and/or positive controls (including dilutions) are being

*Reprinted by permission of the NTP Office of Chemical Health and Safety and the contractor for health and safety support services, Arthur D. Little, Inc., Cambridge, Massachusetts.

handled. After each working session in the hood, this matting will be disposed of as hazardous waste.

7. A non-breakable, secured secondary container will be used for transfer of any test chemical and/or positive controls between laboratories.

8. Any vacuum line used when working with test chemicals and/or positive controls will be protected with an absorbent or liquid trap and a HEPA filter.

9. Eating, drinking, smoking, applying cosmetics, and chewing gum will not be permitted wherever test and/or positive control chemicals are handled. The presence of food or smoking materials will not be permitted in these areas.

10. Warning signs and labels will be used wherever test chemicals and/or positive controls are used or stored (i.e., on primary and secondary containers, affixed to entrances to work areas and on containers holding hazardous waste). These signs and labels will indicate the presence of suspected carcinogenic, mutagenic, or teratogenic hazards, as recommended by *NIH Guidelines for the Laboratory Use of Chemical Carcinogens*, NIH Publication 81-2385, May 1981.

11. The following personal protective clothing will be worn at all times in the restricted access laboratory(s) where the test chemical is stored, weighed, and diluted: (a) disposable Tyvek® (or equivalent) laboratory coat disposed of on a weekly basis or disposed of immediately after any known chemical contact; (b) disposable Tyvek® (or equivalent) sleeves if a non-disposable lab coat is used—disposed of after each use; (c) two pairs of dissimilar disposable gloves (i.e., PVC, latex, natural rubber, etc.)—both pairs will be changed after any known chemical contact and/or after every two hours of use; (d) an approved half-mask respirator equipped with a combination cartridge (this filter is specific for organic vapors, HCl, acid gases, SO_2 and particulate)—these cartridges will be changed once a month and the date of installation will be marked on each new cartridge. All protective equipment used in the restricted access laboratory will be stored in that laboratory.

12. All components of a respiratory protection program will be practiced, as outlined in Appendix II. [Not reprinted here.]

13. Use of disposable Tyvek® full-body jump suits and shoe covers in limited access laboratories can help prevent possible contamination of street clothing and shoes. Any street clothing contaminated with test chemical or positive control (e.g., by a spill) will be discarded as laboratory contaminated waste. Any street shoes contaminated with test chemical will be disposed of.

14. Any contaminated solid or liquid waste generated under the hood will be collected in a leak-proof container. When removed from the hood this container must be closed and placed in a secondary closed container in the limited access area. Disposal containers removed from the limited access area must be stored in an isolated and secured area. This area will be controlled by either the principal investigator or the waste disposal officer. All wastes generated by the testing program will be disposed of in accordance with applicable federal, state, or municipal waste disposal regulations.

15. The chemical-specific Emergency Procedures Document (blue envelope) will be present in the laboratory where the test chemical is used, and all personnel will be aware of its location and purpose. Laboratory personnel will decide in advance what type of incident will result in opening of the Emergency Procedures Document.

16. There will be written general safety policies (Standard Operating Procedures—SOPs) at each laboratory. A written set of emergency procedures to be followed by all project personnel in the event of a spill or leak involving the test chemical and/or positive control will be developed. Personnel will be instructed to call for appropriate help (e.g., in-house emergency group or Poison Control Center) in case of emergency.

17. The location and phone number of the nearest poison control center will be prominently posted in each laboratory.

18. General laboratory safety procedures will be followed, including (but not limited to) the following: (a) use of safety glasses in chemical handling areas, (b) no mouth pipetting, (c) no open toed shoes, (d) no dry sweeping for maintenance or for spill clean-up.

APPENDIX C

National Toxicology Program Health and Safety Minimum Requirements for Pathology Laboratories*

The following precautions will be taken by the pathology laboratories which perform animal necropsy, tissue trimming, and preparation of slides for NTP bioassay studies. These requirements, taken together, are intended to help assure safe conditions at NTP Pathology Laboratories. They will be treated as a group and not taken out of context.

1. An isolated laboratory (or laboratories) separate from other laboratory facilities will be provided for necropsy, tissue trimming, tissue processing, embedding, microtoming and staining.
2. The above isolated laboratory (or laboratories) will have its air supply under negative pressure with respect to connecting laboratories and hallways.
3. An effective exhaust hood for necropsy, tissue trimming, manual tissue processing, manual staining, and weighing and preparation of solid and liquid dye chemicals will provide sufficient contaminant capture velocities (100 fpm +/- 20%), as evaluated by a combination of velometer and smoke tube tests.
4. An effective exhausted enclosure or hood for automatic tissue processing and staining will provide sufficient capture velocities (50–60 fpm minimum), as evaluated by a combination of velometer and smoke tube tests. Exhausted enclosures for automatic processing will be provided with adequate fire protection systems.
5. Exhausted enclosures and hoods, as mentioned above, will be totally vented to the outside and monitored routinely, as described in Appendix I. [Not reprinted here.]
6. Personnel formaldehyde exposures in necropsy, tissue trimming and processing areas will be kept below 1 ppm. Air monitoring for formaldehyde will be performed periodically by NTP.
7. Flammable solvents will be stored in a flammable storage cabinet which conforms to OSHA requirements and NFPA Code 30, and FM approvals. These solvents will be transported between laboratories in leak- and shatter-proof

*Reprinted by permission of the NTP Office of Chemical Health and Safety and the contractor for health and safety support services, Arthur D. Little, Inc., Cambridge, Massachusetts.

secondary containers. Transfer of fresh or waste flammable solvents will be performed in containers which are properly bonded and grounded.

8. Eating, drinking, smoking, applying cosmetics, and chewing gum will not be permitted wherever whole animal, tissue or chemicals are handled. The presence of food or smoking materials will not be permitted in these areas.

9. The following personnel protective clothing will be worn when handling chemicals: a) cloth laboratory coat (knee length); b) one pair of disposable gloves (i.e., PVC, latex, natural rubber, etc.).

10. If during routine or emergency operations respirators are used, all components of a respiratory protection program will be practiced, as outlined in Appendix II. [Not reprinted here.]

11. Residual or archival wet tissues will be double-bagged.

12. Any contaminated solid or liquid waste chemicals will be collected in a leak-proof container. Disposal containers must be stored in an isolated and secured area. This area will be controlled by either the principal investigator or the waste disposal officer. All wastes generated by the testing program will be disposed of in accordance with federal, state, or municipal waste disposal regulations.

13. General laboratory safety procedures will be followed, including (but not limited to) the following: a) use of safety glasses in chemical handling areas, b) no mouth pipetting, c) no open-toed shoes, d) no dry sweeping for maintenance or for spill clean-up, e) removal of ignition sources when handling flammable liquids.

14. There will be written general safety policies (Standard Operating Procedures— SOPs) at each laboratory. These written health and safety policies will include (but not be limited to) issues addressed above (storage, hood monitoring, good housekeeping, etc.), and personnel training, health and safety management responsibility and enforcement, and a written set of emergency procedures to be followed by all project personnel in the event of a chemical spill or leak.

CHAPTER 2

Chemical Containment Design Criteria for Toxicity Testing Facilities

Douglas B. Walters
National Toxicology Program, National
Institute of Environmental Health Sciences,
P.O. Box 12233, Research Triangle Park,
North Carolina 27709

R. Scott Stricoff
Arthur D. Little, Inc., Acorn Park,
Cambridge, Massachusetts 02140

James M. Harless
Radian Corporation, P.O. Box 9948,
Austin, Texas 78766

INTRODUCTION

This chapter emphasizes the need for close interaction between technical personnel and architects in the design of laboratories that use chemicals. This necessitates incorporation of chemical containment principles into design criteria. To build laboratories in which chemicals are to be used, consideration must be given to the chemical, physical, and toxicological properties of these substances. These problems must be addressed on a chemistry level and communicated to everyone involved in the architectural design and construction to provide in-depth understanding and insight into both general as well as particular chemistry concerns. Failure to do so will result in a less safe or even unsafe laboratory of less than satisfactory design which is impractical and inefficient.

The objective of chemical containment design criteria for toxicity testing facilities is simply to achieve the design and construction of safe laboratory buildings. An evolution in the design of laboratory facilities is occurring. Soon buildings will not be built first and then made into laboratories, nor will buildings be designed from the outset as just laboratories. Rather they will be planned, designed, and constructed from the start as *safe* laboratories. The distinctions are significant. The most efficient and effective way to build laboratory buildings is to include safety into the initial planning, development, and design aspects. This is best not only from an employee and environmental standpoint, but it is also the most cost-effective way of accomplishing the goal. Today more and more laboratories, particularly those with special requirements, are being built using this concept.

Advances are being made in new designs for safe laboratories [1-6], but there are no standards or criteria for research facilities using chemicals. This chapter is intended as an introduction to subsequent chapters which address in-depth specific aspects of design and facilities requirements based on containment principles (see Chapters 3, 4, 5, and 7).

TOXICOLOGY TESTING LABORATORIES

In general, toxicity testing laboratories which require special containment facilities can be separated into three categories:

- *in vivo* studies
- *in vitro* studies
- chemistry support

Individual tasks performed in these three categories are shown in Table 2-1 with health and safety toxicology study concerns summarized in Table 2-2.

In vivo studies, which deal with live animals, often are conducted in barrier systems which require shower areas and use of a dual corridor, clean-dirty system. In addition, many diverse functions are usually performed in support of these studies

Table 2-1.   Tasks Performed at Laboratories

Chemistry	Cellular and Genetic Toxicity	In Vivo
Analysis	Receiving	Receiving
Synthesis	Storage	Storage
Repository functions:	Weighing	Weighing
Storage	Dilution preparation	Dose preparation
Handling	Test administration	Dose administration
Weighing	(Cell culture, plating,	Cage cleaning
Shipment	*Drosophila*, etc)	Necropsy
Surplus chemical	Test incubation-duration	Tissue trim
Management	37° C/24-72 hrs.	Histology
	Test evaluation, e.g.	Waste management
	Slide reading	
	Colony counting	
	Drosophila evaluation	
	Waste disposal	

Table 2-2. Toxicology Study Requirements

Chemistry	Cellular and Genetic Toxicity	In Vivo
Large no. of chemicals	Small no. of chemicals	Small no. of chemicals
Varying sample size	Small sample size	Large sample size
Moderate spatial needs	Small spatial needs	Large spatial needs
Single discipline	Single discipline	Multidisciplinary
Localized operations and work area	Localized operations and work area	Dispersed operations and work area
Small-moderate waste	Small amount of waste	Large amount of waste
Small no. of contaminated items of high level	Small no. of contaminated items of low level	Large no. of contaminated items of varying level
Cost effective engineering controls	Can't justify cost of engineering controls	Prohibitive engineering controls cost
Many sources-few paths	Few sources-many paths	Many sources-many paths

such as necropsy, tissue trimming and slide preparation, pathology, histology, dose-chemical mixing and analysis, chemical storage, and waste storage. The result is the manipulation of large amounts of a relatively small number of neat chemicals which are mixed, diluted, and transported throughout the entire facility. Much of the work performed, such as dose preparation, mixing, and administration does not lend itself readily to chemical containment. The primary reasons for these limitations are: extensive spatial needs which usually occupy at least a dozen rooms; multidisciplinary operations in which the contamination is dispersed rather than localized; and substantial amounts of waste with large numbers of contaminated items of varying levels. Hence, there are both many sources of potential contamination and many potential paths for the chemical contamination to reach the receiver, or worker.

In vitro studies, such as those performed in the National Toxicology Program (NTP) Cellular and Genetic Toxicology Branch, include microbial and chromosomal studies as well as cellular transformation. These tasks are usually performed in one or two rooms using small amounts of neat material which are usually diluted during the assay. Operations and work areas are localized and single disciplinary, generating limited amounts of waste with small numbers of items having low levels of contamination. The major problem of *in vitro* laboratories is generally the high cost of sophisticated engineering controls. Hence, engineering controls usually amount to little more than a hood or an occasional glove box. As a result, the safety emphasis is on operational practices since there are relatively few sources of potential contamination but many paths for the contamination to reach the worker. Because engineering controls are costly, often there is no feasible choice but to rely on performing the actual operations correctly, in accordance with standard operating procedures, in proper locations such as hoods.

Chemistry functions that support toxicological testing entail procurement, storage, handling, shipment, analysis, and synthesis of widely varying amounts of neat chemicals which are used in a localized area, often highly specialized in design. Generally there is a moderate spatial requirement, and the work tasks are monodisciplinary. Small to moderate amounts of waste are generated with a small number of contaminated items, often having a high level of contamination. Engineering controls are most effective in this type of operation, because there are many sources of potential contamination but relatively few paths by which the contamination can reach the receiver or worker.

CHEMICAL CONTAINMENT

The underlying principle of chemical containment is the source, path, receiver relationship. Control should take place, to the extent possible, at the source, where potential chemical contamination originates. When this becomes impractical, the path, through operational work practices, must then be controlled. In the event these options are limited, the final reliance is on personal protection. Sole reliance on personal protection should be avoided wherever possible, since it provides no redundancy or backup; relies heavily on the worker's discretion for proper use; and requires periodic upkeep and maintenance to ensure effectiveness.

Figure 2–1 shows the relationship of the source, path, receiver concept to the control techniques employed in each area of toxicology testing studies. The effect of using the chemical containment concepts presented in this chapter for toxicity testing facilities is visualized in Figure 2–2. The overriding purpose of chemical containment is protection of the worker and the environment. This protection can best be carried out using four factors, the first of which is knowledge of the chemistry of what is being used in the facility. This information is essential for a full understanding of the physical-chemical properties of the test substances and is necessary to help determine proper protection against specific hazards. Second, engineering controls, with ventilation of primary importance, should be used for control of contamination at the source, whenever possible. Third, proper chemical storage techniques should be used for source control. Fourth, proper work controls should be instituted through use of standard operating procedures (SOPs) in accordance with good industrial hygiene

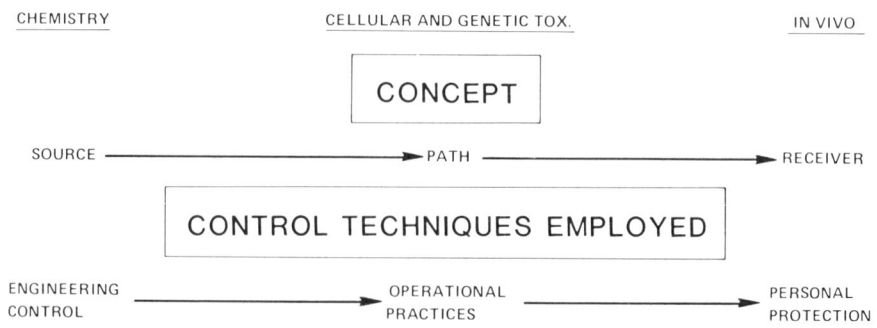

Figure 2–1.   Health and safety concepts and control techniques for toxicity studies.

practices. Such operational practices provide protection from potential contamination along the path to the receiver-worker while the work is performed. In the event that a mishap occurs during work operations, protection at the source (engineering and storage controls) provides backup protection. Personnel protection provides the final redundancy but should not be relied on as an exclusive means of control. The combined use of these four factors serve to protect both the worker and the facility. Similarly, a well-designed, safe laboratory protects both the environment and the workers.

While engineering controls could be designed to provide absolute containment of all chemical hazards, the cost of such a total engineering reliance system would be prohibitive in all but the most crucial circumstances. Control is therefore achieved by combination of work practices and personnel protection with engineering controls. As a result, control at the path employing rigid SOPs is used, but because of the nature of certain types of work and the presence of only partial control at the source, reliance may also fall on the use of personal protection by the worker.

Control of the spread of contamination emanating from the toxicological testing categories listed above is accomplished using principles of chemical containment. As shown in Figure 2–3, the desired goal of this concept is to maximize containment and thereby minimize contamination. To do this, containment must be

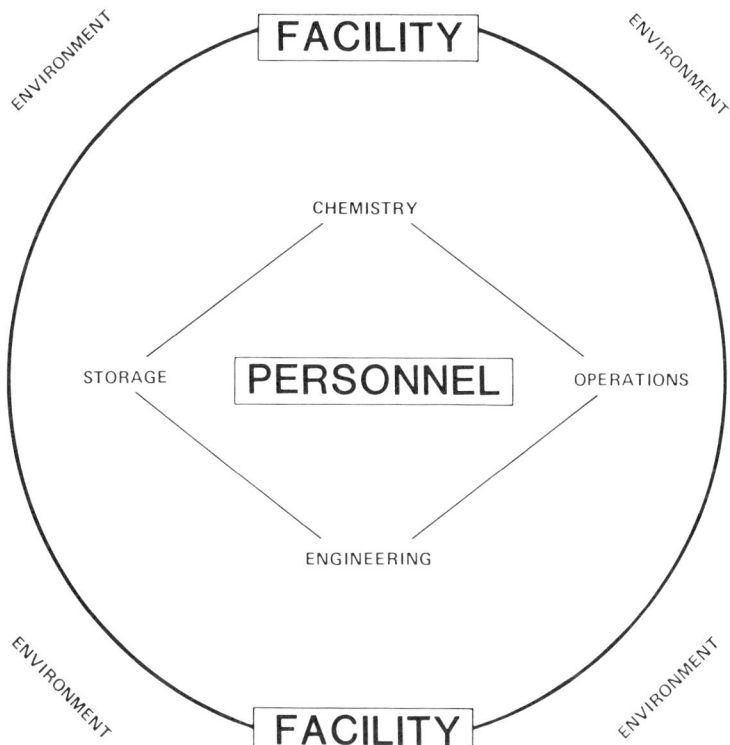

Figure 2–2.   Chemical containment concepts.

designed for the specific chemical or class of chemicals in use, and one must consider the work tasks that will be performed using this chemical. The requirements of a facility used for inhalation studies differ from one used for chronic dosed-feed studies, *Salmonella* or *Drosophila* testing, or chemical synthesis. In addition, accountability of the material is essential. Knowledge of where *all* the material is at *all* times as well as its chemical and physical properties is required for proper control and containment. Hence, an in-depth knowledge of the chemicals one is working with has no substitute. Some of the benefits chemistry knowledge provides include designing laboratories, handling and management of hazardous chemicals, monitoring, spill control, deactivation, waste disposal, and emergency response. In addition chemistry serves other needs, such as: (1) training designed around an understanding of the chemical properties and reactivity of test materials; (2) structure-activity relationships and chemical classification to predict properties and hazards and to provide missing gaps in informational knowledge; and (3) medical surveillance programs with biological monitoring to monitor the presence of test material, its breakdown products, or metabolites in body fluids and tissue samples.

Chemical storage must be given careful consideration in designing laboratories, and redundancy is an important principle which should be applied. This principle begins with the chemical itself and its primary container. For primary or micro containment the chemical must be localized in one place with precautions against spill, breakage, and spread of contamination in the event of a mishap. The next step is proper container storage, employing suitable safeguards such as solvent cabinets, ventilation, and fire alarms. The storage area now becomes a secondary container

MAXIMIZE CONTAINMENT – MINIMIZE CONTAMINATION
DESIGN SPECIFICALLY FOR THE CHEMICAL AND THE TASK
PROVIDE ACCOUNTABILITY AND KNOWLEDGE

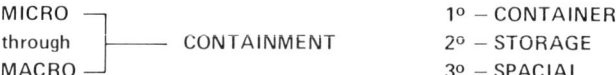

MICRO			1° – CONTAINER
through		CONTAINMENT	2° – STORAGE
MACRO			3° – SPACIAL

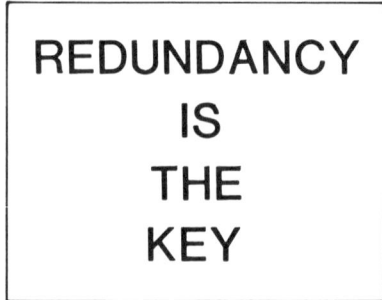

REDUNDANCY
IS
THE
KEY

Figure 2-3.   Principles of chemical containment.

providing backup protection or redundancy. Finally, it must be decided where the storage area should be with respect to the rest of the facility and what protection the area requires. That is, the spatial or building arrangement must be large enough to accomplish and support the operational tasks that are required. Thus, the spatial arrangement now becomes a form of macro container, and the container in a container concept or redundancy is used from the micro to the macro stages. Similar redundancy is necessary in all areas (ventilation, emergency power, filtration, etc.) that support toxicity testing of hazardous materials.

VENTILATION

The primary method of engineering control used for chemical containment is ventilation. Many excellent references exist regarding the theory and application of ventilation [7,8,9,10] (see Chapter 15). The purpose of this section is to present a brief summary of some of the more important concepts of using ventilation for chemical contamination control. Use of ventilation may be perceived as a paradox since it can be used for both dilution and containment. The classical concept is to get fresh air in and to move air through the area, venting it to the outside. Difficulties quickly arise using dilution or general ventilation since large volumes of air may be required; energy cost may be prohibitive; and little containment at the source of the generation of contamination may be possible [8]. An example of an application of dilution ventilation is venting of isolated rooms or areas to achieve a predetermined number of room air changes per hour (e.g., 10–15 changes/hour in NTP animal study rooms). This is effective, however, only when designed to prevent exhaust reentrainment in the facility and when consideration is given to use of proper filtration or scrubbers. Because of these limitations, local exhaust is usually considered a better alternative for consolidation and localization of chemical contamination from hazardous materials. Local exhaust is most commonly used in chemical fume hoods and the many other types of hoods designed for specific tasks. A specialized form of hood is the negative pressure glove box. Such boxes provide containment in the event of a leak and ensure that the flow of air is from the less hazardous to the more hazardous operation and away from the worker. In addition, glove boxes prevent the spread of contamination by instituting control at the source and require less energy to operate effectively.

One example of the creative use of local exhaust for chemical containment is the design of tissue trimming stations in pathology laboratories. This case illustrates the multidisciplinary interaction which is often necessary to achieve effective solutions. The problem is control of formaldehyde, solvent vapors, and potentially hazardous chemical residues from animals used in chemical toxicology studies. Figure 2–4 shows a hood design which can be used for this purpose as well as for necropsy and histology. Mechanical engineering is necessary to determine the proper volume of air flow, duct diameter, and interfacing with the rest of the ventilation system (i.e., fans, filters, exhaust). Important consideration is given to use of gentle bends in the duct system and a taper between the duct and the top of the hood to

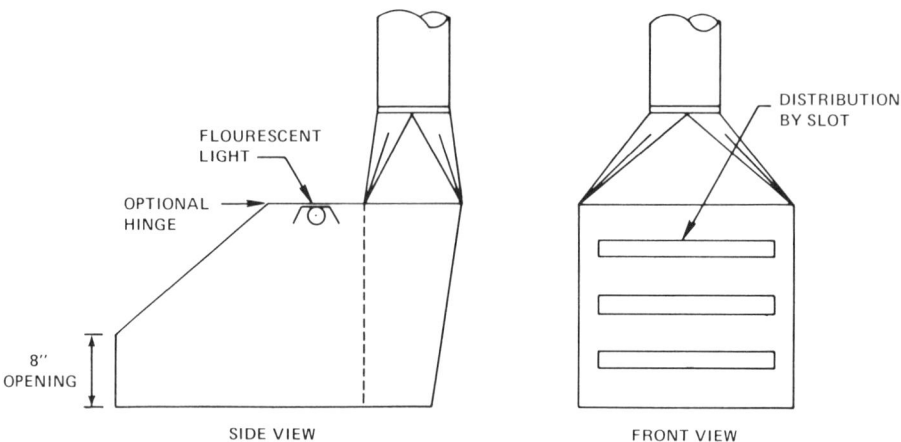

Figure 2–4.   Necropsy, tissue trimming, histology hood.

provide uniform air flow and to minimize eddy currents. The tapered duct is inter-
faced with a tapered plenum containing three slots for uniform air distribution and
capture velocity. The work area of the hood is enclosed in Plexiglas and has a movable
light to minimize glare. The enclosure is hinged at the top to accommodate items too
large to enter through the 8-inch front opening. To construct a useful hood, the
designer should consult with those involved in the work operation. These include a
pathologist to determine precisely what use the hood will serve, a histopathology
technician to describe how the hood will be used and what will be used in it, an industrial hygienist to determine work hazards, a chemist to analyze and determine its
effectiveness, and an industrial or human factors engineer to design safe and efficient
workspace.

DESIGN

Paramount in the development of chemical containment criteria is employee safety
and environmental protection. In addition, maintenance of research integrity to minimize possible chemical cross-contamination helps to ensure that work is performed
safely, efficiently, and effectively. Initial laboratory design decisions require a multidisciplinary approach from experts in the following research fields: health and safety,
architecture, specific engineering areas, and chemistry. A sophisticated knowledge of
chemistry is crucial whenever hazardous research chemicals are to be used. Key roles
are played by the industrial hygienist and health and safety experts with the assistance of other experts, such as engineers, to help assure compliance with federal regulations. In addition, vital input concerning ventilation control is received from
mechanical and electrical engineers. An important aspect of design criteria, often
neglected, is the area of industrial or mechanical engineering referred to as human

factors. The best way to ensure human efficiency and safety in a laboratory is to design human factors into the facility from the start. With existing facilities, problems are often correctable after consultation with appropriate interdisciplinary specialists. Discussions with architects, toxicologists, experts in various disciplines of biology and veterinary medicine, pathologists, and health physicists (if radiolabeled materials are used) are also essential.

Design Phases

Simplified phases in planning the construction of a safe laboratory building are shown in Figure 2–5. The first phase is the definition of the problem, a description of the new facility and what it must provide in order to fulfill program needs. Representatives from all the potential disciplines using the facility must specify their requirements, particularly unique needs such as isolated laboratories, hoods and ventilation, special preparation or mixing areas, barrier areas, and radiochemical laboratories. Often, after the definition phase, the process moves directly to the design phase, and there is no feedback to the scientist and the discussion of requirements is ended. What is essential at this point is inclusion of an interpretation phase. The key person at this stage is an individual who is interested and knowledgeable in both design and health and safety criteria and has an in-depth familiarity with the work for which the facility is being designed. It is this phase which interprets the requirements into the design criteria. This phase allows the architects and scientists, or their representatives, to negotiate and reach agreement over the specific requirements of each scientific discipline. Hence, situations are minimized which require immediate renovations when construction is completed (e.g., avoidance of locating a nuclear magnetic resonance

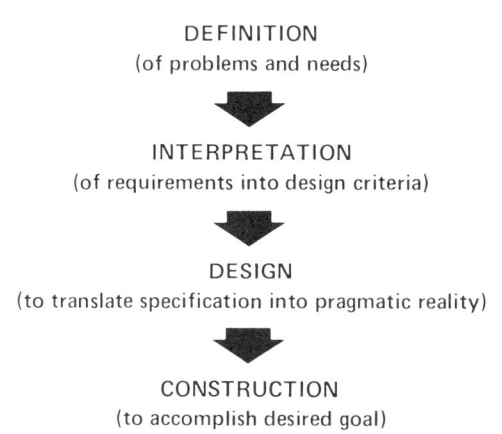

DEFINITION
(of problems and needs)

INTERPRETATION
(of requirements into design criteria)

DESIGN
(to translate specification into pragmatic reality)

CONSTRUCTION
(to accomplish desired goal)

THE GOAL: Design and Construction of Safe Laboratory Buildings

Figure 2–5.   Laboratory development phases.

spectrometer on an upper floor which may subject the instrument to intolerable vibrational effects, relocation problems, and possibly overloading the floor stress). As a result of this step, the architect now has a complete understanding of what requirements are necessary in the facility and he can translate these specifications into pragmatic reality in the design phase.

The final phase is construction to accomplish the desired goal. Inspection and approval of the facility by health and safety personnel, in addition to the typical inspections (electrical codes, etc.), are essential before the facility is occupied. Just as in the initial definition and interpretation steps, it is a lot easier to make changes before people occupy a facility than afterward.

CONCLUSION

The design and construction of safe laboratory buildings necessitate employment of chemical containment concepts. The fundamental principle of chemical containment is the source, path, receiver concept. This concept relies first on the use of engineering controls, usually ventilation, at the source, operational practices during the path, and finally personnel protection by the receiver. Redundancy in all systems is the key to the proper use of these concepts. In chemical toxicology studies, application of sound chemistry knowledge provides the foundation upon which to build.

REFERENCES

1. Everett, K. and D. Hughes. *A Guide to Laboratory Design.* (Somerset, England: Butterworths, 1981).
2. Raab, Martin D. "New Look in Lab Design: It's All About Open Space," *Indus. Chem. News* 3 (11): 1, 24–25, 1982.
3. Walters, D.B., J.D. McKinney, A. Norstrom, and N. DeWitt. "Control of Potential Carcinogenic, Mutagenic and Toxic Chemicals via a Protocol Review Concept and a Chemistry Containment Laboratory," in *Safe Handling of Chemical Carcinogens, Mutagens, Teratogens and Highly Toxic Substances, Vol. 1*, D.B. Walters, Ed. (Ann Arbor, MI: Ann Arbor Science, 1980), pp. 3–30.
4. Harless, J.M., K.E. Baxter, L.H. Keith, and D.B. Walters. "Design and Operation of a Hazardous Materials Laboratory," in *Safe Handling of Chemical Carcinogens, Mutagens, Teratogens and Highly Toxic Substances*, Vol. 1, D.B. Walters, Ed. (Ann Arbor, MI: Ann Arbor Science, 1980), pp. 79–100.
5. Walters, D.B., L.H. Keith, and J.M. Harless. "Chemical Selection and Handling Aspects of the National Toxicology Program," in *Environmental Health Chemistry*, J.D. McKinney, Ed. (Ann Arbor, MI: Ann Arbor Science, 1981), pp. 575–592.
6. Keith, L.H., J.M. Harless, and D.B. Walters, "Analysis and Storage of Hazardous Environmental Chemicals for Toxicological Testing," in *Environmental Health Chemistry*, J.D. McKinney, Ed. (Ann Arbor, MI: Ann Arbor Science, 1981), pp. 593–621.
7. *Industrial Ventilation, A Manual of Recommended Practice*, 17th ed. (Lansing, MI: American Conference of Governmental Industrial Hygienists, 1982).

8. McDermott, H.J. *Handbook of Ventilation For Contaminant Control* (Ann Arbor, MI: Ann Arbor Science, 1977).
9. Caplan, K.J. and G.W. Knutson. "Influence of Room Air Supply on Laboratory Hoods," *Am. Ind. Hyg. Assoc. J.* 43(10): 738–746, 1982.
10. Fuller, F.H., and A.W. Etchells. "The Rating of Laboratory Hood Performance," *ASHRAE J.* 21(10): 49-53, 1979.

CHAPTER 3

Components in the Design of a Hazardous Chemicals Handling Facility

James M. Harless
Radian Corporation, P.O. Box 9948,
Austin, Texas 78766

INTRODUCTION

As chemists, laboratory technicians, and the general public become more aware of the potential health and environmental hazards of toxic chemicals, the demand for appropriate facilities for handling these materials grows. Just as it is irresponsible to eliminate all research using hazardous chemicals, it is likewise irresponsible to conduct such research without maximum protection of laboratory personnel, the general public, and the environment. The fundamental elements in this required umbrella of protection are the design and operation of the hazardous chemical laboratory. Advances in designs of air handling equipment and controls, containment devices, laboratory equipment and the laboratory itself now permit the construction of facilities which can safely support an almost unlimited variety of operations involving hazardous chemicals. Because of the critical protective nature and the extremely high cost of a hazardous materials laboratory, a thorough understanding of the characteristics, design philosophies, and design elements of such a facility is necessary prior to design or operation.

A hazardous materials laboratory (HML) is a protective facility designed to support efficient operations involving hazardous chemicals while providing maximum protection for operating personnel, the general public, and the environment. It may range in size from a small isolation room of less than a hundred square feet to a complex of spaces occupying thousands of square feet. However, the basic HML characteristics listed below are constant:

- The primary protection systems are engineering controls and personnel/operating procedures.
- Personnel protection devices have limited primary roles, but are important in secondary or backup roles.

- The facility operates at negative pressure.
- The locations and methods for handling and storage of chemicals are well defined and controlled.
- Access is rigidly controlled.
- Protective clothing and respiratory protection are required.
- All effluents and wastes are controlled.

These characteristics arise from the basic philosophies for the design and operation of the facility. These philosophies may be summarized by the four "protects":

- Protect the personnel.
- Protect the environment.
- Protect the chemicals.
- Protect the facility.

These four philosophies are the driving forces behind design and operation decisions. As such, they give rise to five goals upon which to base such decisions. These are:

- No chemical shall leave the facility in an uncontrolled manner or in a manner harmful to personnel, the general public, or the environment.
- No person shall ingest, inhale, or dermally contact any chemical.
- No chemical shall change properties in an uncontrolled manner.
- Maximum information about chemical hazards and properties shall be readily available.
- All activities involving toxic chemicals shall be the result of conscious thoughts and decisions.

Unfortunately the intellectual pursuit of ideal HML design and operation soon bumps squarely into reality. Facilities can now be designed to provide virtually 100% protection in all areas; however, their cost would be prohibitively high, equipment would be pushed to operational limits, and personnel would be inefficient and frustrated. Although adherence to the four basic philosophies are paramount in HML design, each decision must be a compromise with such forces as construction and operating costs, work efficiency, and personnel morale. The health and environmental risks associated with handling hazardous chemicals can never be reduced to zero, but the proper design and operation of hazardous materials handling facilities can cost-effectively minimize those risks.

The remainder of this chapter is devoted to defining and explaining the basic elements of HML design. These have been derived from the knowledge and experiences gained during the design, construction, and expansion of Radian Corporation's 5,000-square-foot Hazardous Materials Laboratory and other laboratory facilities. Many of the following discussions are illustrated with examples from the Radian facility.

HML DESIGN COMPONENTS

Design of a hazardous chemicals handling facility requires both design and operations experience with an HML and the independent and collaborative efforts of a technical designer, an architect, and a mechanical engineer. All must be highly qualified, for the design and construction of an HML is probably the most complex undertaking in the realm of scientific laboratory operations.

The participants in the design of such a facility must address the following five basic design components:

- spatial
- mechanical
- structural
- equipment
- safety

These components will be described in the following sections in general terms. They are addressed individually, but all are interdependent. Design decisions can only be made after considering the impact of those decisions within each of the different components. The intention of the following discussions is not to provide answers to specific design questions, but rather to provide a guide for asking the proper questions and ensuring that all critical factors in HML design are considered. Entire chapters and even books could be written if each were to be discussed in depth with all options and combinations considered.

Spatial Design Component

The first task in the design of an HML is to define the spatial configuration of the facility. The principal elements which must be addressed are location, types and sizes of workspaces, and the movement of personnel, materials, and work through the facility. The specifications of each of these elements are determined by the following factors:

- types of technical operations to be supported; e.g., environmental sample preparation, synthesis, analysis, purification, aliquotting
- size of proposed staff
- types and quantities of materials handled; e.g., toxic, explosive, volatile, nonvolatile, liquids, gases, solids
- scope of programs to be supported; e.g., single task, multitask, production-oriented, research-oriented
- management structures and philosophies
- designer preferences

Of these, the first four will have the most direct, quantifiable impact on the spatial design process. The last two will have a significant impact, but it will be more subtle and based upon the personal experiences of the designer(s) and operator(s).

Location

Selection of the location for a hazardous materials laboratory is important in the context of access, physical and psychological security of non-HML personnel, and construction parameters. The ideal HML is a self-contained, freestanding facility, physically separated from other buildings. This configuration minimizes real and imagined risks for non-HML personnel and provides ready access to all areas of the structure. It also provides an element of isolation in the event of an emergency. If the HML must be attached to an existing building, the two structures should have no common walls. This can be accomplished by placing storage and/or mechanical areas ($\geq$6 feet wide) between the two structures.

The least desirable location for an HML is within a larger structure. The ability to isolate the toxic chemicals facility from nonassociated personnel, noncontrolled workspaces and offices, and surrounding utilities and air handling equipment is severely reduced. This situation is at its worst when an HML is built into a remodeled space which was not originally designed for that purpose. Compromises in design caused by restrictions of existing utilities, structural features, etc., can reduce safety factors and personnel effectiveness. The real hazard of this configuration is the potential for release and dispersal of toxic material into other parts of the surrounding structure during or as a result of an emergency equipment malfunction.

Several physical plant parameters will also impact upon the selection of an HML location. The facility must be structurally supported by the ground upon which it is built, and all utilities required for support of laboratory operations must be readily available. Physical security of the facility and access control are also important considerations.

Workspaces

There are seven different types of operational spaces that can be incorporated into a hazardous materials laboratory.

- external access
- shower/dressing
- general laboratory
- isolation laboratories
- chemical storage
- waste storage
- office

All HMLs are developed as combinations of these spaces together with supporting mechanical and storage spaces. However, not all these workspaces need appear in each HML; the selection of specific operational spaces will depend upon the factors determining laboratory specifications discussed earlier. At a minimum, all HMLs contain external access, shower/dressing, and isolation laboratory spaces. In the following paragraphs, each of the above workspaces is described within the context of two possible HML configurations.

A conceptual diagram of a large hazardous materials laboratory incorporating all possible workspaces is shown in Figure 3-1. The key spatial element in this design is the general laboratory which forms the hub for the facility. Primary access to all storage and workspaces is gained via the general laboratory. This concept utilizes the central space as a buffer between the high-risk areas, such as isolation laboratories, chemical storage and waste storage, and the shower/dressing and external access areas. As shown later, this concept also provides for good work/traffic flow and air-flow design.

Personnel access to the HML is provided by an external access area coupled with a shower/dressing area. The external access area contains sign-in logs, lockers, restrooms, and access control spaces. The shower/dressing area contains sufficient clothes-changing and showering areas to accommodate the laboratory workforce. Two changing areas are required: one for changing and storage of street clothes and one for changing and storage of laboratory clothing. The two change areas are separated by the shower area. Two sets of change-shower rooms are usually provided, and additional washrooms, laundry rooms, etc., may be incorporated into this area.

As stated earlier, the general laboratory space is the hub of the full-scale HML; all other laboratory spaces are accessed from this area. Although no chemical handling operations occur on benches in this area, it may contain specialized primary containment devices, such as glove boxes, which are used for handling highly toxic chemicals. In general, this space is used for nonchemical operations such as instrumental analysis, packaging for shipment, and other logistical operations. This space

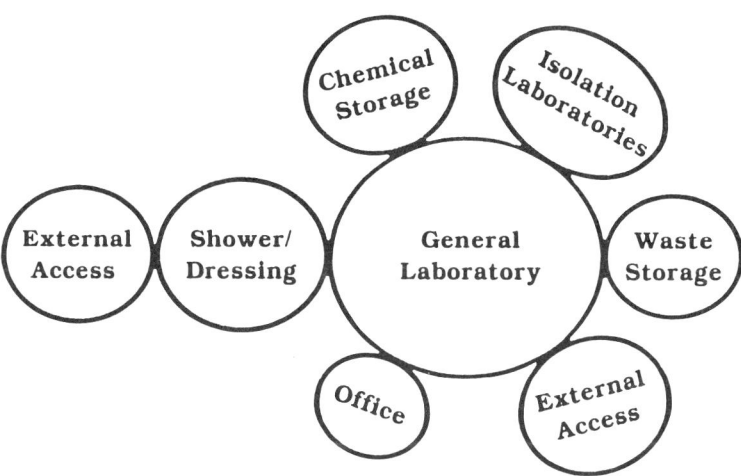

Figure 3-1.   Large HML spatial elements.

also often contains the facility's major safety equipment such as emergency showers, first aid kits, and fire blankets.

The principal chemical handling areas are located in the isolation laboratories. These areas are equipped with the bench space, equipment, and primary containment devices necessary to support the desired chemical activities. Although the isolation laboratories are designed to provide containment of chemicals handled anywhere in the area, most operations are performed in the primary containment device(s), usually a fume hood or glove box. Sufficient floor space and bench space must be provided to accommodate the number of personnel scheduled to work in each isolation laboratory. In general, a 7×11-foot space with a 4–6-foot fume hood is adequate for one person, while a 10×20-foot space with an 8-foot fume hood and 30 feet of bench space is ideal for two people and workable with three. The isolation laboratories must be equipped with all the services, utilities, and equipment needed to support the personnel and the chemical operations.

Another major spatial element in most HMLs is chemical storage. This area has a high potential for contamination and should be isolated from the other areas. It can range in scale from a small, closet-like space to a space large enough for several walk-in storage lockers at a variety of temperatures. Special storage areas such as underground vaults and controlled substance lockers may be included. All chemical storage areas should have vapor- and explosion-proof fixtures and utilities. They spaces should be designed such that accidental chemical spills are contained, and all areas may be easily decontaminated. The recommended packaging for toxic chemicals[1] is rather bulky; therefore, more storage space is required for HML chemicals than standard laboratory samples. Planning for adequate storage space and defining the needed storage conditions, e.g., temperature, humidity, and light, are critical steps in HML design.

All disposable materials generated in an HML must be considered contaminated with toxic chemicals and be disposed of accordingly. A waste storage area is a necessity in a large HML as a place to safely accumulate, segregate, package, and store laboratory wastes prior to disposal. This area should be of sufficient size to handle at least one container for each type of waste generated; this will generally include a waste solvent barrel, aqueous waste barrel, segregated organics containers (e.g., oxidizers, explosives, water reactives), and fiberboard containers for burnable solids such as clothing, gloves, and absorbent paper. Additional storage space may be designed into the waste storage area as needed to store spent air or water treatment filters, etc. The waste area should be equipped with vapor- and explosion-proof fixtures, and should be easily flushed with water and decontaminated. Provision should also be made to electrically ground all barrels containing flammable liquids.

An office area is generally needed in HMLs with a staff of six or more. This area not only provides work space for data collection and reduction, reference materials, and communications, but also provides a space where laboratory personnel can relax without having to endure the rigors of exit procedures. The office area is also designed to serve as a central staging area for responses to laboratory emergencies.

A second external access area is provided to allow movement of chemicals and equipment into the laboratory without having to transit personnel access areas. This access is usually provided into the general laboratory area, but may also connect to chemical, and/or waste storage areas. All external access areas are constructed as air locks so as to prevent direct contact of the laboratory atmosphere with the environment.

Figure 3–2 shows the arrangement of spatial elements in Radian Corporation's Hazardous Materials Laboratory. The floorplan of this facility is shown in Figure 3–3. This 5,000-square-foot facility incorporates all the spatial elements of an HML and is one example of how these elements can be arranged into a working facility. The laboratory is designed to support a staff of 14–17 persons, programs involving large numbers and volumes of chemicals, and virtually all types of chemical manipulations.

Access to the facility by personnel is restricted to a single door into the shower/dressing area. Dual change/shower facilities are provided with access to the "dirty" change area accomplished via the shower stall area. A bypass airlock is incorporated to allow personnel to enter and leave the laboratory when removal of only the outer laboratory protective clothing (Tyvek®) is required [1]. Restroom facilities are provided on the "clean" side only.

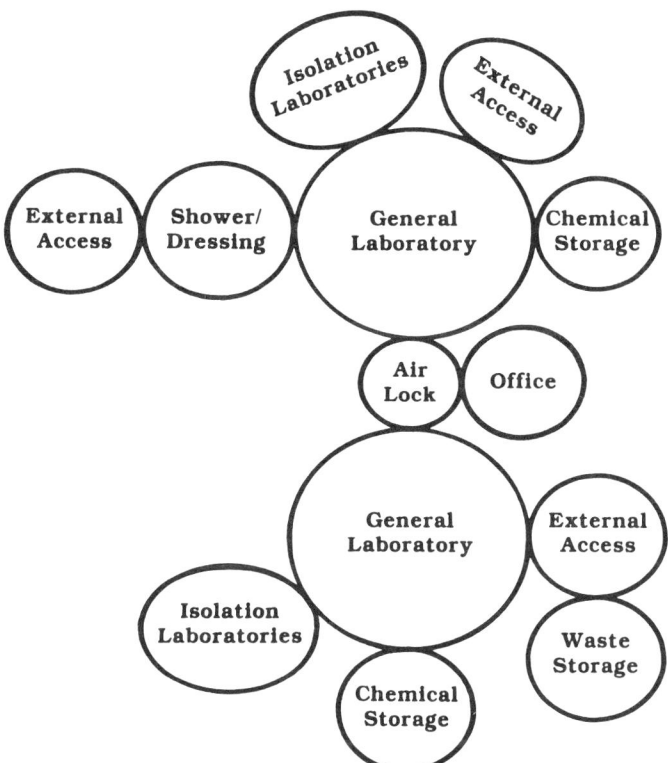

Figure 3–2.   Spatial elements in Radian Corporation's hazardous materials laboratory.

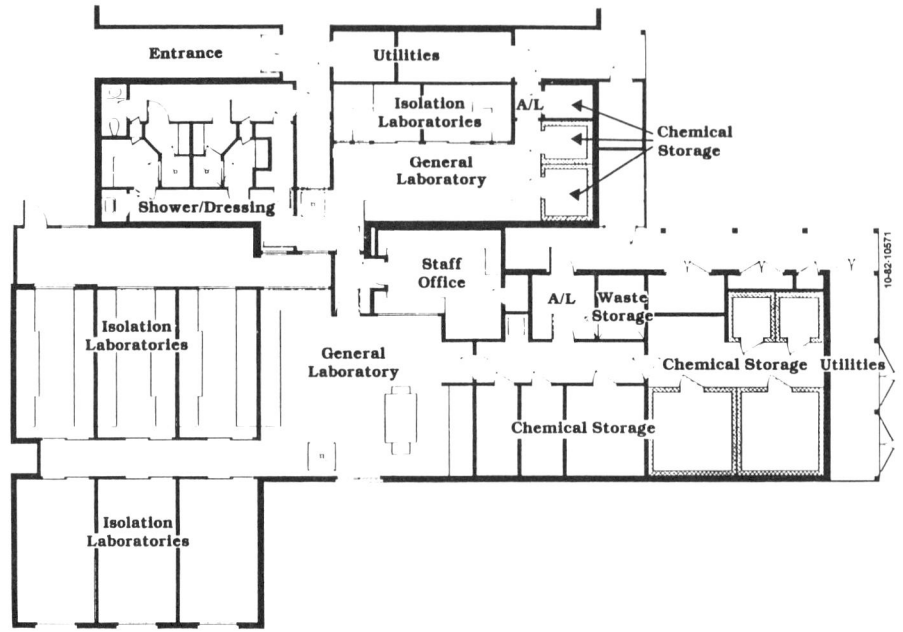

Figure 3-3.   Radian HML facility floorplan.

The core of the HML is composed of two general laboratory spaces occupying ~750 square feet. These areas include general bench and storage space for support for nonchemical operations. Special areas are dedicated for analytical instrumentation and preparation of ampuls of analytical standards. Also housed in the general laboratory area is a $4 \times 9 \times 4$-foot glove box, which serves as the primary containment device for very high hazardous materials. Safety showers, first aid equipment, and major alarms are located in these areas.

The five isolation laboratories are accessed from the general laboratory areas. The facility is equipped with two 7×11-foot one-person areas and six 10×18-foot two- or three-person areas. Each is equipped with a large fume hood and laboratory benches. One laboratory is specially equipped with vacuum and distillation racks to support chemical synthesis operations.

Chemical storage occupies ~15% of Radian's Hazardous Materials Laboratory. The majority of chemicals are stored in walkin lockers maintained at three different temperatures: 25° C, 5° C, and –20° C. Three areas are available at each temperature to provide storage flexibility and segregation of samples. Other chemical storage capabilities include an underground vault, a controlled-substances vault, and upright freezers at –70° C. All chemical storage areas are grouped at the ends of laboratory wings to provide improved isolation and security.

The 55-square-foot waste storage area is located off the primary equipment airlock. This provides additional isolation for the area and allows waste containers to be removed from the facility without passing through other workspaces.

The office area is accessed from an airlock connecting the two general laboratory areas. This serves to isolate the space and protect it from contamination. The office supports a reference library for chemical and chemical hazards data, a computerized hazard and inventory management system, laboratory communications, and general data and records management activities. It also provides a break area for personnel who do not wish to sign out of the laboratory via the standard exit procedures [1].

Chemicals and equipment enter and leave the HML through airlocks connected to the general laboratory spaces. The larger airlock is also used for storage of flammable solvents. Smaller samples and materials may enter or leave the facility through a small airlock chamber connected to the entrance hallway. All airlocks are operated such that only one side is open at any one time.

Utility closets and external storage areas are located around the perimeter of the facility. This allows ready access for maintenance or modification without requiring entrance into the HML itself. Two 6-foot-wide utility areas were used to create a buffer space between the HML and an adjacent building (see Figure 3-3).

These descriptions demonstrate one method of combining the different HML spatial elements into a functioning facility. In many cases, though, a much smaller facility is all that is needed. The other extreme, a two-space HML, is shown in Figure 3-4. The corresponding floorplan is shown in Figure 3-5. In this facility, the external access and shower/dressing areas are combined, and the general laboratories, isolation laboratories, chemical storage, and waste storage areas are combined; no office is needed. The entire facility occupies ~160 square feet and will support one to two people. This type of facility is ideal for laboratories that seldom use hazardous chemicals and use them in small quantities, e.g., analytical standards preparation.

Personnel and Chemical Traffic Flows

Planning for personnel and chemical traffic flows in an HML is another important spatial design activity. Definition of desired flow patterns will indicate the relative placement of the workspaces. Figures 3-6 and 3-7 show examples of primary and alternate personnel and chemical flow patterns, respectively.

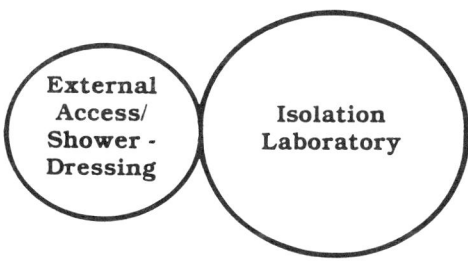

Figure 3-4.   Small HML spatial elements.

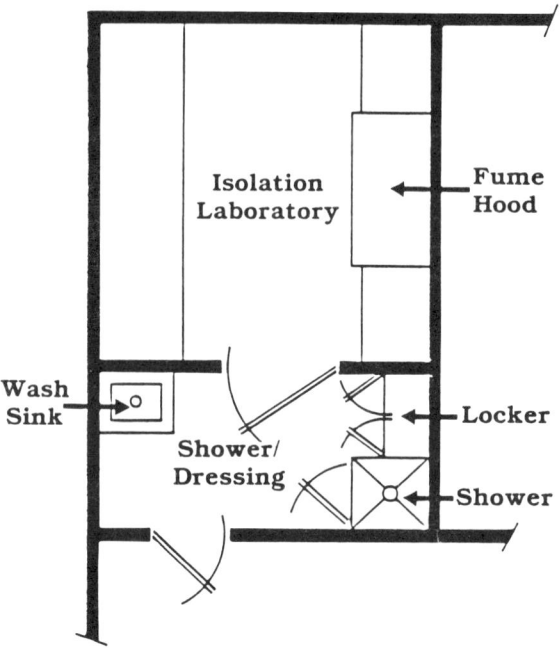

Figure 3-5. Small HML floorplan.

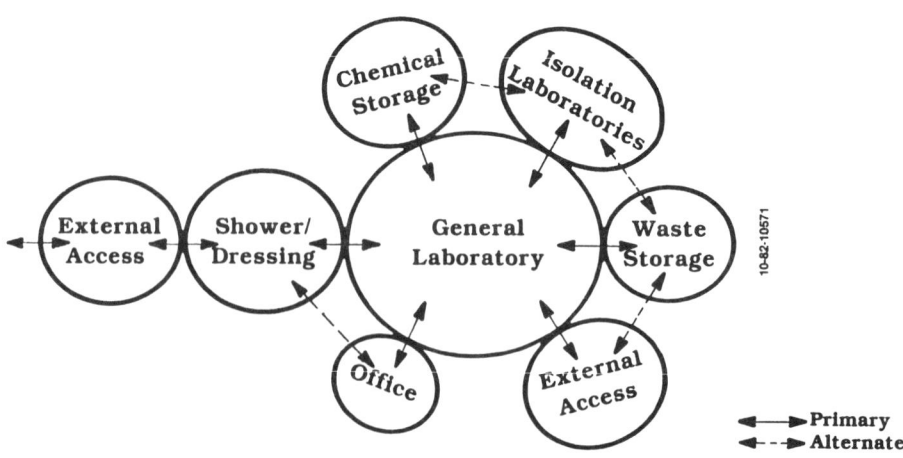

Figure 3-6. Personnel traffic flow.

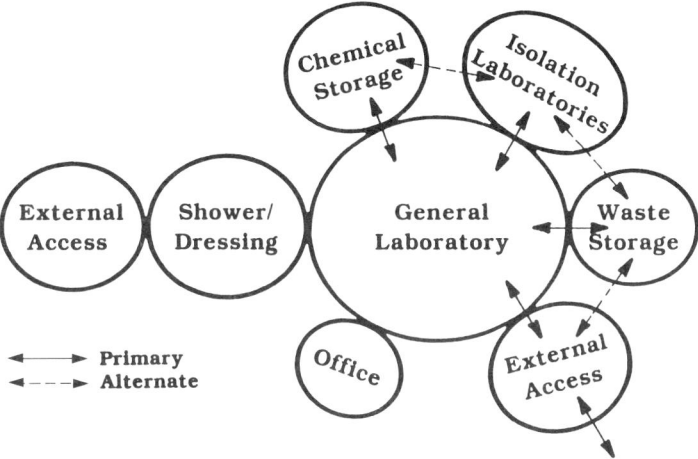

Figure 3-7.   Chemical traffic flow.

The actual traffic patterns chosen for a given facility are highly dependent upon the selection of workspaces, types of operations, and the operational and safety philosophies for the facility. The traffic and chemical flows in the example HML shown in Figure 3-3 is depicted schematically in Figure 3-8. The definition of flow patterns is important in the early phases of HML design because they dictate which workspaces must be contiguous and connected, and which may be situated as "dead ends."

Mechanical Design Component

The design of the mechanical elements of a hazardous materials laboratory is a complex operation requiring highly skilled technical planners and mechanical engineers. These mechanical elements can be grouped into the following four major categories:

- atmospheric control and monitoring
- effluent control
- utilities
- critical systems control and monitoring

The proper design of these systems is the key to the development of a properly functioning, low-maintenance facility. Since engineering controls (i.e., mechanical systems) are the primary safety components of an HML, the health and safety of laboratory personnel, the environment, and the general public depend upon their proper design and operation. Additionally, these elements must function continuously for the life of the facility. The principal methods for achieving this level of security are to select highest quality equipment and to design systems with redundancy, a concept that will occur frequently in discussions of HML mechanical design.

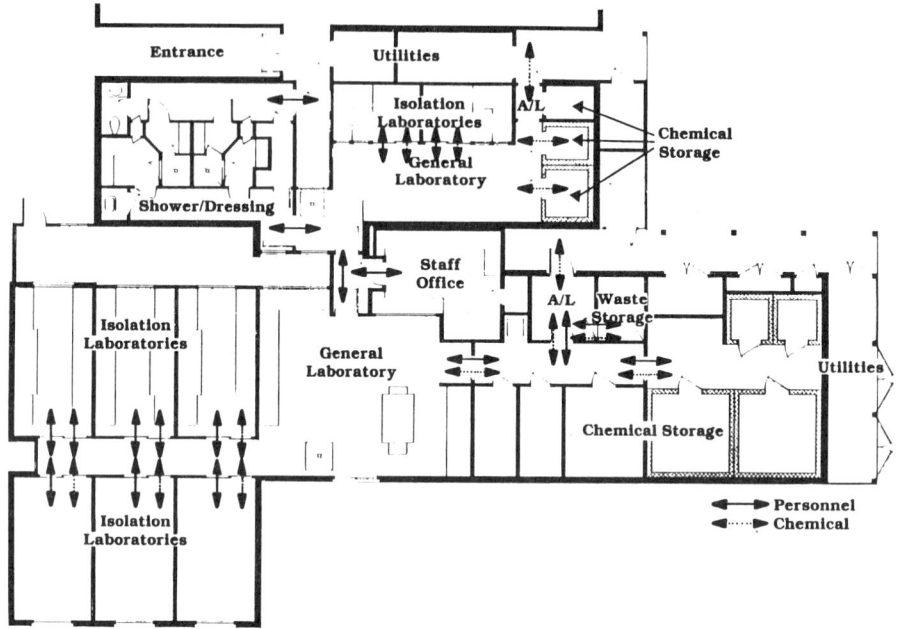

Figure 3–8.   Personnel and chemical traffic flow in example HML.

Atmospheric Control and Monitoring

Atmospheric control within a hazardous chemicals handling facility is the principal engineering control for personnel protection and containment of chemical contaminants. One of the common features of all HMLs is that they operate at a negative pressure with respect to atmospheric pressure. The absolute pressure within the facility is usually –0.1 to –0.2 inches of water. This ensures that air moving through cracks, seals, or open doorways will always flow into the laboratory, toward the area of highest contamination. The negative pressure is maintained in the laboratory while exchanging the building's air volume at least 8, and preferably 10, times per hour.

To add to the complexity of the air handling system, it is necessary to generate varying levels of negative pressure within the facility. The goal is to always have laboratory air moving from areas of lower contamination potential to areas of higher contamination potential. This concept is illustrated in Figure 3–9 using the conceptual HML spatial design developed earlier. The shower/dressing, office, and external access areas are low contamination areas, whereas the isolation laboratories, chemical storage, and waste storage areas have high contamination potential. The general laboratory spaces have an intermediate contamination potential.

All air leaving the facility is exhausted from the areas of highest contamination potential, hence lowest absolute pressure. This is necessary for maintenance of the pressure differentials, and it minimizes the residence time and traverse distance of

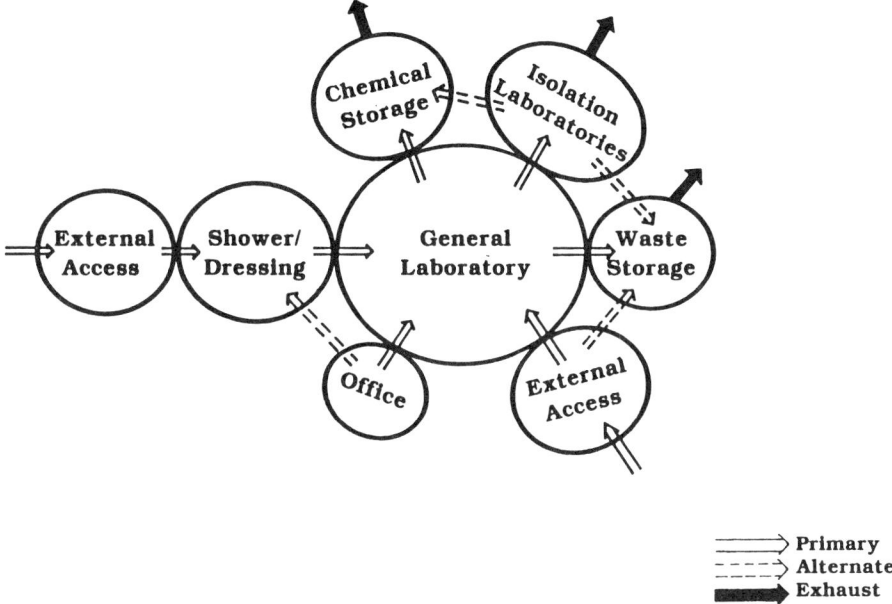

Figure 3-9.   HML airflows.

chemical contaminants within the laboratory. Additional air may be exhausted from specialized containment devices (e.g., glove boxes) or vent hoods over analytical instrumentation.

An example of the application of these principles is shown in Figure 3-10. Overlaid on the floorplan of Radian Corporation's HML are the airflow directions and absolute pressures within the various workspaces. It should be noted that the airlock in the center of the facility separates two portions of the laboratory, each having its own separate air handling systems.

The design of such a complex air handling system requires that the airflows through every vent and exhaust be calculated precisely. In the above example, this means managing a total facility airflow of ~16,000 cubic feet per minute (cfm). Airflow through each laboratory space must be designed to assure an exchange rate of 8-10 times per hour. Air enters the laboratory system through the air conditioning/ distribution system, but additional air required for the proper functioning of fume hoods and other devices may be added directly to those systems as makeup air. This helps reduce some of the massive utility costs associated with the HML air handling system. For the facility shown in Figure 3-10, ~9,000 cfm of air is delivered through the air conditioning system and ~7,000 cfm is delivered as makeup air.

As a footnote to these discussions, it is reasonable to expect that the cost of an HML air handling system will be at least one-third the cost of the entire facility. This system is clearly not only a significant technical challenge and critical safety element, but it is also a significant investment. It should receive utmost attention during the HML design phase.

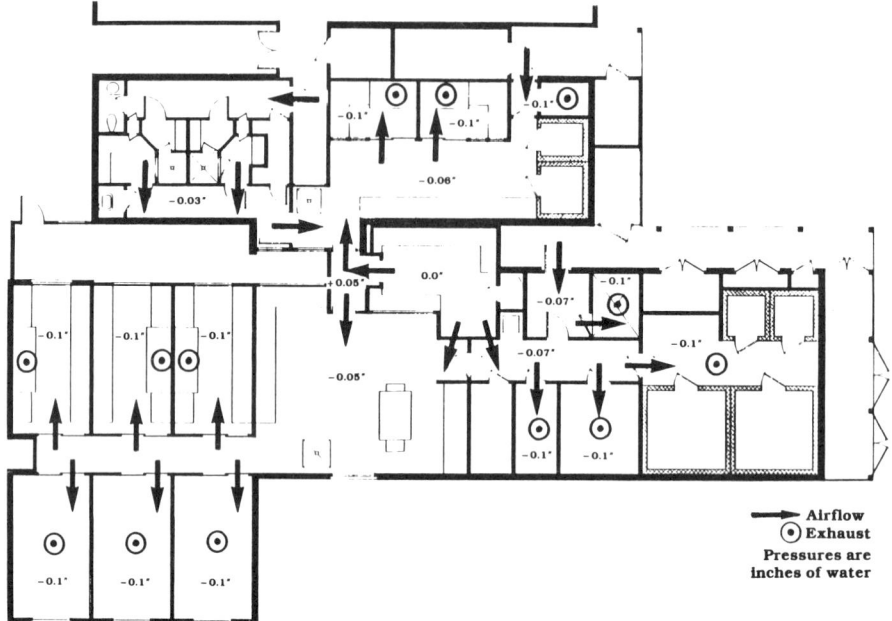

Figure 3-10.   Example HML facility airflows and static pressures.

Effluent Control

The operation of a hazardous materials laboratory results in the generation of three effluents: exhausted air, wastewater, and laboratory wastes. Laboratory wastes generally exit the facility packaged for disposal and are not subject to design considerations other than in the spatial component. Exhausted air and wastewater are high-volume effluents which must be managed by engineering controls. Since no chemicals are to leave the facility in an uncontrolled manner, all contaminants in the air and water effluents must be removed and contained for disposal.

Exhaust Air.   The contaminants of concern in the air effluent streams are particulates, aerosols, and chemical vapors. A filter system must be installed on each exhaust stream to ensure that none of these contaminants enters the atmosphere. A typical exhaust filtration system is shown schematically in Figure 3-11 and photographically in Figure 3-12. It consists of a rough particulate filter—high efficiency particulate (HEPA) filter is optional—absorption bed(s) of activated carbon, and a high-efficiency HEPA filter. The prefilter will trap most particulates, the carbon beds will collect most organic vapors (limited by the absorption isotherms of each compound), and the terminal HEPA filter will collect aerosols, fine particulates, and contaminated carbon fines. The exhaust filtration system is also designed to include an auxiliary exhaust fan to ensure continuous operation in cases of primary fan failure.

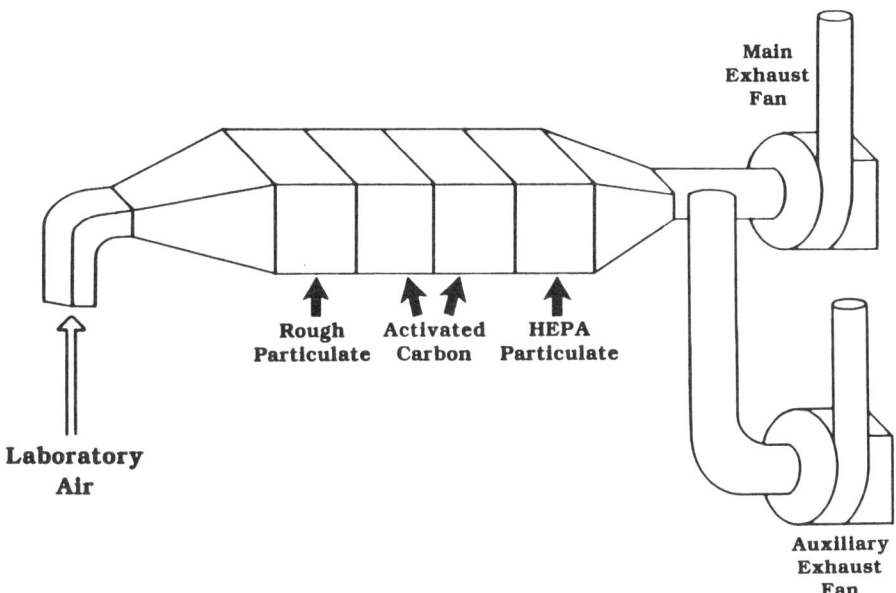

Figure 3–11.   HML air effluent treatment.

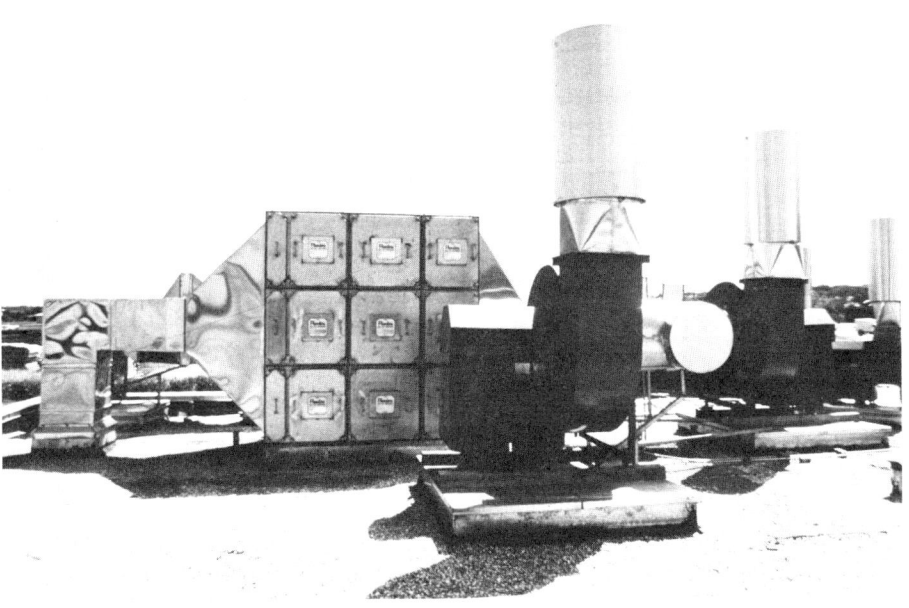

Figure 3–12.   Exhausted air treatment system.

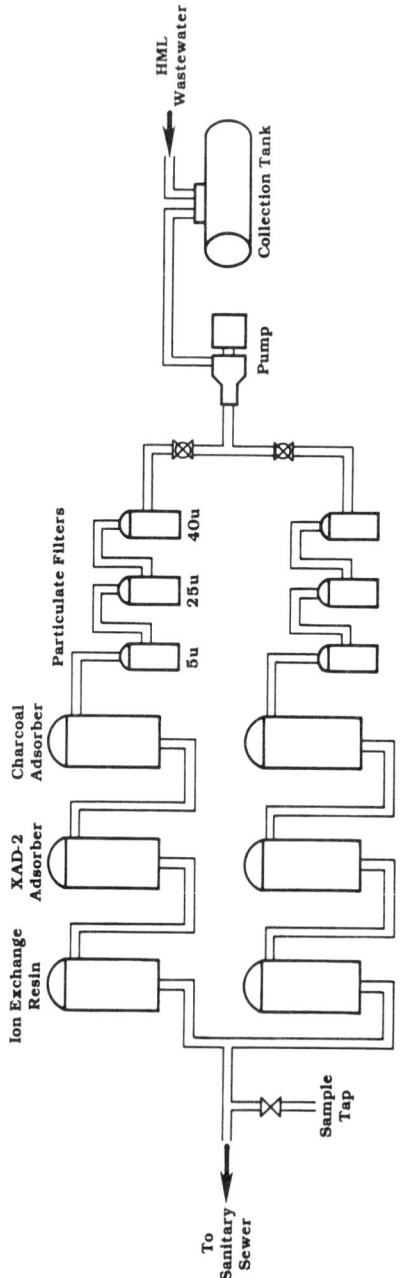

Figure 3–13. HML wastewater treatment system.

To increase the protection of personnel and the environment while filters are changed, the use of "bag-out" filter housings is recommended. These devices allow the extraction of filters into heavy plastic bags without direct contact with personnel. The bags act as crude "glove bags" and may be heat sealed around the filter. An example of such a system is the Flanders Model E–4 Bag-Out Housing (Figure 3–12).

Wastewater.   The HML wastewater treatment system is designed to remove particulates and dissolved and undissolved chemical contaminants from the facility's wastewater. A typical treatment system [2] is shown schematically in Figure 3–13. It is composed of a collection tank, pump, particulate filters, and chemical adsorbers. Effluent from the system is suitable for discharge into a sanitary sewer.

Since the wastewater must be moved through the system under pressure, it must first be collected in a holding tank, then pumped into the treatment stages. The wastewater is pumped through a series of successively finer particulate filters to remove suspended solids. It then enters the organics removal section, which is composed of an activated carbon adsorption chamber followed by a polymeric resin (e.g., XAD-2) chamber. Ionic species are then removed by one or more ion exchange resins. The organic or ionic species treatment stages may be omitted if those species are not utilized in laboratory operations; however, this reduces versatility and is not recommended. The system is always designed with two complete trains so that one is available for use if the other fails or is exhausted.

A typical system designed to support a 5,000-square-foot facility is shown in Figure 3–14. This system is composed of a 500-gallon collection tank, small centrifugal pump, and commercial water purification filters and adsorbers. Only organic

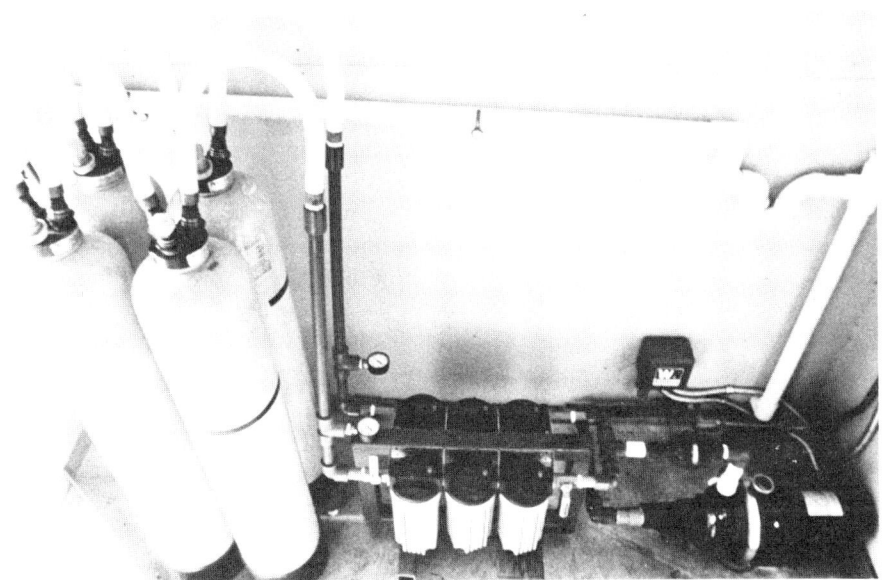

Figure 3–14.   Water effluent treatment system.

adsorbers are used in this facility, and they are prepared by replacing the ion exchange resins in commercial deionizing cannisters with activated carbon and XAD-2 resin.

Utilities

A third mechanical design concern is utility service. The types, quantities and placements of utility services are critical to the efficient operation of a hazardous materials laboratory. The following is a list of typical services that appear in general-purpose HMLs:

- electricity
- hot, cold, and deionized/distilled water
- natural gas
- inert gas
- vacuum
- instrument gases
- compressed air
- breathing air

Planning the electricity, water, natural gas, and compressed air services involves definition of demand levels and locations and determination that adequate service is available to the facility. Inert gases are generally supplied only to laboratory areas and may be heavier than air (e.g., argon), lighter than air (e.g., helium or nitrogen), or both.

A central vacuum system operated at 20–50 mm Hg is preferable over water aspirators for use in the HML. Chemical vapors are contained more effectively, and the wastewater treatment system is placed under less demand. The exhaust from the vacuum pump must be filtered through activated carbon prior to release to the atmosphere.

Supply manifolds for all gases delivered from compressed gas cylinders should be designed such that the cylinders are located outside the controlled areas. Gas cylinders should not be taken into an HML because they are difficult to manage, often interfere with laboratory operations and movement, can be a safety hazard, and must be decontaminated prior to removal. Since it is often difficult to add gas service once a facility is operational, it is imperative to accurately predict and design for present and future needs. Installation of one to three extra gas service lines is advisable.

Breathing air can be supplied from compressed gas cylinders or breathing air compressors. The latter is recommended as the primary source, with gas cylinders readily available for immediate use if the compressor fails. Oil-free compressors are the best choice for breathing air systems, but oil-sealed compressors may be used if a downstream purification and monitoring system is used. Each laboratory outlet should be equipped with a filter, pressure gauge, and regulator (if demand pressure differs from system pressure).

Primary utilities distribution systems should be located outside the controlled laboratory space to facilitate repair and maintenance. Utilities should enter the laboratory at a minimum number of locations, and those locations should be near the laboratory terminus of the utility line. All traverses of laboratory walls and ceilings must be carefully sealed to prevent air leakage. All distribution systems (pipes, conduits, etc.) within the laboratory should be enclosed in utility chases to reduce contamination and cleaning problems.

Critical Systems Control

One major problem facing the mechanical designer is the creation of a mechanical system which ensures that the HML will provide the maximum level of protection at all times under all circumstances. This requires that the facility operate at design specifications 24 hours a day every day, that operational parameters are not significantly affected by mechanical failures, and that the physical structure is preserved. The operation of the following critical systems is key to this goal:

- electrical power
- air exhaust
- chemical storage refrigeration
- fire control
- effluent treatment
- breathing air

The successful accomplishment of this requirement is based upon redundancy and monitoring.

Redundancy is the key to continued operation of an HML at design specifications in the event of mechanical failure. Critical systems such as electrical power, air exhaust, and effluent treatment are responsible for containment of the toxic materials and protection of the environment. Each HML facility should be equipped with an auxiliary generator of sufficient size to support the air handling system, chemical refrigeration, effluent treatment system, and partial lighting in case of primary power failure. The generator should be equipped with automatic start and system interconnect features. An auxiliary exhaust fan should be co-ducted with each primary fan. The fan system should be designed with sensors to detect an increase in duct pressure and automatically activate the auxiliary fan. The wastewater treatment system should be designed with dual filter/adsorber trains.

Redundancy in the breathing air system is necessary for protection of laboratory personnel. Combinations of two compressors or one compressor and multiple compressed gas cylinders with either automatic or manual switchover systems are effective solutions to this design challenge. If manual switchover is used, controls must be placed inside the laboratory in a readily accessible location.

Operation and failure monitoring are other components of critical system control. Quick response to a system failure requires an awareness of the failure. For this reason, all the critical systems listed above should be continuously monitored by devices which will detect a failure and activate audible and visible alarms. Alarms should be placed such that personnel inside and outside the facility are alerted, and they should be continuously monitored during evenings, weekends, and other non-working periods. All systems control, monitoring, and alarm functions should be centralized in a master control panel located outside the controlled laboratory areas. It should be noted that the design of the control and monitoring system for a large HML is a significant technological undertaking in itself.

Structural Design Component

The structural component of HML design generally belongs in the realm of the architect. This component comprises construction techniques and materials specifications. These are common to most laboratory design and construction and are generally not of special concern to HML design. However, four areas which are of special concern to HML design are listed below:

- floorplan design
- utilities access
- equipment placement and loadings
- surface treatments

Each of these areas is particularly important to the overall success of any hazardous materials laboratory design.

Floorplan design is important in two respects. First, it is the way by which the spatial design component is translated into the facility structure. Placement and orientation of workspaces is important to assure proper access, traffic flow, and utilization. Placement of spaces with respect to each other and placement of external access areas, interior walls, exterior walls, utilities access, etc., must be considered.

Floorplan design is also important when planning for the expandability of the facility. The extreme cost ($\geqslant$\$500 per square foot in 1983) of hazardous chemicals facilities inhibits the building of excess space for future growth. Therefore, it is very important to design these facilities so that they may be expanded by additional, adjoining construction. Proper planning involves the following:

- Utilities should be sized and located for easy connection to and support of the additional space.
- The building shape should be designed for easy expansion and compatibility with the additional spaces.
- Future walkways and portals to connect new and old spaces should be designed into the facility.
- Foundations and other structural elements must be compatible with expansion plans.
- Expansion should be accomplishable without creating a facility with excessive distances between interactive operations areas.

Utilities access is another element of HML structural design that requires significant attention. Utilities may be distributed to spaces in the laboratory from inside or outside the controlled laboratory unit. Distribution from within the laboratory is difficult since all laboratory surfaces must be sealed (no false ceilings) and utilities must be exposed at the ceiling or placed inside the permanent ceiling or wall spaces. The former is not advisable because exposed pipes, conduits, etc., may become surface-contaminated, and they are difficult to clean. Extensive utilities distribution inside finished walls, ceilings, or floors is not desirable because repairs or modifications require laboratory shutdown, wall or ceiling surface destruction, and movement of maintenance personnel inside the facility.

Distribution from outside the facility is the method of choice. All major runs of pipes, conduits, etc., are made external to the laboratory spaces as much as possible, then distributed into the facility at a minimum number of places. This leaves the majority of utilities accessible for maintenance and modification without disrupting laboratory operations or having maintenance personnel inside the facility. Two techniques for designing a structure to accomplish this goal are shown in Figure 3–15. The optimum structural technique for external utilities access is to provide a 6–8-foot high interstitial space above the entire facility. This is a more expensive type of construction, but it will provide space for utilities, air distribution equipment and ducts, and special equipment such as vacuum pumps and compressors. An alternate method is to provide utility "alleys" or hallways at floor level within the facility or around its perimeter. These have to be isolated from the controlled spaces and can serve as buffers between spaces.

Equipment placement and the corresponding structural loadings are significant concerns when designing an HML. The large amount of equipment, particularly air handling, required to support a hazardous materials laboratory results in a large structural loading. The air handling equipment, exhaust filters, fans, and air condi-

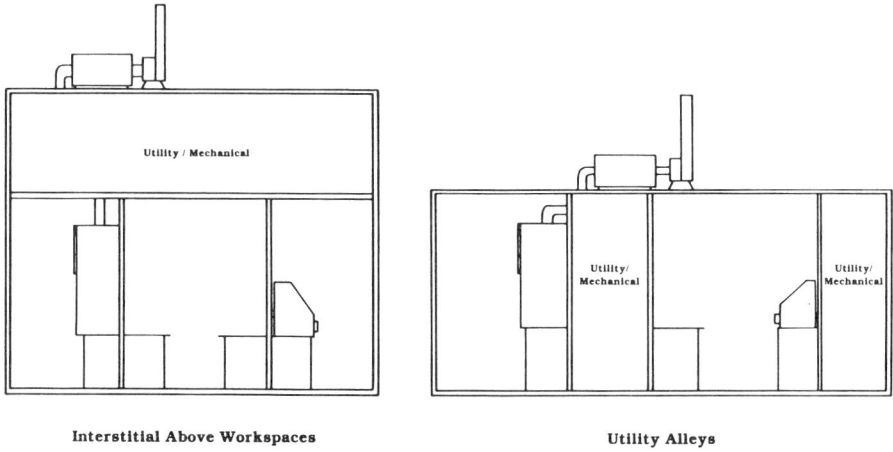

Interstitial Above Workspaces   Utility Alleys

Figure 3–15.   Utility distribution techniques.

tioning units are usually placed in an interstitial above the facility or on its roof. The structure must be designed to efficiently transmit these loads to the foundation. If other equipment such as breathing air compressors or vacuum pumps are to be placed in one of the above areas, their weight must be considered in the structural design.

A key element in the protection afforded by a hazardous materials laboratory is the method of sealing the interior surfaces. These treatments must be designed to prevent chemicals from passing into the environment and from penetrating into the foundation, walls, or ceiling materials. This protection must be effective even in the event of a major spill. Otherwise, large portions of the structure might have to be removed due to contamination, a difficult and expensive task. The optimum wall treatment is three coats of epoxy paint. Wall surfaces should be as smooth as possible for easy cleaning and decontamination. Floors should contain no seams and be coved at least 6 inches onto the walls. This creates a dish to contain spilled materials and allows for easy cleaning and decontamination. Several types of welded-seam sheet floorings are currently available and are excellent for HML use. They also provide the added advantage that damaged or contaminated sections of flooring may be removed and a new piece welded into place.

Equipment Design Component

Selection and placement of equipment in a hazardous chemicals handling facility comprise a fourth design concern. In general, each piece of equipment in an HML should be designed and constructed so that:

- It is easy to clean (e.g., coved or rounded corners, accessible, smooth surfaced).
- It is durable.
- It is resistant to adsorption or permeation of chemicals.
- It is adequately sized.
- It meets the highest standards of laboratory safety (e.g., electrical, mechanical).

Once an HML becomes operational, it is very difficult to remove, modify, or replace major equipment items. For that reason it is imperative that major equipment be considered early in the design of a hazardous materials facility. The major items of concern are containment devices, laboratory furniture, chemical storage units, safety equipment, and special operations equipment.

The primary chemical containment devices in a hazardous materials laboratory are fume hoods and glove boxes. Fume hoods are generally satisfactory for most hazardous chemicals operations provided they are properly designed, installed, and operated. The ideal fume hood has a single-unit, stainless steel interior with welded seams and coved corners. The work surface should have at least a 0.5-inch lip on the front to prevent runout of spilled liquids. The face velocity should be 125 ± 10 fpm at all points with the sash in the fully open position. Most regulatory specifications for face velocities are 150 fpm when handling carcinogens, but hood manufacturers and ventilation authorities generally agree that this is too high and causes excessive turbulence and backflow. Auxiliary air hoods are acceptable for toxic materials operations, but the makeup air should be ≤60% of the total hood exhaust. Fume hoods ≥ 8-ft wide should have multiple vertical or horizontal sashes. Laminar flow hoods are designed primarily to control hazardous agents with particulate-like properties (e.g., bacteria) and not chemical vapors. They may be used in hazardous chemical laboratories if the hood exhaust air is not recycled; however, fume hoods are the hoods of choice because they are specifically designed to handle chemical vapors and dusts.

The placement of fume hoods is very important to their proper operation. In fact, the placement of the fume hood, room doors, and room air inlets are the most critical factors affecting modern fume hood performance. The complexity of the problem defies easy answers, and research is continuing to more accurately define all the parameters. In general, the fume hood should be placed in the middle of a space, either against a wall or free standing, and away from doorways. Room air vents should be located as far as possible from the hood, and the air velocity should be as low as possible.

Extremely hazardous materials such as toxic gases (e.g., phosgene and hydrogen cyanide), volatile toxic liquids, and very toxic materials (e.g., acetylcholinesterase inhibitors and 2,3,7,8-TCDD) should be handled in glove boxes rather than fume hoods. Glove boxes, either controlled atmosphere or negative pressure, offer significant, additional personnel protection. Glove boxes that operate at negative pressure with respect to the surrounding laboratory space are applicable to most operations. They may be sized to accommodate one person and small operations ($\sim 3 \times 2.5 \times 2.5$ feet) or several people and large operations ($\sim 6 \times 4 \times 4$ feet) as illustrated in Figure 3–16. All such devices should be operated at –0.2 to –0.3 inches H_2O relative to the laboratory and be equipped with pressure monitoring equipment and equipment to prevent backflow of contaminated air should the glove box pressure become positive. Exhausted air must be handled as contaminated effluent as described earlier. Controlled atmosphere glove boxes are to be used only when handling air or moisture-sensitive chemicals. Gloves used in glove boxes should be selected for resistance to both degradation and permeation by the chemical(s) being handled.

Laboratory furniture and benchtops selected for use in an HML must not absorb chemical contaminants. Steel cabinetry is preferred, and wood is not acceptable. Countertops made of epoxy resin are the best for HML use, while wood and plastic laminate are the worst. Cabinets should be installed so as to provide a utility chase, and all in-laboratory utility distributions should be made in this space. Dishwashing sinks should be provided in all chemical handling areas to prevent transport of contaminated glassware.

The aspects of chemical storage which must be addressed early in the HML design process are temperature, size, and special features. Storage spaces at three temperatures, 25°C, 5°C, and –20°C, are needed in almost all facilities, and additional storage at lower temperatures (e.g., –76°C) may be required. The scope of planned operations and the chemical packaging techniques will define the sizes of each storage area. They may range from 15-cubic-foot refrigerators, freezers, and closets to 1,000-cubic-foot walkin units. No matter what the configuration, all chemical storage equipment must be vapor and explosion proof. Examples of special storage equipment that may have to be considered are vaults for controlled substances,

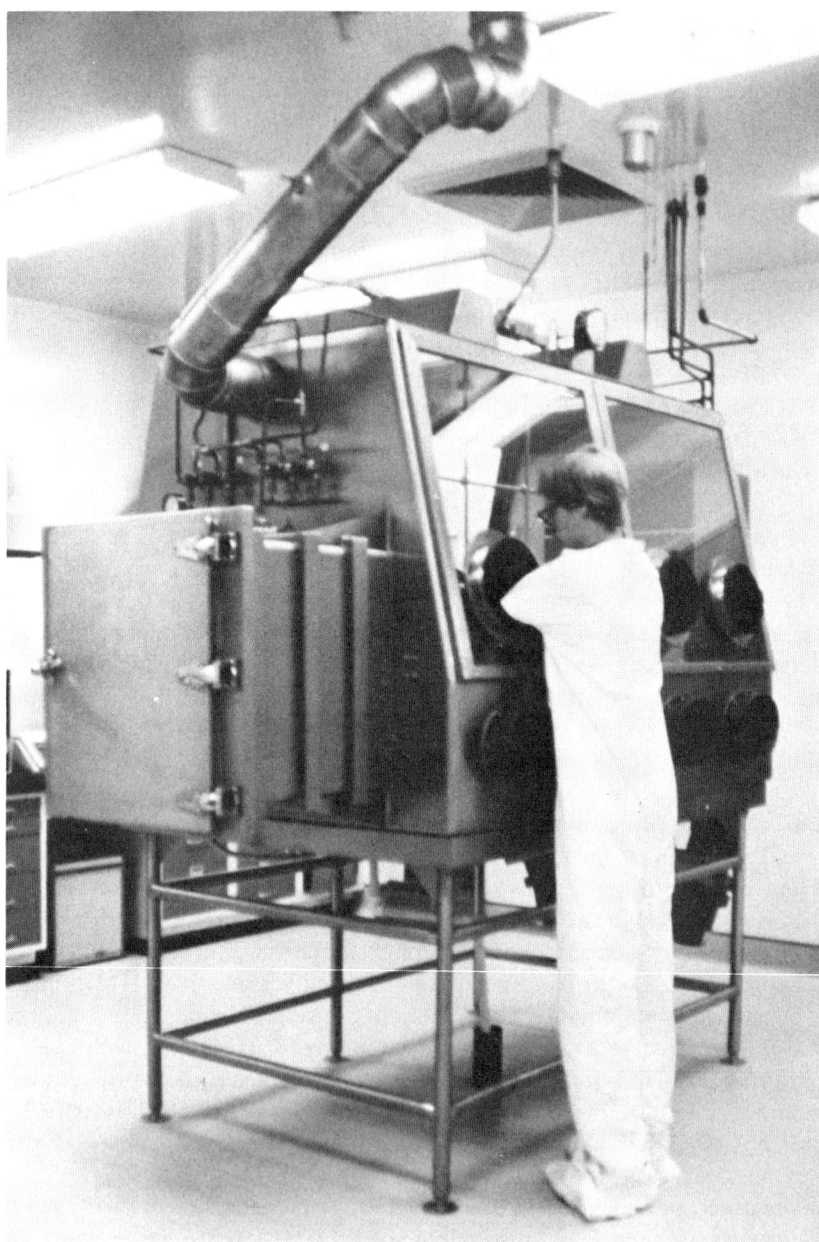

Figure 3–16. Large glove box for highly toxic materials.

subterranean vaults for highly toxic materials, and special ultra-low-temperature freezers. The final selection of chemical storage equipment will define the scale and configuration of the chemical storage space discussed earlier.

Major safety equipment selection and placement are additional design considerations. First aid centers, fire blankets, decontamination stations, self-contained breathing apparatus, and safety showers are usually placed in the general laboratory spaces. Here they are most centralized and away from chemical handling and storage areas. Safety showers should be multinozzle (up to 16) deluge stalls with foot-treadle or push-valve actuators. They must be accessible from chemical handling areas and visible from inside and outside the facility. These showers require a large volume of water, mandating adequate plumbing and drain design. Eyewash stations are most practically attached to the emergency shower. The selection and location of additional safety equipment outside the laboratory must also be considered. Fully enclosed suits, air lines, and self-contained breathing apparatuses must be available for entry into the facility in case of a major accident.

Some chemical operations, such as synthesis, membrane permeation testing, and ampul filling and sealing, require equipment large enough and specialized enough to necessitate consideration during the HML design phase. Since each is a unique item, specific discussions are not warranted, but some general considerations may be useful. First, the size of the equipment, its physical support requirements (e.g., floor, benchtop, ceiling suspension), and its access requirements (front only, all sides, etc.) will define the type of location and amount of space needed. Next, the type of operation for which it will be used will define the spatial elements into which it may be placed (e.g., isolation laboratory, general laboratory, waste storage). Finally, the utility requirements of the equipment must be defined and incorporated into the utility design.

Safety Design Component

Very few aspects of the safety design component can be discussed as separate entities. Every element of HML design described thus far has a major safety component; indeed, the ultimate objective of an HML design is safety. However, there are some design topics that warrant discussion as purely safety matters. These are the development of lines of vision, access control, design of fire protection, communication and alarm systems, and provision for information access.

One of the key safety elements in an HML is visibility. Hence a large amount of wall space is occupied by glass. Visibility from the outside is important for monitoring laboratory operations and recognizing problems. External visibility is also important in emergency situations to allow for assessment of the situation from a safe vantage point prior to committing personnel to a response. Clear vision within the laboratory into all work areas is important for monitoring personnel safety. Early recognition of problem situations is critical to the safe operation of an HML. The laboratory staff must continually monitor each other and recognize and respond immediately if someone is accidentally contaminated or injured.

Access to an HML is strictly limited to only those personnel who are qualified to work in the facility and who are properly medically monitored. Access should be limited to only one door with an externally activated lock. All other doors should be locked from the inside at all times. The facility should be secured from approach from the outside, e.g., fenced, and all critical utilities and equipment should be tamper-proof. Intrusion alarms may be installed within the facility if deemed necessary due to location or type of research being conducted.

All hazardous chemical facilities should be equipped with a fire alarm and control system. The dispersion of unburned toxic chemicals in the smoke plume of a fire would be a major disaster. The best fire control system currently available uses Halon 1301 as a fire retardant. Halon 1301 will not damage equipment and is not harmful to humans. Carbon dioxide systems are harmful to humans, and water systems can spread chemical contamination and destroy electronic equipment. The control system should be designed with cross-zoned detection; ionization detectors should be used in temperature-controlled areas and thermal detectors in areas subject to high, low, or widely varying temperatures. The Halon 1301 discharge should be sufficient to provide a 5–6% concentration throughout the facility. All spaces including utility closets, interstitials, and storage areas should be protected.

Intralaboratory communication is vital to the efficient and safe operation of an HML. The system should be designed to provide two-way voice communication between all work and storage areas and the external viewing areas. Audio sensitivity and tone quality are important because many conversations must be conducted through respirators. The system should also be designed so that all transmissions are heard at all stations in case a request for help is being made.

An important aspect of operating a hazardous materials laboratory is knowing when something is amiss. Critical mechanical systems are continuously monitored, and an alarm system alerts the HML staff to a failure. An additional alarm system necessary in an HML is the personal injury or accident alarm. Highly visible alarm actuators should be placed in each laboratory and storage area and near each safety shower. They should be large, visible, and located near doorways or in readily accessible areas. Critical alarms such as personal injury, fire, and intrusion should be distinguishable from mechanical failure alarms. Alarms should sound in the laboratory itself, surrounding work areas, and in other office and laboratory areas as necessary to alert response personnel. The alarm system must be monitored 24 hours a day, and a system must be in effect to notify responsible personnel when an alarm is registered.

One of the primary personnel protection systems within an HML is knowledge of the properties, hazards, and emergency responses associated with the chemical(s) being handled. Provision for supplying this knowledge should be designed into each HML facility. Information may be stored in a reference library, in files or on computer, but the method(s) must be defined during facility design. An area should be dedicated for storage and retrieval of hard copy information, and a space should be set aside for a computer or terminal if that type of system is to be used. If a remote computer system is to be accessed, communication linkages must be designed into the facility.

CONCLUSION

The design of a hazardous materials handling facility is an incredibly difficult and complex undertaking and should be attempted only by highly skilled planners, architects, and engineers. However, during the coming years, many technical and management personnel will be faced with the realization that such a facility is needed for adequate protection of their personnel. This realization will be coaxed into being by the growing body of knowledge about chemical hazards and the increasing monetary and social liabilities wrought by lawsuits for real and potential harm due to chemical exposure. It is hoped that this chapter will serve as a guide to those technical and management personnel who are responsible for overseeing the design and operation of an HML and for those persons who must actually perform the design functions.

REFERENCES

1.   Harless, J.M., K.E. Baxter, L.H. Keith, and D.B. Walters. "Design and Operation of a Hazardous Materials Laboratory," in *Safe Handling of Chemical Carcinogens, Mutagens, Teratogens and High Toxic Substances,* D.B. Walters, Ed. (Ann Arbor, MI: Ann Arbor Science, 1980).
2.   Nony, C.R., E.J. Treglown, and M.C. Bowman. "Removal of Trace Levels of 2-Acetylaminofluorene (2-AAF) from Wastewater," *Sci. Total Environ.* 4: 155–163, 1975.

CHAPTER 4

Health and Safety in the Design of Toxicity Testing Laboratories

R. Scott Stricoff and E. Robinson Hoyle
Arthur D. Little, Inc., Acorn Park,
Cambridge, Massachusetts 02140

Douglas B. Walters
National Toxicology Program, National Institute of
Environmental Health Sciences, P.O. Box 12233,
Research Triangle Park, North Carolina 27709

INTRODUCTION

Toxicity testing laboratories require many features not commonly found in the traditional laboratory design. In designing a toxicity testing laboratory, the prospective user is often called upon to provide insights to the architect and engineer regarding important design considerations. Since the architect and engineer are unlikely to be familiar with the scientific requirements, the degree to which a safe laboratory is designed will be a function of the quality of the prospective user's input. This chapter represents a discussion of some of the important considerations which should be recognized in the specification of a toxicity testing laboratory.

The laboratory can be thought of as a compilation of several functionally oriented areas. Depending upon the type of testing to be conducted, these areas may include chemical receiving and storage, dose preparation, dose administration, necropsy, histology, analytical and clinical chemistry, and waste handling and utilities. (An animal testing laboratory might contain each of these areas, while an *in-vitro* lab might have only a few.) Each of these areas should be designed with consideration for the activities which will take place within that area.

RECEIVING AND CHEMICAL STORAGE

The receiving area should be isolated from traffic within the building, and should be near the chemical storage area. The receiving area should be equipped with fire protection (e.g., sprinklers, fire extinguishers, standpipes for hose connection, alarms),

73

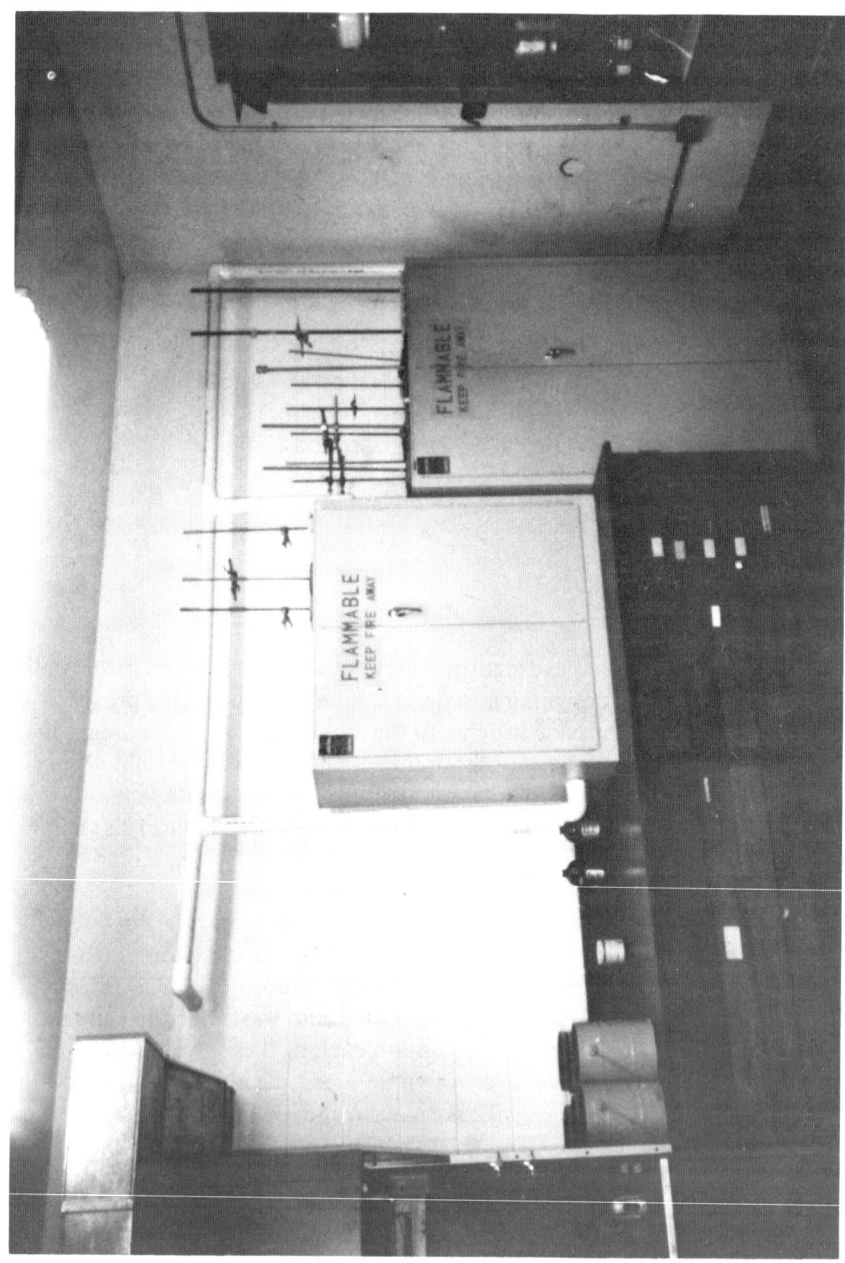

Figure 4–1.   Flammable liquid storage cabinets connected to an exhaust system.

and should be designed to facilitate cleanup of spills such as those resulting from incoming leaking packages. Providing a diked area with a chemically resistant floor treatment will simplify the rapid containment of leakage from packaging which loses its integrity. There should be adequate space to permit storage of packages away from activities that could lead to breakage (e.g., lift truck movement).

The area which will be used for bulk chemical storage should be designed to have negative air pressure relative to the adjacent space. Exhaust inlets at floor level are suggested to prevent the accumulation of heavier-than-air vapors. Explosion-proof electrical fixtures should be incorporated into the design of this room, and provision for the grounding and bonding of flammable liquid drums and cans should be made [1,2]. For smaller quantities of flammable liquids, solvent storage cabinets (see Figure 4–1) should be provided, and these cabinets should be exhausted at all times (with roughly 10 air changes per hour recommended). Provision should be made for storage of some materials at subambient temperature, and the refrigerator(s) and freezer(s) provided, whether walkin size or smaller, should be explosion-proof. The bulk chemical storage room should have automatic fire detectors connected to both visual and audible alarms, and the audible fire alarm should sound different from alarms used for freezers, incubators, air handling systems, etc. [3,4].

DOSE PREPARATION AND ADMINISTRATION

The dose preparation and dose administration areas should be designed as a barrier facility within which clearly segregated "clean" and "dirty" areas exist, and the potential spread of chemical contamination is limited by the physical design. The two-corridor arrangement for animal laboratories, shown in Figure 4–2, provides clear-cut physical separation of clean and dirty areas. An integral part of a barrier facility is the shower/locker area. As Figure 4–2 indicates, in the barrier facility the shower area provides the only point from which one can exit the dirty side of the facility. The shower/locker room itself should have physically separate clean and dirty sides, with pass-through lockers to permit the movement of noncontaminated inner garments (e.g., underwear and shoes which have been worn within jump suits). Provision should be made within the locker/shower area for both the storage of personal respirators and their cleaning [5]. Cleaning of respirators requires a sink and adequate space for air drying. Figure 4–3 shows one acceptable approach, although the provision of shelves instead of hooks would minimize deformation stress in respirator facepieces and straps, prolonging respirator life.

In developing the layout of the locker/shower area, it is important to consider carefully the traffic patterns that will be used when the facility goes into operation. In many cases, inadequate consideration of these factors has resulted in locker/shower facilities which require the user to continuously move back and forth between the nominally clean side to the nominally dirty side in order to change in or change out. It is also important to consider the direction of airflow within the locker room. Air should flow from the clean side to the dirty side.

Within the barrier facility, workers are generally required to wear disposable overgarments, and these items can place a heat load on the user after prolonged wear.

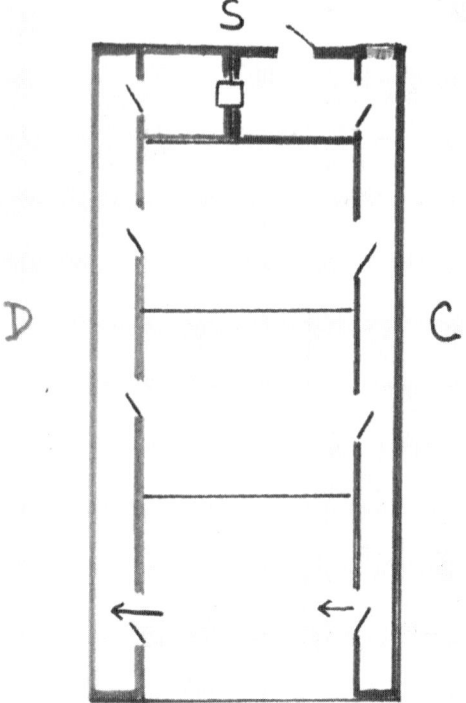

Figure 4-2.   Schematic representation of a two-corridor barrier facility.

In recognition of this, and within the constraints imposed by the animal care requirements of experimental protocols, it is desirable to keep the environment relatively cool and dry. It is also important to provide a clean room in which workers can spend break periods without wearing respirators, gloves, and other outer layer protective equipment.

The dose preparation area is the place within the toxicity testing laboratory at which the most potential for personnel exposure to chemicals exists. In this area, undiluted test chemicals and positive controls are handled regularly. The dose preparation area should be located as close as possible to chemical storage. Vented enclosures should be provided for both weighing and mixing bulk chemicals. Although one often hears the complaint that weighing within a hood or glove box on an analytical balance cannot be done with precision, design of an enclosure which provides exhaust near the balance while isolating the balance from all sources of vibration has been shown to be an effective approach. Figure 4-4 shows an analytical balance routinely used within a chemical fume hood. The absence of turbulence-creating clutter within the hood helps in the success of this arrangement. Figure 4-5 shows a pair of "V" blenders used by the National Toxicology Program bioassay laboratories, with these blenders situated within a small, exhausted room. When the doors to the

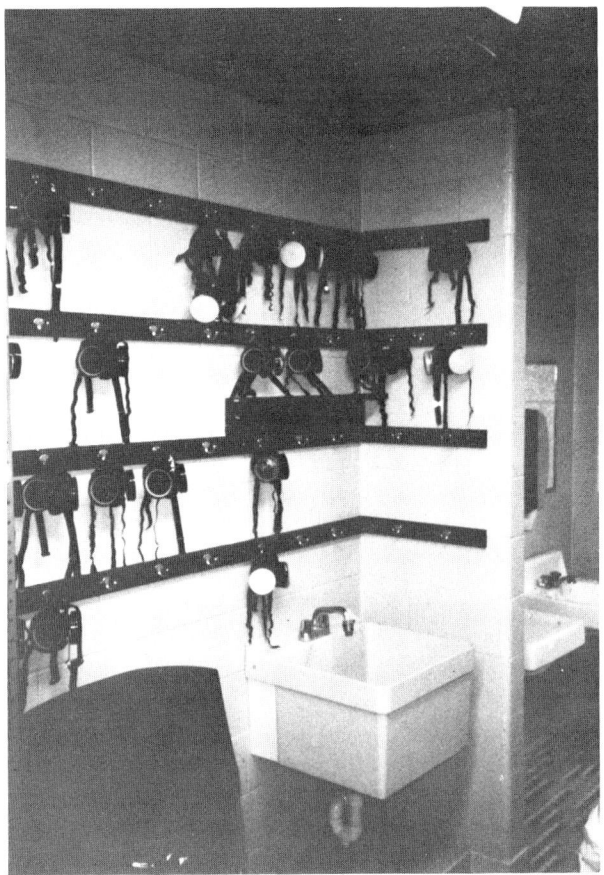

Figure 4–3.   Respirator cleaning station.

blender enclosure are closed, the blenders are within a small, isolated space under negative pressure relative to all surrounding spaces.

The dose preparation area should be under negative pressure relative to all adjacent spaces; in fact, this area should be the most negative area within the entire laboratory. A static pressure gauge should be present to allow workers to confirm that negative pressure is being maintained.

It is advantageous to provide connection to breathing air for supplied air respirators within the dose preparation area so that this equipment can be used when the chemical being handled requires a high level of protection. The dose preparation area should have access to the clean side of the barrier so that prepared dose ready for administration can be readily provided to technicians preparing to enter the administration rooms. Figure 4–6 shows a pass-through refrigerator which allows dose preparation area workers to drop off material from the dirty side and dose administration workers to pick up material from the clean side.

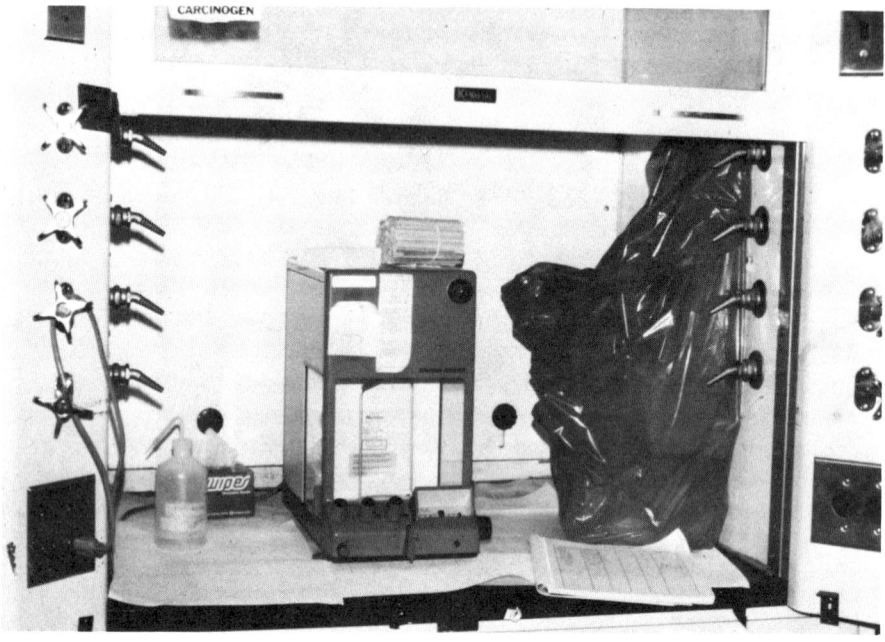

Figure 4-4. Analytical balance located within a chemical fume hood (with a plastic bag for waste collection at right).

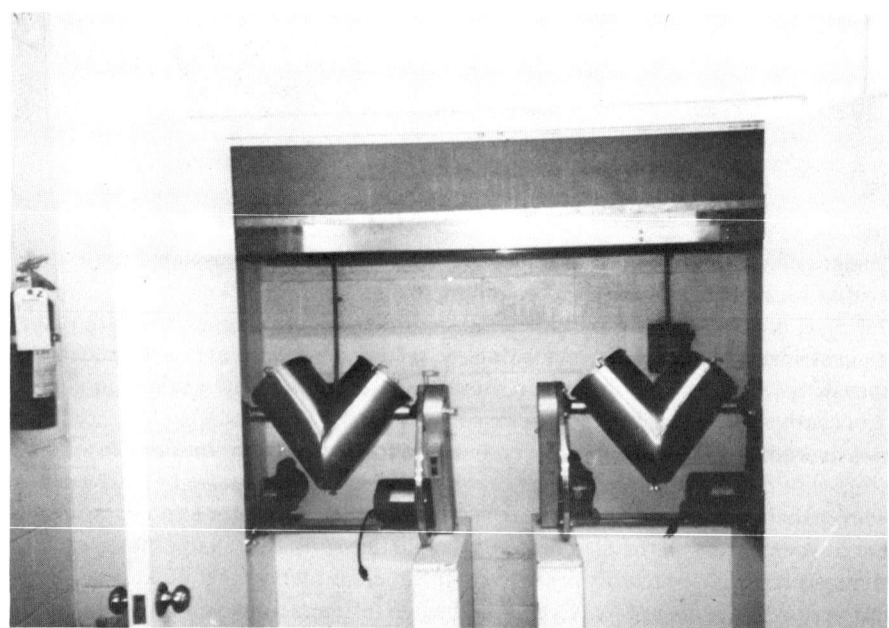

Figure 4-5. Feed blender located within a vented walk-in enclosure.

The dose administration area should have access to both clean and dirty corridors and be designed so that it is under negative pressure relative to the clean side, and under positive pressure relative to the dirty side. It is desirable to provide a static pressure gauge for each room in each corridor to facilitate checking the maintenance of desired airflow directionality. Animal care considerations dictate that 10 to 15 air changes per hour be provided within each animal room. Each room should be provided with communications to other locations within the facility, either through an intercom system or with a telephone.

A vented work station with each study room provides a place in which to do dose administration by gavage, injection, skin painting, etc. Several approaches to providing vented work stations while maintaining desired air change rates have been successfully employed. In some laboratories, all air exhausted from a study room

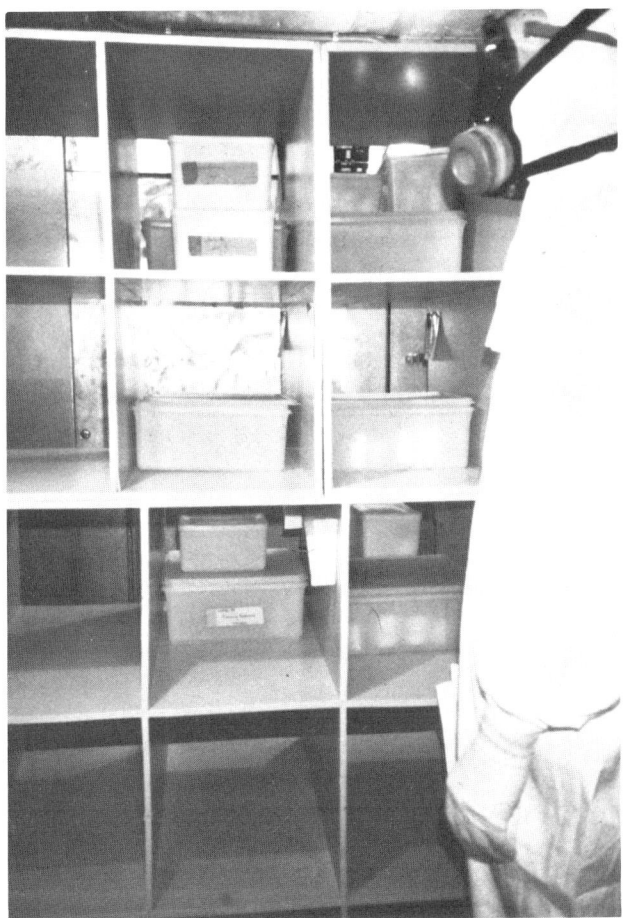

Figure 4-6.   Pass-through refrigerator (looking from "dirty" side toward "clean" side of facility).

flows through a fixed work station (Figure 4-7). In other labs, portable work stations are designed to be connected to the room exhaust duct when the work station is needed (see Figure 4-8). When inhalation studies are to be done, inhalation chambers (vented through appropriate filters) should be present in the animal room, and the challenge atmosphere generator should be within a vented enclosure.

The doors of the study room should have windows within them, so that someone working inside the room can be observed by those in the corridor. Study room floors should be a monolithic material such as epoxy-painted concrete or heat-welded PVC, and walls should be epoxy-painted. Providing breathing air connections can enhance the flexibility of the facility to accommodate a wide variety of types of work.

One of the newer problems encountered in toxicity testing laboratories is associated with the growing use of computer terminals for data collection and review in the study room. This application of automated data handling creates the dilemma that when a computer terminal is to be removed from a study room, the terminal must somehow be decontaminated. In a newly designed lab, this problem could be overcome by putting a terminal outside the lab (in the clean corridor) accessible to

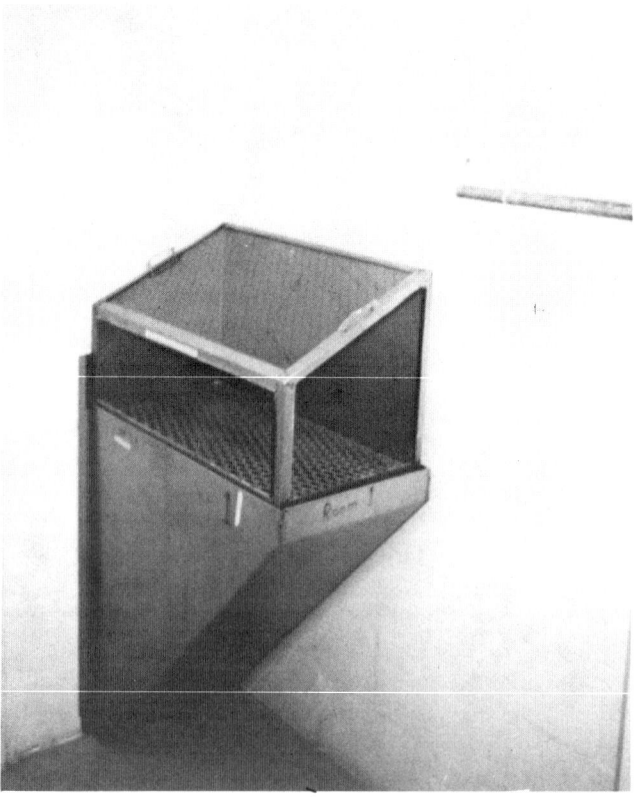

Figure 4-7.   Vented work station for dose administration.

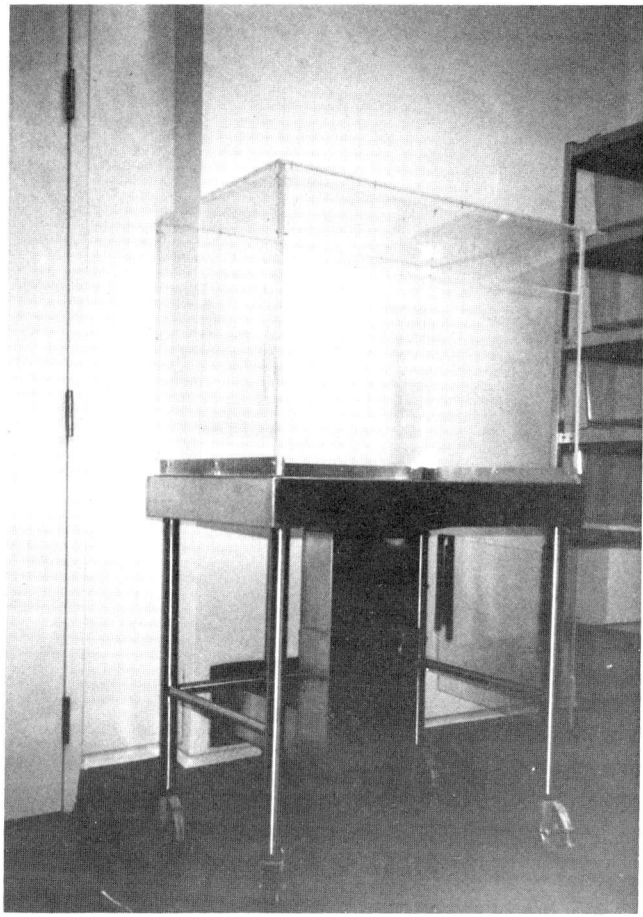

Figure 4-8.   Portable vented work station for dose administration.

the worker inside the lab. This would require a window properly positioned to permit viewing of the terminal screen, and a "plastic window" (a rectangular wall cutout fitted with a piece of heavy-gauge, flexible plastic) through which the keys of the terminal can be pressed.

NECROPSY AND HISTOLOGY

In the areas where necropsy and histology work are to be done, it is particularly important that an exhausted work station be provided since the potential for exposure to formaldehyde exists. Figure 4-9 shows one type of work station. Consideration should also be given to how formaldehyde will be supplied to the laboratory. Piped-in systems are sometimes operationally convenient but demand continual vig-

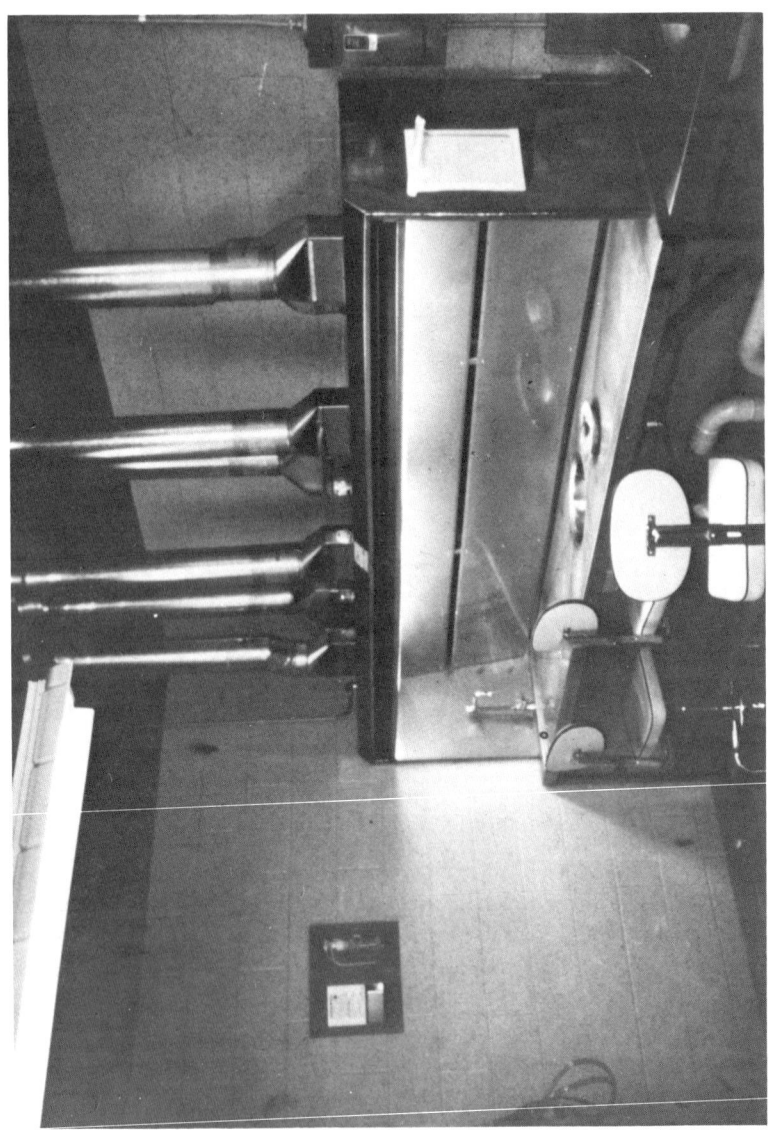

Figure 4-9.   Local exhaust necropsy work table.

ilance to ensure that leaking fixtures do not become an unrecognized source of formaldehyde exposure.

In the histology area, it is not unusual for large quantities of flammable solvents to be required. Appropriate flammable liquid storage locations should be allowed for, and vented enclosures should be provided for the equipment which utilizes flammable solvents. Where tissue samples are to be stored, a room with adequate air changes rather than an unvented closet should be provided. The histology area is also one in which a fire detection system should be considered. In particular, there should be a vented enclosure provided for automatic staining and processing equipment, and this enclosure should have an automatic fire detection and suppression system (e.g., an automatic carbon dioxide deluge system).

CHEMISTRY LABORATORIES

Chemistry laboratories should contain fume hoods which are properly located within the room and are engineered according to good ventilation principles [6]. Special operations which cannot conveniently be performed in standard lab hoods (e.g., extractions which require especially tall apparatus) may require specially designed hoods (e.g., those in Figures 4–10 and 4–11). Analytical equipment which produces effluent should also be vented (see Figure 4–12). An adequate amount of chemical storage should be provided, and an eye wash and a safety shower should be designed into each room (see Figure 4–13).

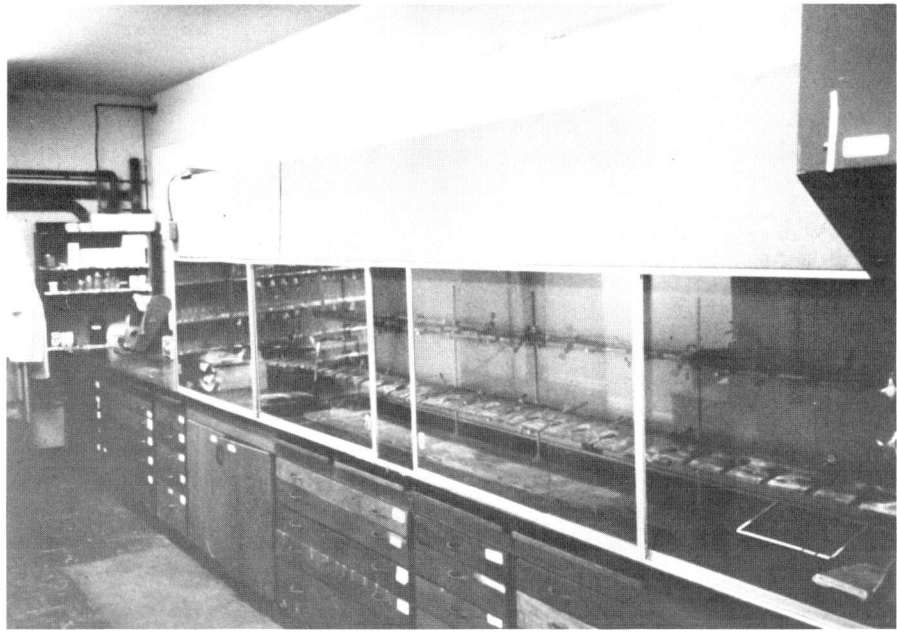

Figure 4–10. Chemical fume hood for extraction operations.

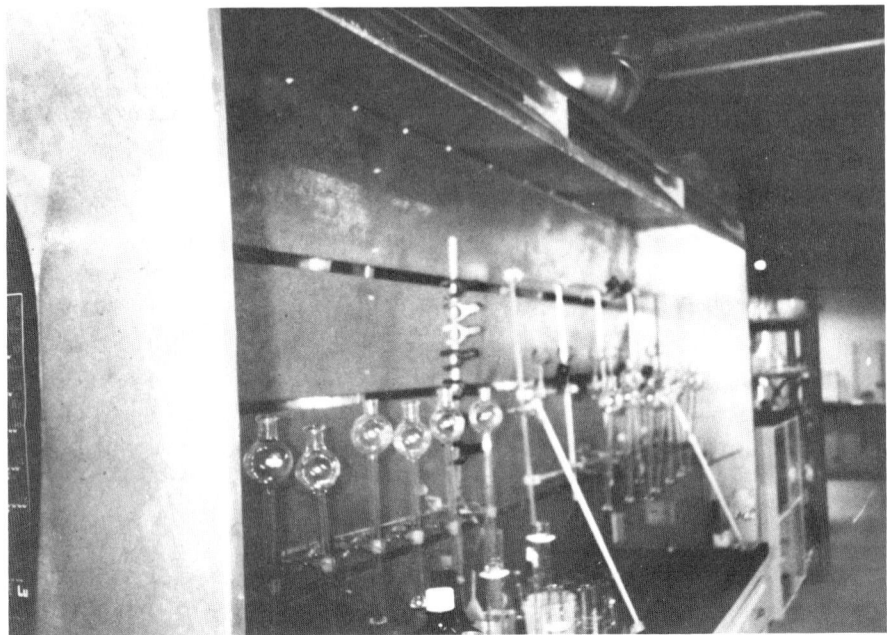

Figure 4-11.   Slot hood for extraction operations.

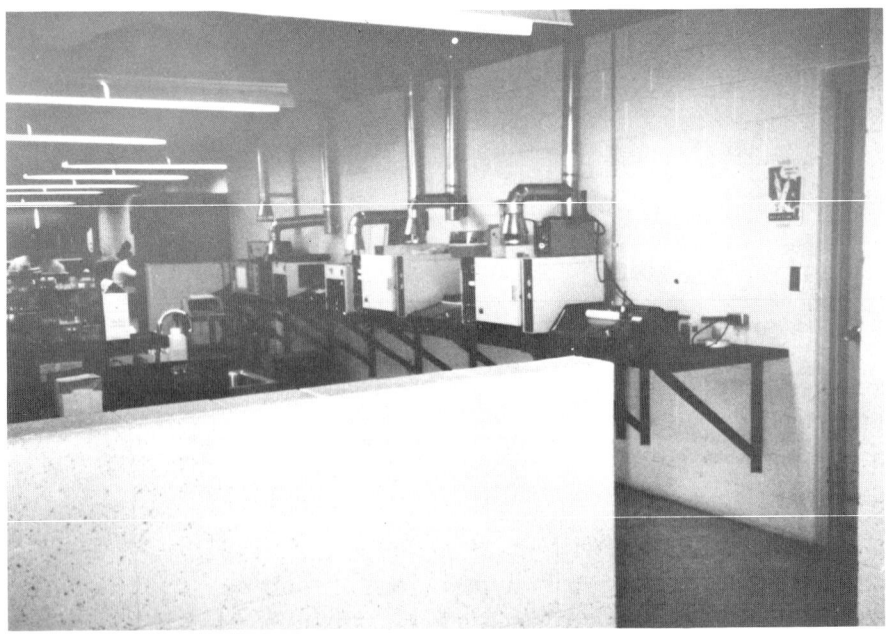

Figure 4-12.   Analytical chemistry equipment with vented effluent.

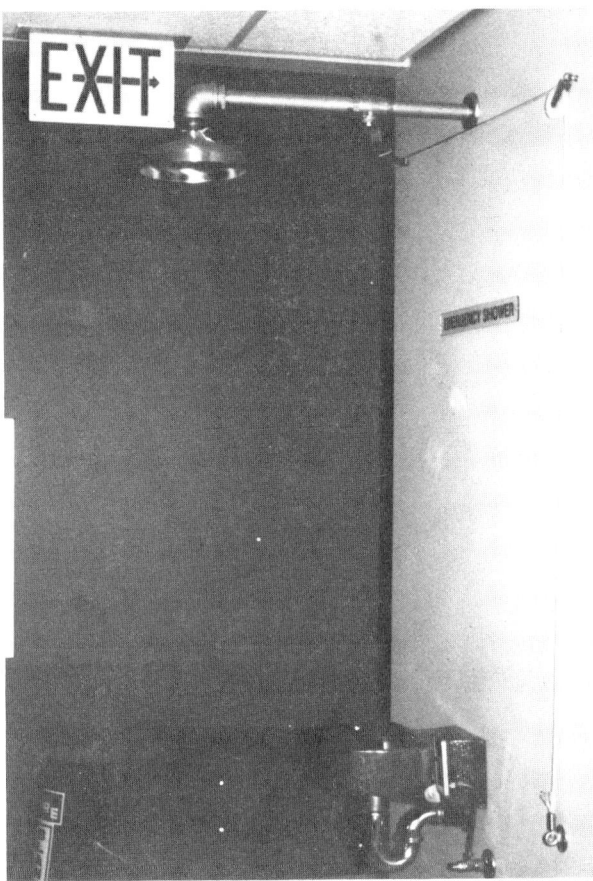

Figure 4-13.   Safety shower and eyewash station.

GENERAL CONSIDERATIONS

Several facility design considerations relate to waste handling. An isolated, vented, secured storage area for wastes that are to be taken off site or are to be stored pending incineration should be provided. The interim storage area should be immediately accessible to the dirty side of the barrier facility. Where animal cages are to be dumped prior to washing, a vented cage dump station, like those shown in Figures 4-14 and 4-15, should be included. It is also desirable to provide an incinerator capable of burning both animal and chemical wastes. The incinerator should be located relatively close to the lab area (to minimize the distance that waste must be transported within the facility) and should have adjustable operating temperature, ideally with a range of 1,500-2,200° F. It should meet all local permit requirements.

The facility should be provided with utilities support appropriate to the tasks at hand. Plumbing should include vacuum breakers and accessible traps. Drains which

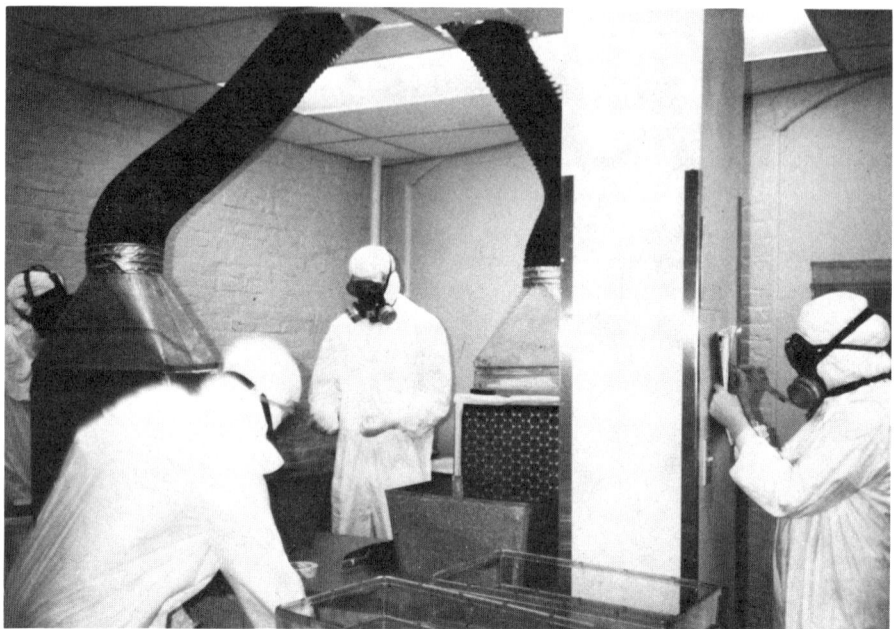

Figure 4-14. Cage dump station with backdraft exhaust.

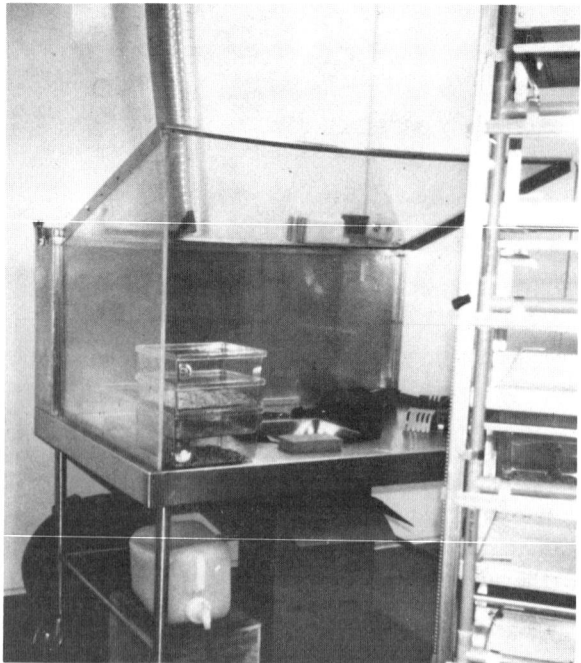

Figure 4-15. Enclosed cage dump station.

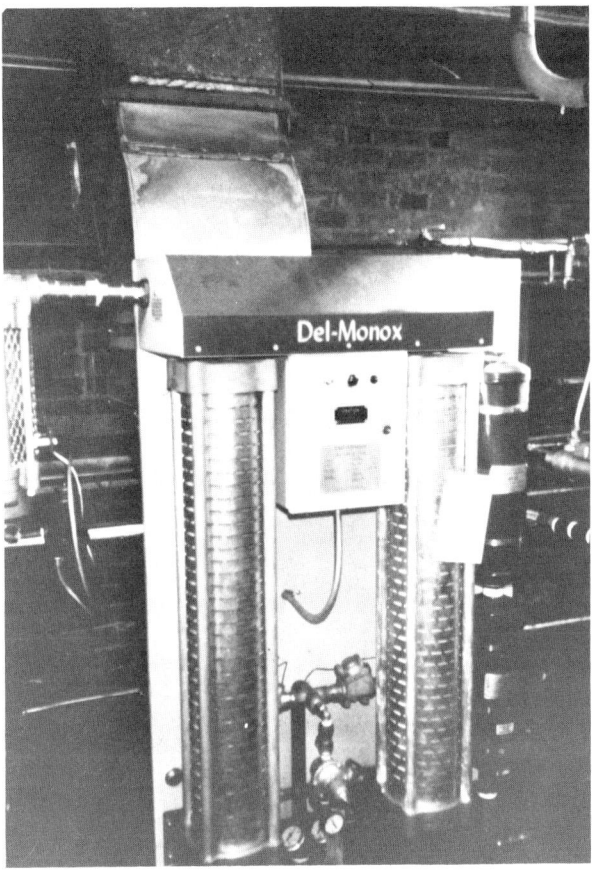

Figure 4-16.   Filter for compressor outlet of breathing air system.

may collect contaminated water, either normally or in case of a chemical spill, should be connected to holding tanks to provide the option of water treatment. Eyewashes and safety showers should be located throughout the facility. An emergency electrical generator should be connected to the air handling systems and some lighting fixtures. The air handling systems should be alarmed to permit rapid detection of fan failures, filter clogging, and other malfunctions. The source of breathing air should ideally be an oil-less compressor with a low-pressure alarm, a filter at the compressor (e.g., Figure 4-16), and a final filter at each potential connection point (e.g., Figure 4-17). Utility shutoffs (for electricity, gas, compressed air, water, etc.) should be located outside the barrier area to simplify emergency response. In addition, a control panel with gauges indicating the status of ventilation systems and with shutoffs for these systems should be located outside the barrier facility, readily accessible to maintenance personnel.

Exhaust stacks should be elevated above the roof level of the laboratory (see Figure 4-18) to minimize the chances of reentrainment, and air intakes should be

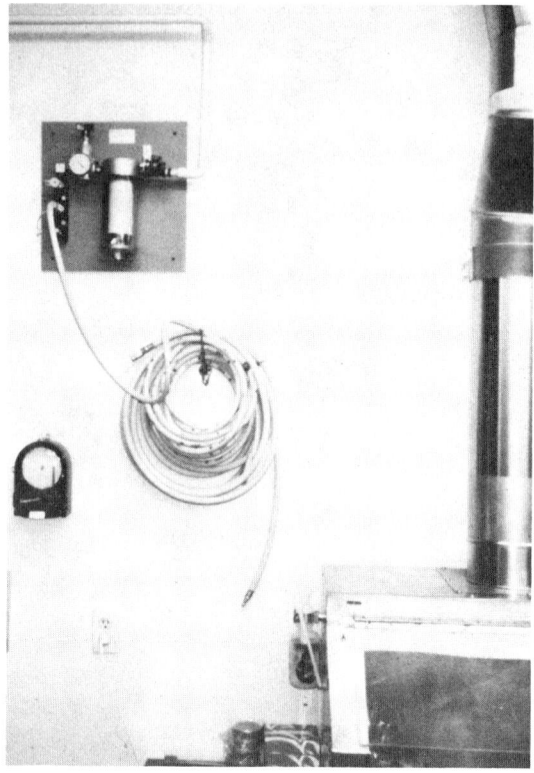

Figure 4–17. Breathing air connection with final filter.

located on the leeward side of the building rather than the roof. Exhaust air should be filtered with both HEPA and charcoal filters, with a bag-in, bag-out system provided to minimize exposure to maintenance personnel. The exhaust fan should be located outside the facility (e.g., on the roof) so that the positive pressure duct work that follows the fan is not indoors. It is desirable to have a backup fan which can be switched on-line in case of primary fan failure in each exhaust system. Taps should be provided in the filter housing to allow for monitoring of air before and after the charcoal filter, so that break-through can be evaluated. Installing tubing to these taps and running the tubing to a panel within the lab (see Figure 4–19) greatly simplifies the task of charcoal bed evaluation.

Walls and ceilings should be flat (i.e., without surface-mounted conduit, boxes, fixtures) and monolithic with lighting recessed to minimize the number of locations at which dust can accumulate (especially important in dose preparation and dose administration areas). Electrical fixtures should be waterproof so that areas can be hosed down for cleaning. This, of course, also requires a floor drain, and it is desirable to have holding tanks for drained water so that contaminant can be captured in

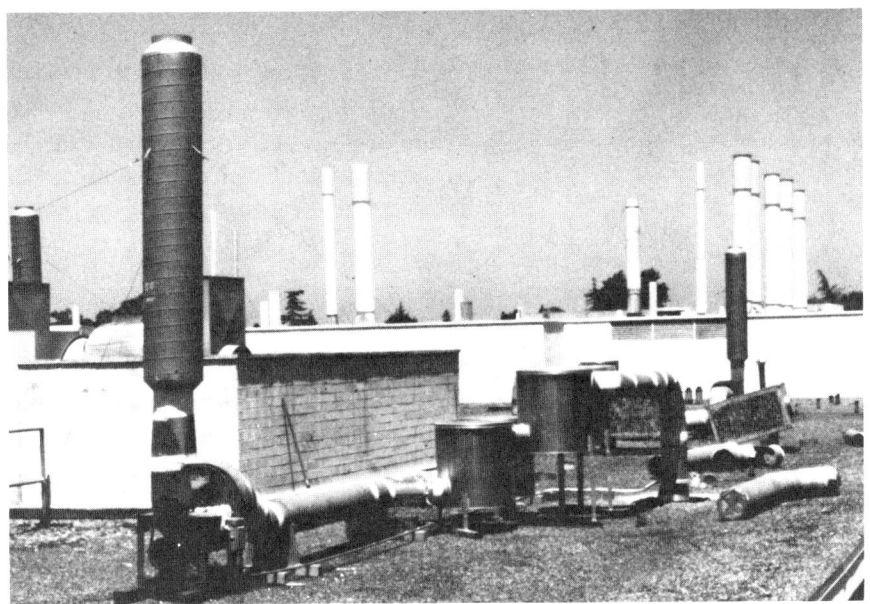

Figure 4–18.   Exhaust stacks elevated above roof level.

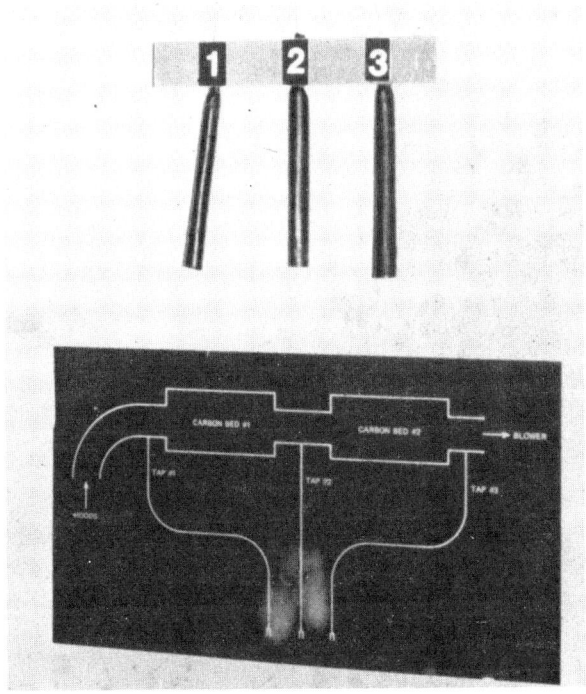

Figure 4–19.   Carbon filter testing panel.

of a spill. Incorporation of a central vacuum system facilitates floor cleaning within the facility.

Because an animal toxicology laboratory typically has a complex interior arrangement with many doors and corridors and sophisticated ventilation systems, some consideration should be given to fire protection of the facility. Providing standpipes and fire hose within the facility can greatly enhance response time in case of a fire. Also, emergency egress should be carefully considered to ensure that two well-marked means of egress are provided for each area [4]. All wall, floor, and ceiling penetrations (such as for water pipes or electrical lines) must be sealed, both to prevent potential fire spread and to preserve biological separation between adjacent areas.

CONCLUSION

The design of a toxicity testing laboratory should incorporate prospective health and safety concerns that may arise during the laboratory's use. While health- and safety-enhancing features may modestly increase the initial cost of the facility, these incremental initial costs tend to be much less than the costs of either retrofitting at a later date or using special operating procedures (e.g., extra personnel protective equipment) to compensate for a poorly designed facility.

REFERENCES

1. "Fire Protection for Laboratories Using Chemicals," NFPA 45-1982 (National Fire Protection Association, Quincy, MA, 1982).
2. *National Electrical Code*, NFPA 70-1981 (National Fire Protection Association, Quincy, MA, 1981).
3. *National Fire Codes*, sections 71, 72A, 72B, 72C, 72D, 72E (National Fire Protection Association, Quincy, MA, 1982).
4. "Life Safety Code," NFPA 101-1981 (National Fire Protection Association, Quincy, MA, 1981).
5. *Code of Federal Regulations*, Title 29, Section 1910.134, "Respiratory Protection," Occupational Safety and Health Administration.
6. *Industrial Ventilation, A Manual of Recommended Practice*, 17th ed. (Lansing, MI: American Conference of Governmental Industrial Hygienists, 1982).

CHAPTER 5

Barrier Laboratory Facilities: A Fire Control Manager's Perspective

Robert G. Nemchin

Office of Occupational Safety and Health,
Litton Bionetics, Inc., 5516 Nicholson Lane,
Kensington, Maryland 20895

INTRODUCTION

The barrier or containment laboratory commonly used for toxicology studies presents special problems for firefighting specialists. The fire control aspects of barrier facilities have emerged as a high-priority item to the fire control manager because of the increasing number of these types of facilities and of the number of people working in them. This increase principally has been a result of federal legislation affecting the safety testing of chemical substances (e.g., Toxic Substances Control Act[1]). Additionally, the concern for fire safety is heightened by the variety and quantities of the chemicals to be found in the barrier facility, especially in connection with chronic toxicological testing such as inhalation and feeding studies, which require large quantities of the test chemical. Some categories of chemical substances commonly found in toxicology laboratories are as follows:

- cosmetics, health, and hygiene products
- food additives, preservatives
- plastic intermediates
- rubber and elastomer intermediates
- pharmaceutical intermediates and products
- biocides
- fuels: natural and synthetic
- explosives, propellants, and initiators
- carcinogens, genotoxins
- solvents, lubricants
- wood and paper additives
- adhesive, coating materials

- fibers, textiles
- flame retardants

Because of the potential hazards associated with these substances, it is essential, in the design and operation of these types of laboratories, to be especially concerned with fire and explosion prevention, fire control and mitigation, and hazardous materials control as integrated program components of the overall building design and operation. It is also essential that the facility incorporate adequate structural features and protective systems to minimize fire and smoke development and spread, to permit easy removal of heat, smoke, and toxic (and sometimes explosive) products of combustion, and to facilitate firefighting operations and evacuation of personnel.

THE BARRIER CONCEPT

The particular architectural design and contamination control features found in barrier facilities depend upon what function the facility is to serve. Many barrier facilities are designed to confine and manage hazardous agents such as pathogenic microorganisms, toxic chemicals, and radiation within the laboratory in order to prevent accidental release of these agents and exposure of laboratory personnel or of the environment external to the laboratory. The toxicology laboratory is included in this category. Some types of barrier facilities may have as their principal objective the exclusion of external contaminating agents which may affect the scientific studies contained therein. Examples of this type of barrier facility would include bioclean assembly of spacecraft components, packaging of sterile pharmaceuticals, and axenic, specific pathogen-free, or germ-free studies. Still other barrier facilities are designed to satisfy both types of containment criteria through a complementary combination of architectural design features, carefully defined operating practices, specialized safety equipment, and contamination control systems.

Despite the purposes for which the facility is used, containment of a hazard (or exclusion of contamination) is customarily achieved through the use of well-established physical and administrative principles of contamination control [2–6]. The physical controls consist of primary, secondary, and tertiary levels of containment. *Primary containment*, the first line of defense for the protection of laboratory personnel and the immediate laboratory environment from exposure to hazardous materials, is provided by safety equipment such as chemical fume hoods and biological safety cabinets. The exhaust air from these devices is filtered or treated prior to discharge in order to remove the contaminant. *Secondary containment*, the protection of areas external to the laboratory, is provided by the laboratory structure itself, corridor and room construction and arrangement (the box within a box concept), airlocks, a ventilation system that provides unidirectional airflows, clothing change-rooms and showers, and facility effluent air and water treatment systems to remove contaminants from these waste streams prior to discharge from the facility. *Tertiary containment* is provided by isolating the entire barrier within a segregated or remote area of an existing facility or within a building which is physically separated from

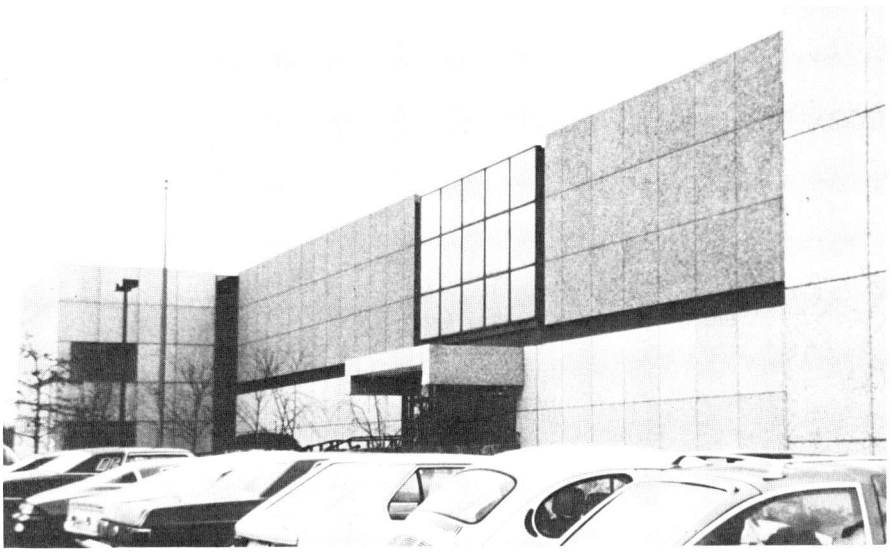

Figure 5-1.   Typical windowless laboratory design.

other structures. In order to maintain the internal laboratory environment (temperature, humidity), within tightly controlled limits the building is frequently windowless (Figure 5-1).

Regardless of the type of barrier facility, it is these architectural, structural, and contamination control features—essential for assuring the integrity of the scientific study and safeguarding the worker and the environment—that may actually become a liability in the event of a fire. Collectively, these features conspire to contain the heat and toxic products of combustion, impede rapid egress and access, hamper search and rescue, delay firefighting and ventilating operations, and prolong overhaul (locating and extinguishing spot fires in concealed spaces) and salvage operations (protection of laboratory equipment from water and heat, removal of water, debris, and hazardous materials). Firefighting in these kinds of facilities takes its toll by its demand for large numbers of fire suppression personnel and results in extensive property losses because of the difficulties in setting up and initiating an effective and timely attack.

GENERAL FIRE SAFETY CONSIDERATIONS

The occupants of barrier facilities, especially those involved in planning and design functions as well as architects and engineers should view these problems from the standpoint of personnel who have to deal with them during a fire. In order for these individuals to appreciate the magnitude of the problems confronting both the fire control manager and the firefighter, a review of the following fundamental building fire safety considerations is appropriate:

- ignition sources and fire propagation
- smoke, fire, and heat movement
- movement of occupants and firefighting personnel
- detection, alarm, and communications systems
- fire suppression systems
- firefighting operations
- maintaining structural integrity
- site factors

At the outset designers should be cognizant of the possible types and locations of potential ignition sources and the means by which fire can start and be propagated within such a facility. They should be knowledgeable in the fundamentals of fire behavior, aspects of which are not generally known outside of the firefighting sector, so that smoke, fire, and heat movement can be previsualized. They should also be concerned with the movement of occupants out of, and of fire suppression personnel into, the facility. This will dictate corridor and exit layouts. Designers should be sure that appropriate detection, alarm, and alternative communications systems have been provided in order to alert occupants and to provide for the coordination of firefighting activities, whether they are provided by the barrier facility's emergency organization or a municipal fire service. Fire suppression systems should be installed, even though they may not be required by local building codes. Selection of the specific system(s) should be done with due regard to the types and quantities of hazards. Building design should incorporate features that will facilitate firefighting operations as well as ensure structural stability throughout the evolution of a fire incident. Similarly, well-planned facility siting provides adequate access to all structures for emergency vehicles and to water supplies for exposure protection. Moreover, the designer should consider how to minimize environmental contamination by chemicals in firefighting water runoff. Each of these general considerations is examined in greater detail below.

Ignition Sources and Fire Propagation

Building fire safety is attained through fire prevention (i.e., isolating ignition sources from the fuel load) or, once a fire occurs, by minimizing its effect through knowledgeable building design and specialized control systems. Although fire prevention is considered to be the most important part of fire safety, it is obvious that fire safety cannot totally rely on fire prevention since it so intensively involves the human element.

Elements of ignition sources and fire propagation include:

- equipment
- human error

- chemicals
- arson
- fuel load and distribution
- finish materials
- architectural design features
- construction defects

The first five items in this list are principally under the control of the building occupant. Fires can start as a result of overheated equipment, electrical short circuits, or friction. Electrical equipment is the largest single cause of fires in the industrial sector, accounting for approximately 25% of the total number [7].

Preventive maintenance programs are a proven means of minimizing ignition due to faulty electrical or mechanical equipment. Providing training together with appropriate facilities reduces careless handling and storage of chemicals and minimizes this potential ignition source. Security measures designed to minimize vandalism lessen arson as a significant factor. Although arson is rare in the laboratory setting, the greater public profile that toxicology laboratories have today imparts a visibility that may engender a reaction by dissident environmental, political, or economically depressed groups, especially if chemical surety agents are being evaluated. Fire propagation, i.e., extension from the point of origin, depends upon the fuel load. The fuel load (anything that will burn) and its density and distribution are highly dependent upon the nature of the operations, storage capabilities, and housekeeping practices of the building occupant. Poor housekeeping practice is ostensibly one of the leading contributors to recorded property losses.

In addition to test chemicals, chemical reagents, and flammable liquids, the fuel load within the toxicology laboratory consists of furnishings, paper bags of bedding and feed, cardboard or plastic boxes of records, slides, and paraffin blocks (paraffin burns with a high Btu output and an intense black smoke), plastic rodent caging, and cases of filter tops, to name just a few items. When ignited these items may release one or more of the following toxic gases: carbon monoxide, hydrogen cyanide, hydrogen chloride, oxides of nitrogen, hydrogen sulfide, sulfur dioxide, acrolein, ammonia, and in some cases, phosgene.

The last three items in the above list are under the control of the building's designers and builders. It is these features which the planners, using clearly defined fire safety objectives, can anticipate and provide for in the final design criteria. Architectural design features like pipe chases and plenums, open stairwells, decorative facades, long and complex corridor systems, and windowless construction make fire extension more probable, access and ventilation difficult, and fire suppression more dangerous. Interior finish materials comprise floor and wall coverings (carpeting, drapes, wood or plastic paneling), coatings (paints, varnishes), wallboard, cabinetry, doors, ceiling tile, and insulating materials. Although finish materials are not normally the first items ignited, they often become involved and can contribute extensively to the spread of fire. Careful selection of finish materials with due regard for flame spread ratings greatly reduces property loss (and the hazards to life safety). In many municipalities, selection of finish materials must be approved by local building or fire authorities.

Fire safety features embodied within the fundamental architectural design are largely a function of the applicable building and fire codes that apply *and economics.* These codes may vary from state to state and even in different communities within a particular state. Compliance with minimum codes in communities which have not had major building code revisions within the past 10–20 years seriously shortchanges the occupants of the modern laboratory regarding fire safety. In these localities, designing beyond code is almost essential. However, designing a building that goes beyond minimum code may be difficult to justify to the occupant and/or owner since cost can be an overriding factor.

In some states with "mini-max" building codes [8,9], designing beyond code is actually illegal. A mini-max building code provides that a local code cannot be more restrictive than the state code. In effect, the state code is not only the minimum code but is also the maximum code allowed. This constraint does not permit local jurisdictions to have the latitude needed to require additional built-in fire protection beyond that called for in the state code. For example, the local jurisdiction could not require certain structural features to limit the spread of smoke and fire, sprinkler protection, smoke detectors, or other fire protection devices if such requirements exceed those of the state's mini-max building code. It is prudent for laboratory planners (and owners) to determine whether their state has such a mini-max building code and to determine whether this code is adequate to protect their investment in people and property.

Unfortunately the fire safety features embodied within the best designed barrier laboratory (or any building for that matter) may be seriously compromised during the construction phase. Barrier facilities are, by their very nature, complex structures with multiple subsystems. These characteristics and a host of factors relating to the level of skill and experience of the contractors, the pressure of completion schedules, and the quality of inspections all conspire to create a facility that most certainly will have some defects. Many of these defects may be corrected during the shakedown phase of the facility. However, the ones that remain are frequently those that are part of the building's structure and relate to the features that would confine fire and smoke to the room or area of origin. Unsealed penetrations in floors, walls, and ceilings where plumbing, electrical conduits, or mechanical systems pass through and missing fire stops or dampers are examples of defects that are often overlooked because they are found principally in concealed locations such as partitions, closets, and interstitial utility spaces. These openings become insidious routes of travel for fire, heat, and the products of combustion.

Smoke, Fire, and Heat Movement

Fire and the products of combustion travel vertically at first and then horizontally when meeting resistances such as ceilings and partitions. Unless the fire is extinguished in the incipient stage (as with a sprinkler system), smoke, heat, and carbon monoxide (itself a flammable gas) will travel both vertically and horizontally for considerable distances from the point of origin if there are any openings in partitions.

Corridors, shafts, concealed utility service spaces above the ceiling, and openings into pipe and duct chases spread the products of combustion throughout the barrier network. Depending upon the size of the fire, the facility's ventilating system may be adequate to initially control the buildup of smoke and heat. As the fire develops beyond the incipient stage the ventilation systems become overwhelmed and may fail entirely if the fire involves the electrical and mechanical control systems. Room compartmentation, a feature of the barrier facility, may initially help to confine the fire and provide occupant protection until extinguishment can be effected, but frequently doors are left open during the evacuation phase, thereby nullifying this control. The situation is exacerbated by the construction defects mentioned.

As the ventilating capability fails, fires in windowless buildings become excessively smoky as oxygen levels are depleted, and heat buildup is unusually rapid and intense. Firefighters must then endure greater punishment as they advance into the building unless adequate supplemental ventilation can be brought into play. In firefighting procedures, ventilation must be done early in order to release smoke, heat, and toxic gas buildup. Roof ventilation, where it can be done, obviously is most effective if the fire is on the top floor. Barrier facilities have ceilings below the roof which may be constructed of poured concrete. Ventilating through the roof then may not be a practicable means of rapidly relieving the burden and danger to firefighting crews. In large multistory buildings, ventilation frequently must be done horizontally, i.e., using the corridor system. This becomes dangerous to the occupants if evacuation and firefighting operations are progressing simultaneously, since the same corridors are used.

Heat can be conveyed to remote parts of the building either by conduction through unprotected steel structural members and piping or by air conditioning or hot-air heating ducts. These ducts usually penetrate firewalls in order to provide services throughout the building. Smoke and toxic gases also are transmitted in this manner. Many building codes permit air conditioning ducts to connect all sections of a building.

Movement of Occupants and Firefighting Personnel

The first consideration of the architect/designer for any building are form and function. The first consideration for the fire control manager and the firefighter is life safety. In many cases these two aspirations are not mutually served. Building designers (and their clients) are content to meet the minimum safety standards of the building code. Frequently both assume incorrectly that these codes provide completely adequate measures rather than minimal ones. The occupants are thus lulled into a false sense of security with respect to fire safety. Barrier facility designs often utilize the double-corridor concept of containment. This type of barrier results in a network of parallel (or dead-end) corridors which may be confusing to those who are not familiar with the layout (Figure 5–2). In a fire, with its smoke and toxic gases, even veteran employees may easily become disoriented and may not find their way to the exits. The barrier facility must be designed so that adequate numbers of clearly

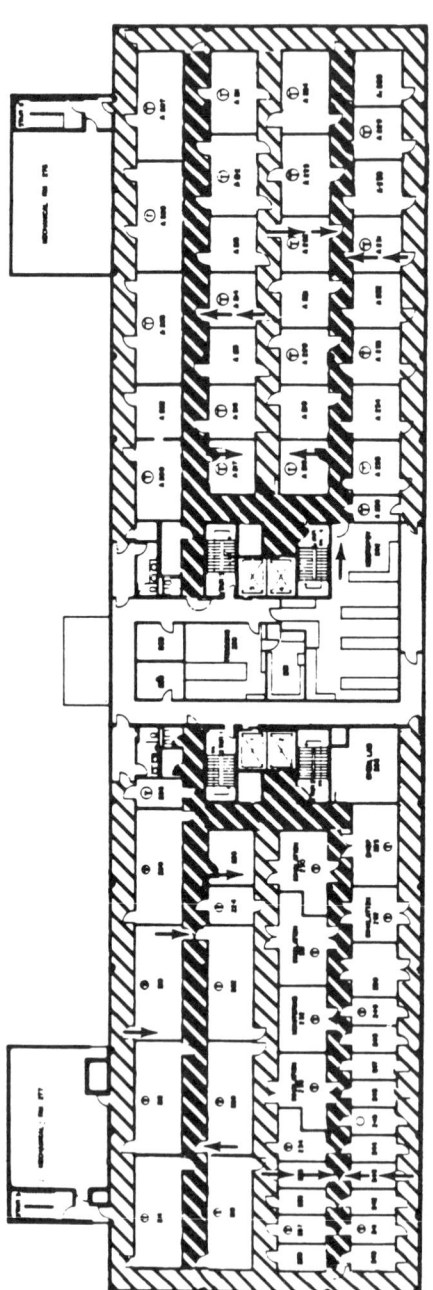
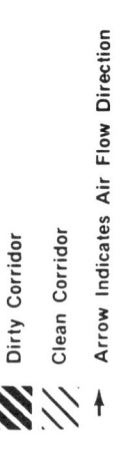

Figure 5–2.   Schematic of a typical toxicity testing barrier facility.

marked exits are distributed throughout the corridor system. Since smoke normally rises to the ceiling, exit signs mounted over doors are the first things to become obscured. A better approach to the identification of exits would be to provide arrows on the floor, or on the walls approximately 1 to 2 feet above the floor, leading to the exits. Under heavy smoke or heat conditions, smoke can bank down to floor levels. Building occupants are advised to stoop low, or better yet, crawl to the exits to avoid breathing superheated air and toxic (invisible) combustion products. When mounted as suggested, the exit markers can still be easily seen. Firefighters also can become lost within a large facility and may use these exit markers to find their way out if they become separated (as in search and rescue) or if fire conditions worsen so as to make parts of the building untenable.

During the day toxicology laboratory facilities are congested with caging, cage racks, water bottles, and other equipment which may obstruct rapid occupant egress and firefighter access. In older buildings corridor widths may be barely adequate to handle the traffic loads of normal operations. These narrow or congested (or both) corridors considerably delay the setup operations for advancing to and extinguishing the fire. For buildings with no internal firefighting water supply such as standpipes or sprinklers, firefighters have to extend hose lines for considerable distances from the street to reach the fire. The congestion in the corridors substantially hinders this operation and may even become dangerous if conditions worsen. In heavy fire situations the firefighter cannot see beyond the facepiece of his breathing apparatus and must find the fire by feel or sound. Rarely have building designers or occupants actually experienced a fire where they can truly appreciate the firefighters' problems and how building design and operation can be a hindrance.

Life safety design considerations [10] could conceivably provide for safe refuge areas to be designated so that in very large or multistory facilities all the occupants do not necessarily leave. This approach has been used in the past in occupancies such as high-rise office buildings and hospitals, where large numbers of people cannot be moved easily to the outside. This concept aids worker evacuation from the fire area and interferes less with firefighting operations both inside and outside the building.

Detection, Alarm, and Communications

It is essential that employee safety be foremost in our minds. Providing the means for early detection of the fire and alerting of the facility occupants is the best way to show this concern. Products of combustion or heat detectors should be situated in all areas where fire can reasonably be expected to start and propagate. Chemical storage, combustible commodity (feed, bedding, caging) storage, custodial closets, office and mechanical spaces, and incinerator and boiler rooms are typical locations for detector placement. Detectors in exhaust ventilation ducts should shut down supply air while continuing to provide exhaust for initial smoke and heat control. Audible and visual signaling systems should be used for alerting all occupants. Special care should be taken to ensure that workers in high-noise areas, such as cage washing and laundry rooms, can be alerted. A backup alerting capability such as a public address system is useful in the event that the alarm system malfunctions. Depending upon the building's construction, fire service portable radios may not be able to transmit effectively out of or within the various areas of the building. This public address system then may be used by the fire department for their own communications or for evacuation instructions to occupants. A desirable feature found in many newer high-rise buildings is the fire control room which serves as the detection, alarm, and communication control center for the entire facility. This capability provides to the fire command officer a way to monitor the fire protection systems in the building from a central point and to communicate instructions to the occupants and facilities engineering personnel, and to direct fire service operations.

Fire Suppression Systems

Up to this point, it should be apparent to the reader that for various reasons relating to design, construction, and contents, many buildings (laboratories included) are deficient in their ability to withstand the initiation and propagation of fire. These shortcomings, however, may be offset by the installation of fire suppression systems. In fact, the National Fire Protection Association's (NFPA's) "Life Safety Code" [10] recognizes the value of certain fire suppression systems, such as automatic sprinklers, by permitting longer travel distances to exits and interior finish of higher combustibility when a sprinkler system is present.

Fire suppression systems fall into three broad categories:

- manual
- automatic water sprinklers
- special systems

Manual systems comprise portable fire extinguishers and internal standpipe and hose stations. Unfortunately, the effectiveness of these items is a function of someone's being present at the time of the fire to use them and of the level of training that the workers have received in using them. Thus, these items are considered only as a first aid approach and generally should not be relied upon solely for fire protection. For those times when personnel are not in the facility or for unattended hazardous operations such as those involving tissue processing equipment (which use large quantities of flammable liquids) in histology laboratories, a full-time fire extinguishing system is a prudent approach.

If the designer and client are truly concerned with protecting the substantial investment involved in constructing, equipping, and operating a barrier facility, an automatic fire extinguishing system is a cost-effective measure for ensuring continued operation. Automatic sprinklers are the equivalent of a firefighting team on duty 24 hours a day. Depending upon the material involved, the five to eight minutes it takes the fire department to reach the facility may be enough time to develop sufficient fire to destroy a substantial portion of the operation. Properly installed and maintained automatic sprinklers operating at the incipient stage (usually two to five minutes, depending upon the material involved in the fire) could make (and historically have made) the difference between a $100 loss and a $1 million loss.

Automatic sprinkler systems may not always be found in older (and in some newer) barrier facilities, especially if the facility was built to minimum building code. This places an inordinate burden on fire suppression personnel to extend hose lines for long distances within the facility from the available water supply. Depending upon the type of fire service available to the facility, especially in rural areas, there may not be adequate personnel available for the placement of long interior hoselays just when it is needed most, i.e., during the initial attack phase. Thus one can expect greater property losses, and consequently, delays in recovery of operations.

Automatic water sprinklers are remarkably effective for life safety since they not only warn of the existence of fire by sounding an alarm but also apply water to the fire. The downward force of the water cools the area and lowers the smoke level, permitting easier access for firefighters to the seat of the fire. Historically automatic sprinklers have compiled an impressive, cost-effective performance record approaching a 100% reliability factor. However, this reliability is obtained only when these systems are properly sized, installed, and maintained.

The third category, specialized systems, comprise carbon dioxide, foam, and dry chemical flooding systems for specific applications such as flammable liquids. Halogenated extinguishing agents (Halons) are useful for delicate electrical equipment found in computer installations and for scientific instrumentation. Although these systems are effective, their reliability factor does not approach that of automatic water sprinklers.

FIREFIGHTING OPERATIONS

Most people outside the fire service do not truly understand and appreciate the activities performed by and the difficulties facing firefighters during a building fire. Building designers, owners, and occupants are numbered among them. One can speculate that perhaps the incidence and severity of building fires would be reduced substantially if buildings were designed instead by firefighting personnel. In order to gain an appreciation of these difficulties, it is necessary to introduce the reader to the fundamentals of firefighting operations.

Over the years, firefighting professionals have developed a strategy which has changed somewhat with the modernization of buildings, operations, materials, and firefighting equipment but has changed little conceptually since the introduction of the fire hose in Holland in 1672 [11]. This firefighting strategy can be broken down into the following discrete tactical elements applicable to all fire situations:

- access
- rescue
- locating, confinement, and extinguishment
- exposures
- ventilation

- salvage
- overhaul

These tasks are listed in order of priority, although several may be performed simultaneously depending upon the type of structure involved, fire conditions at the time of arrival, and personnel availability during the initial sizeup and attack stages.

It is widely accepted by firefighting and fire prevention specialists that in any type of fire situation, the first five minutes in fire development are the most critical. National surveys [12] have shown that the response time for urban and suburban fire departments, after receipt of the alarm, averages approximately two to six minutes. The response time for rural departments can be considerably longer (i.e., ten minutes or more). Delayed alarms increase this time factor and may exacerbate the losses.

Access

Ready access to the premises is of vital importance for fire department operations to commence swiftly and efficiently, and in recent years has become even more difficult. The problem has two aspects: access not only to the interior of the building but accessibility to the structure itself. Employee and service vehicles, building setbacks, landscaping, and high-voltage power lines make the approach and deployment of emergency vehicles difficult. Aerial ladders and platforms cannot be used because the apparatus cannot be brought in close enough to the building. Ground ladders and hose lines must be handcarried long distances to the building.

Access to the interior of the building is not as easy as it once was. Because of an increase in the crime rate, the use of sophisticated locks and security devices has burgeoned. Entry in this regard is equally critical at night and weekends unless there are security or engineering personnel present to admit firefighters and direct them to the fire. In many communities, the fire departments are given keys to various unattended businesses so that forcible entry is unnecessary. Interior access is also hampered by windowless construction, decorative facades, solar panels, and signs covering large areas of the exterior. These obstacles make it difficult for firefighters to initiate a timely attack. This means that the fire has ample opportunity to become well established even when reported promptly, possibly spreading into the extensive network of concealed spaces commonly found in the barrier facility.

Rescue

Firefighting personnel are trained that the first consideration in any fire is life safety and that search and rescue operations may have to be performed. If personnel is limited on the initial response to a fire incident, depending upon the number of victims, rescue may be the only possible task in the first few minutes. Extinguishment, ventilation, etc., must be left to later arriving engine and ladder companies, again creating delays in extinguishment (if there is no fixed automatic fire protection system operating in the facility).

Fortunately, loss of life is relatively infrequent in the industrial setting so that the danger extends not so much to the building occupants as it does to the firefighter. The greatest hazards to the firefighter are smoke and heat, structural failure, and explosion, either from chemicals or backdraft conditions.

Smoke is hazardous because of its toxic components and because it obscures vision. The heat associated with the fire is dangerous to firefighters not only from the view of burns but also from heat exhaustion through extended exposure to moderately high temperatures. This can cause internal injuries to those not promptly treated. Firefighter clothing and breathing apparatus provide a good deal of protection but are not the perfect solution.

Structural failure is perhaps the greatest hazard in firefighting. Some buildings can collapse quickly and with little warning. In some cases, floors or roofs will collapse within the walls of the structure. In other situations, the walls will fall outward, endangering personnel and fire equipment. It is probably not well known outside the architectural engineering and firefighting sectors that structural steel starts to weaken at 1,200° F and loses 90% of its strength at 1,400° F. Under certain fire conditions, this temperature can be reached in 10–15 minutes. At this temperature, a steel beam or girder will expand 5 inches in a 50-foot span; enough to push away its supports [13]. The floors or roofs of many laboratory structures are constructed of steel bar joists and behave in this way when subjected to fire impingement if unprotected.

Backdrafts or "smoke explosions" represent a recognized life hazard to firefighters if ventilation of a fire building cannot be initiated early enough. Under conditions where the flammable gases produced during combustion (principally carbon monoxide) cannot be released, they may ignite suddenly with explosive force upon the introduction of air (as when opening doors). The energy released from a long smoldering fire where large quantities of carbon monoxide have accumulated can be sufficient to cause structural damage, blowing out windows and doors and frequently injuring or killing firefighters in or near the building. The difficulties in rapidly ventilating barrier facilities may create the conditions for this kind of life hazard to occur.

Locating, Confinement, and Extinguishment

In a large barrier facility, locating a fire may be difficult because of the complexity of rooms and corridors, and because of the ventilation airflow patterns. In windowless buildings, the number of floors is not readily apparent from the outside to first arriving units unless they are familiar with the facility and have actually been through it. During normal business hours, employees can inform the fire department of the exact location and of the materials involved. However, during nonworking hours, locating the fire is not so easy. Providing the fire department with building plans in advance, showing the locations and types of hazardous and combustible materials, utility shutoffs, service valves, fire protection systems, control valves and panels, and emergency power outlet locations, and marking stairwell doors to indicate floor or wing location considerably enhance the fire department's ability to find the fire and start extinguishment that much sooner.

If the fire has developed to the point where the compartment where it origi-nated was insufficient to contain it before water could be applied, then the fire officer must determine how much, and into which areas the fire may have extended. Obviously extension of the fire, heat, and products of combustion depends upon the type of construction (frame, masonry, steel, concrete); penetrations in the room or area of origin such as unprotected ceiling or wall openings, pipe chases, elevator shafts, and ventilating ducts; the quantity and type of fuel that is burning or can become involved; and the presence or absence of an automatic extinguishing system. For large, difficult fires, the fire department must judge what areas it can afford to give up to the fire in order to make an effective stand, i.e., writing off a portion of the facility. Confinement then constitutes the strategic placement of hose lines (usually on four sides and above the fire) in order to protect uninvolved areas, property, and personnel. By this action confinement then is synonymous with exposure protection.

Exposures

Exposure protection refers to protecting employees, firefighters, and property adja-cent to the fire area inside and outside the building. The use of hose lines for protect-ing routes of egress for evacuating employees and nearby equipment or structures from radiant heat and flying brands minimizes the extension of fire. In some cases, there might not be sufficient staff to cover all exposures when it is needed, and priori-ties must be established. This may mean initially foregoing neighboring building pro-tection if there is a distinct life hazard to be considered. Protection of exposures then must be done according to a prearranged plan that is tailored to the particular labor-atory. This requires a coordinated effort between the laboratory management and the fire department. Effective coordination can only be achieved by prefire incident planning between the laboratory management and the fire department.

Ventilation

Ventilation of a fire-involved building should begin as soon as possible after arrival of the fire department. Again this depends upon the number of people available at the fire scene in the initial stages. Next to rescue, ventilation is perhaps the most impor-tant firefighting operation. It is so important that in most fire departments special teams of firefighters are assigned this task as their primary function (ladder compan-ies or, as they are known in fire department terminology, truck companies), although they do perform other functions such as rescue and raising ladders. Ventilation involves the *controlled* removal of smoke, gases, and heat from the building by mak-ing or using openings in roofs, walls, floors, and ceilings. These actions serve the fol-lowing important functions:

1. Protect life by removing or diverting heat, smoke, and toxic gases from locations where the building occupants may have found temporary refuge.

2. Improve the environment in proximity to the fire by removal of smoke and heat. Removal of heat and increased visibility enable firefighters to advance closer to the fire and extinguish it with a minimum amount of water and time, thus minimizing damage.
3. Control the spread or direction of fire by setting up air currents that cause the fire to move in a desired direction.
4. Allow the release of flammable combustion products before they can accumulate to levels which could create backdraft (explosion) conditions.

Architects and designers must be aware of these conditions, which can develop rapidly during a fire. The installation of smoke vents, panels, or skylights that open automatically during the initial stages of a fire, pressurized stairwells that keep these routes of egress free of smoke, and automatic closing doors for confinement of smoke and fire pay for themselves in their reduction of life hazard, property damage, and firefighting efforts.

Salvage

Salvage operations should begin with the arrival of the fire department. Salvage is defined as any operation designed to protect property not already involved in the fire. Such operations constitute protection of property from smoke or water by tarpaulins or removal (if possible) of the property from the building, and of water and debris removal after the fire has been extinguished. In the case of hazardous materials, salvage may also involve removal or decontamination operations. Usually these operations are left to, or are performed in conjunction with, the building occupants. Laboratory building designers would do well to consider the provision of drains or scuppers (drainage ports in the building's outside walls) to channel water used for extinguishment away from expensive equipment and to shorten the cleanup time. Scuppers are preferred since drains have a tendency to clog frequently in laboratory animal facilities. With dry-housed animals there may be no drains available.

Overhaul

Overhaul is a thorough examination of the involved structure after the main body of the fire has been extinguished in order to locate and extinguish small fires in concealed spaces. This operation ensures that no embers are left to rekindle later on and involves opening up partitions, floors, ceilings, and roofs to inspect for extension of fire into these spaces. The construction of many barrier laboratories, with their interstitial spaces, could mean extensive overhaul operations unless these spaces are well isolated and protected (e.g., with automatic sprinklers).

MAINTAINING STRUCTURAL INTEGRITY

The stability of any structure and the integrity of the interior compartmentation are vital design considerations for any building. Unfortunately, architects (generally not knowledgeable in fire behavior) tend to develop design criteria which frequently overlook the additional stresses imposed upon the compartmentation and the load-bearing structural members if a fire occurs in the building. In order to minimize the probability of structural collapse and compartmentation failure during a fire, the designer must incorporate adequate fire resistance materials for partitions, ceilings, and support members which take into consideration the fire loading (i.e., the type, quantity, and distribution of items that will burn). In order to do this effectively, the designer must be knowledgeable of the changes that occur in the physical and chemical characteristics of common structural materials at elevated temperatures. As mentioned previously, steel load-bearing members will start to fail at about 1,200° F. Additionally, prestressed concrete loses 20% of its strength at 600° F and is permanently weakened at 800° F, and masonry will lose its integrity at approximately 800° F due to calcination (water loss) of the mortar in the joints [13,14]. The time to failure of each of these materials depends upon several factors, such as the type of material involved in the fire. A high Btu output fuel can cause unprotected steel to fail in as

Table 5-1. Design Deficiencies Responsible for Spread of Fire, Heat, and Smoke

Throughout a building

Lack of adequate vertical and/or horizontal fire separations.

Unprotected or inadequately protected floor and wall openings for stairs, doors, elevators, escalators, dumbwaiters, ducts, conveyors, chutes, pipe chases, and windows.

Concealed spaces in walls and above ceilings without adequate fire-stopping or fire divisions.

Combustible interior finish, including combustible protective coatings and insulation.

Combustible structural members (beams, girders, and joints) framed into fire walls.

Improper anchorage of structural members in masonry bearing walls.

Explosion or pressure damage to the building due to lack of or inadequate explosion venting where required.

Damage to unprotected framing resulting in weakening or destruction of floors and walls used as fire barriers.

Lack of means to ventilate fire gases.

From one building to another

Lack of adequate fire division walls between adjoining buildings.

Unprotected or inadequately protected openings in fire division walls between adjoining buildings or in fire walls between detached buildings.

Exterior walls with inadequate fire resistance.

Inadequate separation distance.

Combustible roofs, roof coverings, roof structures, overhanging eaves, trim, etc.

Lack of protection at openings to passageways, pipe tunnels, conveyors, ducts, etc., between detached buildings.

Explosion or pressure damage to adjoining or detached buildings.

Collapse of exterior walls.

little as 8–10 minutes. Concrete and masonry withstand heat substantially better (one or more hours) and in many cases, are the material of choice. However, the fire resistance of steel structural supports can be increased considerably by simply encasing the supports in concrete, gypsum board, cementitious materials, sprayed-on mineral fiber or intumescent paints (coatings that char and swell up, increasing the thickness of the coating and concomittantly the fire resistance factor). The fire resistance of steel can be increased up to five hours depending upon the encasement method utilized [14].

Another important consideration in designing for structural stability is floor loading. Floor loading factors are considered by the architect for the normal operations within the building plus a safety factor. However, during a large fire, thousands of gallons of water can be applied through both the automatic sprinkler systems and hoselines. If drainage to a particular area is insufficient to carry water away faster than it is being applied, it will accumulate. The weight of this water (8.34 pounds per gallon) may exceed the designed floor loading characteristics, resulting in collapse.

Design and construction deficiencies play the major role in the spread of fire, heat, and smoke throughout a building. Table 5-1 summarizes those deficiencies which can affect structural stability [7].

Careful consideration by the architect and building planners of the factors shown in Table 5-1, together with detailed and competent inspections during the construction phase, are the fire control manager's and the firefighter's greatest allies. These considerations can mean the difference between rebuilding a few laboratory rooms and rebuilding the facility.

SITE FACTORS

Selection of a site for barrier facilities involves a number of factors: possible hazards to the community and their relationships to climate and terrain, space requirements, type and size of buildings, special facilities, transportation, business market, and labor supply [15]. The importance of siting for access to the buildings for emergency apparatus was discussed previously. Additionally, consideration must be given from the fire protection standpoint of access to readily available water supplies. The availability of water, next to rescue, is of vital concern to both the fire control manager and the fire officer, not only for firefighting in the primary structure but to cover exposures. Those exposures may represent a more serious problem than the fire structure itself in that laboratory facilities may be situated close to other laboratory buildings, chemical storage facilities, compressed gas cylinder storage, fuel gas tanks (propane, butane), and hazardous waste storage facilities. Site planning must consider obtaining sufficient property to provide the spacing (and/or fire protection systems) necessary to protect these facilities if one or more of them are involved in fire.

Site planning must not only take into account the environmental impact of normal operations of the toxicology laboratory on nearby sewers, rivers, streams, public parks, and bathing areas, but the impact of the building's contents which may be released during firefighting operations. During a major fire, considerable water runoff occurs. This water may be contaminated with flammable liquids or toxic chemicals originally contained within the facility. Under these conditions, the incident may develop into a potential major public danger rather than a localized one as the water runoff enters sewers or nearby streams. In order to circumvent some of these problems, the NFPA's "Flammable Liquids Code" [16] requires that containment diking or tanks be provided for certain storage installations and that they be of sufficient size to contain not only all material stored therein but the water used in firefighting operations. The collected runoff then can be disposed of after firefighting operations have been concluded. This requirement not only protects the environment but also protects nearby exposures from fire involvement if there is the possibility that the runoff could travel toward other structures.

DISCUSSION

In planning, designing, and constructing a containment facility, integrated design for fire safety must be done as a part of the architectural design process if it is to be effective and economical. The building design team should anticipate emergency fire conditions by considering the following fire-safe building design elements: the type of fuel load, its distribution, and the chance of fire initiation (ignition sources), possible routes of smoke and fire movement; detection and alarm systems during the incipient stage of fire development; communications; the horizontal and vertical movement of people, both employees that are leaving and firefighters entering; fire suppression systems; firefighting operations (access, rescue, venting, extinguishment, overhaul, salvage, protecting exposures); confinement and removal of hazardous materials; building structural members and stability; and a host of other factors. It is imperative that the building designer become knowledgeable in the basic operations of the fire service during fire emergencies in order to incorporate the features that will assist, not hinder, firefighting operations. Experience has demonstrated that the efficiency of these operations is a direct function of building access, design and layout, finish materials, engineering services, and fire suppression capabilities. Architects and planners should use existing fire-safe design and fire protection technology concepts and explore innovative approaches to barrier laboratory design.

Scientists work to improve the quality of life in the world at large. On the other hand, safety professionals work to improve the quality of life in the workplace. If we consider the factors discussed here we can provide a safe workplace for a highly specialized population of workers. But we must also be mindful of designing, constructing, and maintaining these laboratories to minimize the dangers to another highly specialized resource: the firefighter.

SUMMARY

The barrier or containment laboratory facility, commonly used to conduct toxicology studies on a wide array of chemical substances (many of which may be hazardous), is specifically designed to manage and confine hazardous agents within the facility in order to protect laboratory personnel and the environment. This protection is afforded by a combination of building design features and contamination control systems to prevent hazardous material release and to process facility effluents in case of an accidental release. Unfortunately, these features actually become a liability during a fire. Windowless facilities and inadequate ventilation entrap heat, smoke, and toxic gases, making fire attack difficult. Complicated corridor systems and room compartmentation impede access, hamper rescue and firefighting operations, and prolong overhaul and salvage. These problems and others relating to building design and operation in fire control management and recommendations for aiding, not hindering, firefighting efforts are discussed.

ACKNOWLEDGMENT

I wish to express my appreciation to the management and staff of Litton Bionetics, Inc., for their support in the preparation of this manuscript.

REFERENCES

1. Toxic Substances Control Act, Public Law 94-469, enacted September 28, 1976 and 15 USC 2602.
2. Runkel, R.S. and G.B. Phillips. *Microbial Containment Control Facilities* (New York: Van Nostrand Reinhold, 1969), p. 25.
3. Chatigny, M.A. and D.I. Clinger. "Contamination Control in Aerobiology," in *An Introduction to Experimental Aerobiology*, L. Dimmick and A.B. Akers, Eds. (New York: John Wiley and Sons, 1969), pp. 194-263.
4. Kuehne, R.W. "Biology Containment Facility for Studying Infectious Disease," *Appl. Microbiol.* 26:239-245, 1973.
5. U.S. Department of Health, Education and Welfare. "Design Criteria for Viral Oncology Research Facilities," DHEW Publication No. (NIH) 75-891 (Washington, D.C.: U.S. Government Printing Office, 1975).
6. Phillips, G.B. and R.S. Runkle. "Design of Facilities for Microbial Safety," in *CRC Handbook of Laboratory Safety*, 2nd ed., N.V. Steere, Ed. (West Palm Beach: CRC Press, 1971), pp. 618-632.
7. *Fire Protection Handbook*, 14th ed., G.P. McKinnon, Ed. (Boston: National Fire Protection Association, 1976), Chapter 6.
8. *Managing Fire Services*, J.L. Bryan and R.C. Picard, Eds. (Washington, D.C.: International City Management Association, 1979), pp. 168-194.
9. *Fire Protection Through Modern Building Codes* (Washington, D.C.: American Iron and Steel Institute, 1971).
10. "Life Safety Code," NFPA No. 101, *National Fire Codes* (Boston: National Fire Protection Association, 1980).
11. Clark, W.E. *Firefighting Principles and Practice* (New York: Donnell Publishing Corp., 1974), Chapter 5.
12. *America Burning: A Report of the National Commission on Fire Prevention and Control* (Washington, D.C.: U.S. Government Printing Office, 1973).

13. Brannigan, F.L. *Building Construction for the Fire Service* (Boston: National Fire Protection Association, 1971), Chapter 2.
14. *Handbook of Industrial Loss Prevention,* 2nd ed., Factory Mutual Engineering Corporation (New York: McGraw-Hill, 1967), Chapter 3.
15. *Accident Prevention Manual for Industrial Operations,* 7th ed. (Chicago: National Safety Council, 1974), p. 368.
16. "Flammable Liquids Code," NFPA No. 30, *National Fire Codes* (Boston: National Fire Protection Association, 1980).

CHAPTER 6

Hazard Containment in an Inhalation Toxicology Laboratory

W.B. Reid, J.R. Klok, and B.K.J. Leong
The Upjohn Company, Kalamazoo, Michigan

INTRODUCTION

Until recently the pharmaceutical industry was concerned primarily with protecting drugs intended for human consumption from contamination by employees during the manufacturing process. However, the industry is increasingly aware that workers should be protected from the possible harmful effects of overexposure to drugs. The Occupational Health and Safety Act of 1970 made a safe environment for the workers a legal obligation of the employer.

The Upjohn Company's standing policy and practice has been to comply with the law and to minimize the environmental impact of drug manufacturing on employees and the surrounding community. For the evaluation of hazards and toxic effects from exposure to drugs and chemicals in the workplace, the company built an industrial toxicology laboratory with the most up-to-date facilities for conducting inhalation toxicology studies.

PLANNING

Before the drawings for the inhalation toxicology laboratory were started, the effects of working with potentially hazardous materials had to be considered [1,2]. First, The Upjohn Company engineering staff, already quite experienced with the unique requirements of designing pharmaceutical laboratories, and the inhalation toxicology personnel had to establish communications. The inhalation toxicologist

Reprinted with permission from Leong, Basil K.J., Ed., and The Upjohn Company in *Inhalation Toxicology and Technology* (Ann Arbor, MI: Ann Arbor Science, 1981), pp. 1–10.

111

explained to the engineers the philosophy of inhalation toxicology and reviewed the techniques for testing gases, liquid aerosols, and dust generation and procedures for performing inhalation experiments. The detailed explanation was in terms that people outside the field readily understood.

The design team visited several inhalation laboratories, discussed their function with the scientists using them, the problems encountered, and the changes the scientists would make. The latest technology and planning were incorporated in the layout drawings. Following careful review and discussion between the inhalation toxicologist and the design team, the design approved for field work was developed.

HAZARD CONTAINMENT

Floor Plan

The inhalation toxicology laboratory suite was built in an isolated corner of a research building. The building's general traffic pattern is outside the suite which has only one entrance, and yet other facilities like the building ventilation system, utility service shafts, animal waste disposal, and cage-washing are convenient. Furthermore, a floor-to-floor dimension of 14.5 feet in this section of the building permits all service conduits or cables to be installed overhead, keeping the floor traffic and work area free of obstacles.

Traffic flows from the clean to the contaminated parts of the suite (Figure 6-1). The clean areas include rooms for animal quarantine before experiments begin, office space, the rooms housing analytical equipment for exposure chambers and the corridor that connects the suite with the rest of the building. The dirty areas include the exposure chambers, the postexposure animal holding rooms and the corridor connecting the holding rooms with the elevator to the waste disposal and cage-washing areas on the floor below.

The animal exposure facilities follow the one-room one-experiment and the double-corridor concepts [3,4]. Animals from each exposure chamber can be isolated in separate holding rooms after each daily treatment. The temperature and humidity of each holding room are controlled by zone thermostats and humidistats.

LABORATORY VENTILATION

One air-conditioning unit serves the inhalation toxicology laboratory. Air drawn from the outside of the research building is filtered and regulated to 74° ±2° dry bulb and rehumidified to 50% ±5% relative humidity before being distributed to other sections of the laboratory. All animal holding rooms are provided with 20 air changes per hour. A pressure gradient is created so that all air flows from clean to dirty areas in a one-pass system (Figure 6-2). Within the laboratory suite in the rooms designed for handling and preparing chemicals, conditioned air flows through the perforated

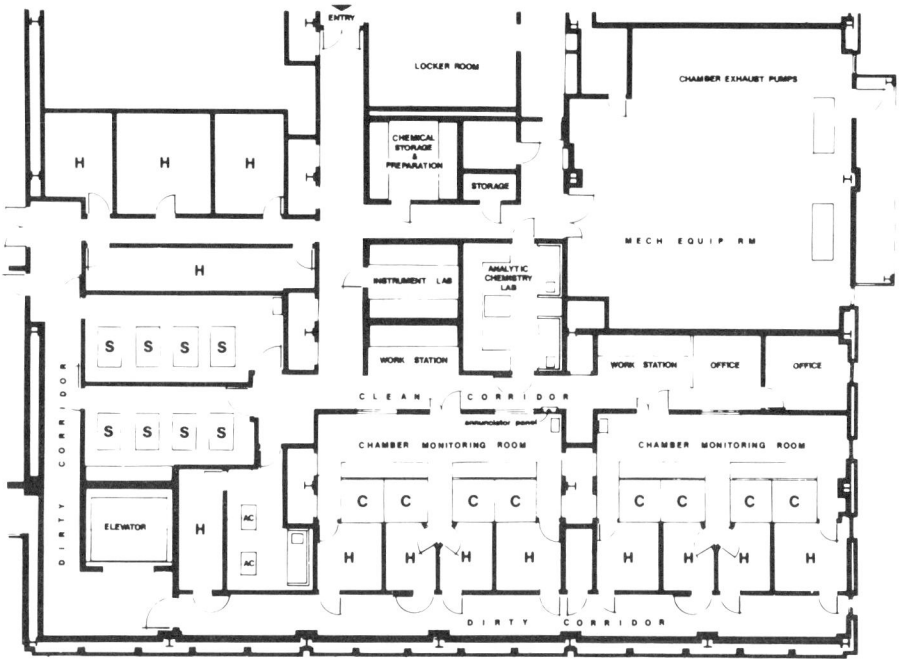

Figure 6-1.   Floor plan of the Upjohn Company inhalation laboratory.

ceiling toward the laboratory benches. All the air entering from the ceiling is exhausted through hoods equipped with two-stage filtration systems consisting of bag-out filter housings. The first-stage filter is 90–95% efficient according to the ASHRAE (American Society of Heating, Refrigerating, and Air Conditioning Engineers) test, and the second-stage filter is 95% efficient according to the DOP (dioctyl phthalate test).

All exhaust hoods also have airflow-sensitive alarm systems which are activated when the linear velocity of airflow across the face of the hood drops below a specified ft/sec value [5]. Exhaust hoses which we fondly call "elephant trunks" are provided for local removal of waste gases generated by analytical instruments such as gas chromatographs and chemical storage cabinets.

The air exhausted from the laboratory suite is discharged into the central exhaust system. Then it passes through the heat exchanger for energy recovery before being released outside.

EXPOSURE CHAMBER VENTILATION

Air from the laboratory air-conditioning system is drawn through branching ducts into individual chambers. At each branch, an additional heating and cooling system

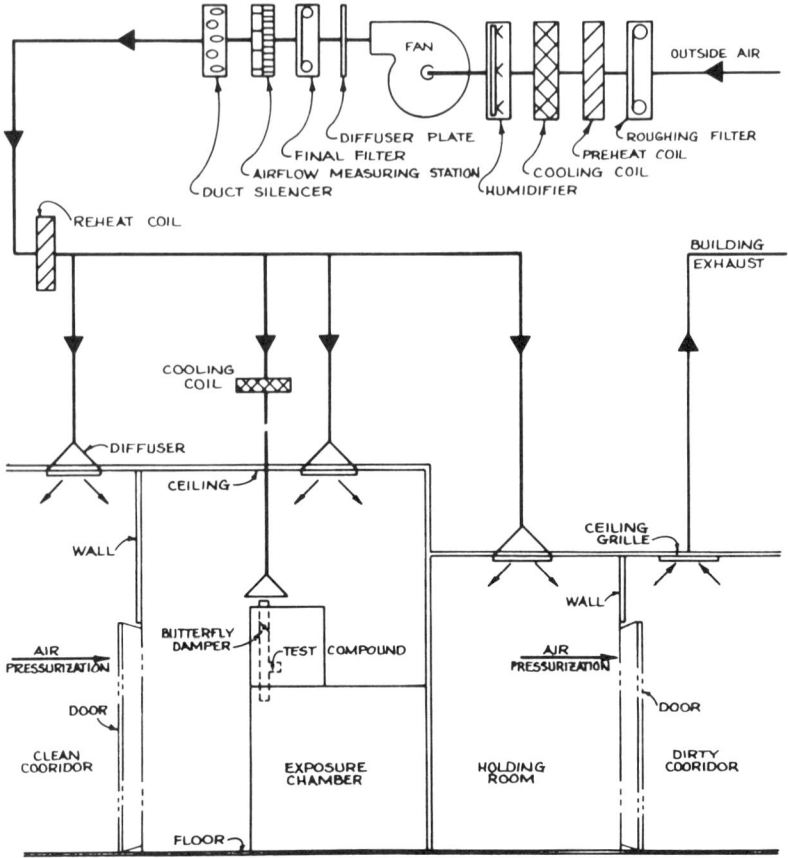

Figure 6-2. Schematic diagram showing the direction of airflow within the inhalation toxicology laboratory.

permits further adjustment of temperature and humidity to meet the needs of individual experiments (Figure 6-3). The design temperature points are 55° F dry bulb temperature for the supply air, 54° F wet bulb for the cooling coil and 75° F for the reheating coils. Temperature in the chamber is monitored by a high and low thermostat connected to an automatic pneumatic controller with manual override.

If the temperature varies from the range selected for a particular experiment, a signal is sent to the microprocessor which triggers an alarm in the work and office areas. The light flashing on a panel indicates the chamber which caused the alarm. While the alarm can be silenced by pushing the silence button, the pilot light will continue to flash until the problem has been corrected. During the silence, failure of another chamber will sound the alarm as before.

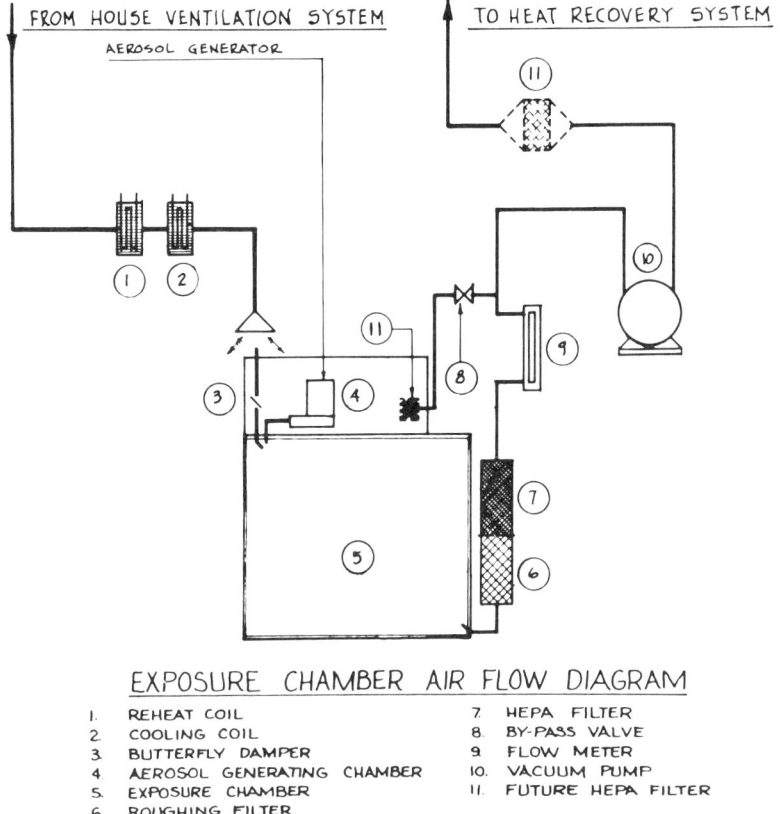

Figure 6-3. Schematic diagram showing the air supply and exhaust for an exposure chamber.

CHAMBER PRESSURE CONTROL

All chambers operate under dynamic air flow at a negative pressure of 0.1 to 0.2 inches of water. This is accomplished by restricting the air supply entering the chamber by throttling the butterfly damper in the chamber air inlet. The total chamber airflow equals the sum of the volume of air ejected from an aerosol or dust generator and the volume of air drawn into the chamber to make a specified concentration of test compound. Airflow is read on the flow meter and adjusted to the proper rate (cubic feet per minute) by throttling the manual bypass valve. Two differential pressure switches (DPS) within the chamber monitor the pressure. The first DPS is wired to the microprocessor alarm system. If, for any reason, the chamber is not properly sealed and the negative pressure is not within the proper limits, the first

DPS will sound a local alarm within 30 seconds, depending on the specified program (Figure 6–4). If a pump fails, a back-up pump can be switched on manually to restore airflow and the slightly negative pressure in the chamber.

CHAMBER EXHAUST PUMPS

Rotary sliding-vane pumps [6] with the capacity to create various vacuums exhaust the animal exposure chamber atmosphere. This type of exhaust pump has a stable volumetric efficiency over a wide range of vacuum pressure and, therefore, reliably maintains a constant airflow in each chamber. The pump is also durable for continuous operation for a long period of time. One pump is used for each chamber so that the chamber airflow can be individually regulated.

EXPERIMENTAL ATMOSPHERE GENERATION

A compartment at the top of the chamber houses all vapor or aerosol-generating equipment. The compound to be tested is added to the air stream entering the air inlet at an upper corner of the specially designed chamber [7]. This compartment also operates under a slightly negative pressure relative to the ambient pressure to ensure total containment of the test compound. A DPS connected to the exposure chamber controls the power supply to the generating equipment. All generating equipment operates only when the chamber atmosphere reaches a specified negative pressure. Thus, the hazard from accidental dispersion of airborne toxicants can be eliminated.

CONTAMINANT AND WASTE CONTROL

For ease of decontamination, the wall and ceiling finishes in the animal and chamber rooms are coated with epoxy paint. The floors are made of inlaid epoxy. All doors, frames, case work and exhaust hoods are enameled steel. Thus, all the finishes used are based on durability, ease of maintenance and impermeability.

The airborne toxicant in the experimental atmosphere is exhausted through a filtering system which consists of successive filters of fiberglass, foam, high efficiency particles and activated charcoal. The filtered waste air is then discharged into the central exhaust system previously described. The entire filtering system can be disassembled easily, and the various filters can be pushed into a bag and disposed of by incineration without contaminating personnel.

The nonairborne wastes such as deposited particles, excreta and fur of animals in the exposure chambers or the animal holding rooms can be hosed into drains leading to the company sewage disposal system. If necessary, the drainage can be diverted to a holding tank in which a hazardous compound can be neutralized, inactivated or retained until being pumped into suitable containers for further treatment.

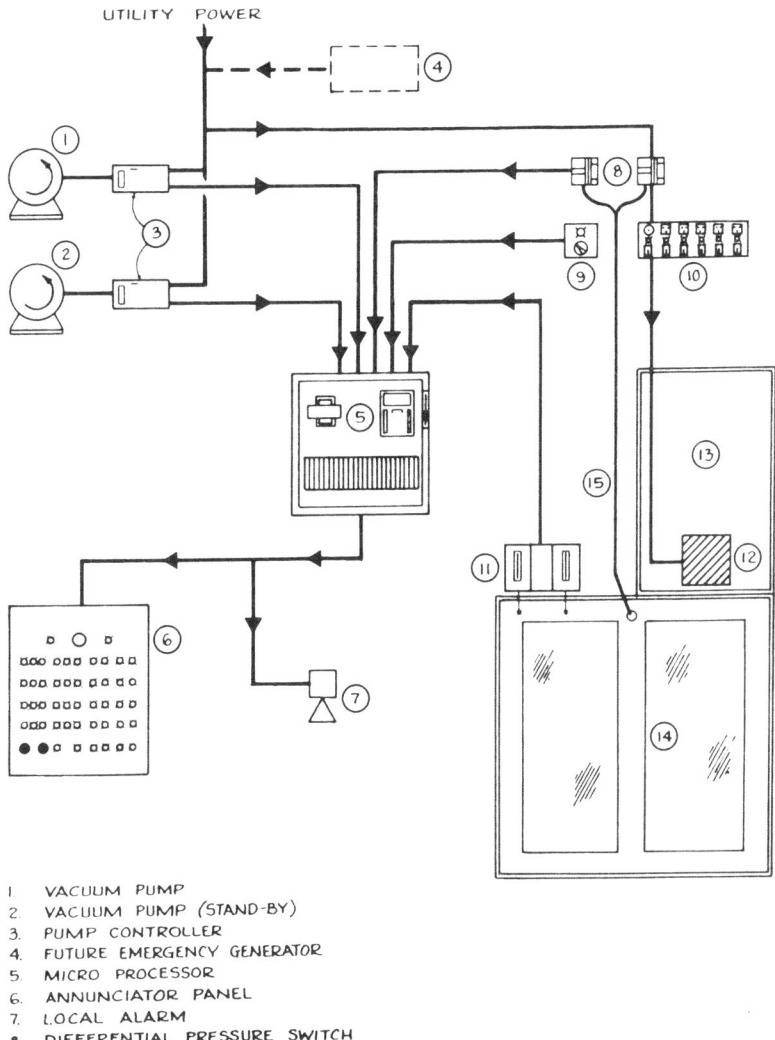

1. VACUUM PUMP
2. VACUUM PUMP (STAND-BY)
3. PUMP CONTROLLER
4. FUTURE EMERGENCY GENERATOR
5. MICRO PROCESSOR
6. ANNUNCIATOR PANEL
7. LOCAL ALARM
8. DIFFERENTIAL PRESSURE SWITCH
9. REMOTE START/STOP VACUUM PUMP SWITCH
10. EQUIPMENT OUTLETS FOR AEROSOL GENERATING CHAMBER
11. HIGH - LOW THERMOSTAT
12. AEROSOL GENERATOR
13. AEROSOL GENERATING CHAMBER
14. EXPOSURE CHAMBER
15. PRESSURE SENSOR PROBE

Figure 6-4. Schematic diagram of chamber temperature and pressure monitoring alarm system.

SAFETY

In general, the safe operation procedures follow the guidelines for chemical laboratories [1,2,8,9]. Standard safety equipment such as fire extinguishers, eye washers and emergency showers are provided at strategic locations in the laboratory. In addition, all emergency showers are connected to pneumatic horns which sound when the shower is turned on. Furthermore, all the inhalation exposure rooms and the corridors are provided with breathing air supply lines and hood attachments to be used routinely during animal transfer and chamber cleaning or during emergencies.

SUMMARY

The Upjohn Company has built and is operating an inhalation toxicology laboratory which has incorporated the most up-to-date technology of floor plan, exposure chamber designs, animal and chemical wastes control for safe operation and personnel protection.

ACKNOWLEDGMENT

We gratefully acknowledge the contribution of J.O. Haeger, S.N. Moerman, and R.C. Patel, members of the Engineering Design Team; J.R. Cushman, the Field Engineer; and the editorial assistance of S.K. Moyer of the Scientific Publications unit of the The Upjohn Company.

REFERENCES

1. Steere, N.V., Ed. CRC *Handbook of Laboratory Safety,* (Cleveland, OH: Chemical Rubber Company, 1971).
2. Sansone, E.B. (Particulate and vapor contamination in experiments with carcinogens), in *Generation of Aerosols and Facilities for Exposure Experiments,* K. Willeke, Ed. (Ann Arbor, MI: Ann Arbor Science, 1980), pp. 541–551.
3. Leong, B.K.J. "The current state of chamber design and inhalation toxicology instrumentation," in *Proceedings of the 7th Annual Conference on Environmental Toxicology,* pp. 141–149. (AMRL-TR-76-125 National Technical Information Service, 5285 Port Royal Road, Springfield, VA, 1977), pp. 141–149.
4. Sansone, E.B. and A.M. Losikoff, "Potential contamination from feeding test chemicals in carcinogen bioassay research: Evaluation of single- and double-corridor animal housing facilities," *Toxicol. Appl. Pharmacol.* 50:115–121, 1979.
5. Witheridge, W.N. *Ventilation in Industrial Hygiene and Toxicology,* Vol. 1., F.A. Patty, Ed. (Interscience Publishers, New York, 1967), pp. 307–310.
6. Furtado, V.C. "Air movers and samplers," in *Air Sampling Instruments for Evaluation of Atmospheric Contaminant,* 5th Ed. (American Conference of Governmental Industrial Hygienists, Akron, 1978), p. K5.

7. Leong, B.K.J., D.J. Powell, G.L. Pochyla, and M.G. Lummis, "An active dispersion inhalation exposure chamber," in *Inhalation Toxicology and Technology*, Basil K.J. Leong, ed. (Ann Arbor, MI: Ann Arbor Science, 1981), pp. 65–76.

8. Manufacturing Chemists Association. *Guide for Safety in the Chemical Laboratory* (New York: Van Nostrand Reinhold, 1972).

9. McKusick, B.C. "Prudent practices for handling hazardous chemicals in laboratories." *Science* 211:777–780, 1981.

CHAPTER 7

Human Factors Considerations in the Handling of Toxic Chemicals

Eileen J. Phelan
Westinghouse Electric Corp.,
Baltimore, Maryland 21203

Carla M. Snyder
Arthur D. Little, Inc., Acorn Park,
Cambridge, Massachusetts 02138

Douglas B. Walters
National Toxicology Program, National Institute
of Environmental Health Sciences, P.O. Box 12233,
Research Triangle Park, North Carolina
27709

INTRODUCTION

Human factors engineering, or ergonomics (from the Greek for "laws of work"), is an approach to design that permits the individual to perform operations, services, and supportive tasks with a minimum of stress and a maximum of efficiency. This goal is accomplished through an integrated approach to design that considers the user as a part of the operating system. Although humans are the most adaptable feature in most systems, it is important to design within human capabilities and limitations, thus avoiding compromising the objectives of safety, productivity, and comfort. By meeting these goals, the individual's adaptability will permit him to respond in an emergency situation, perform his task(s) accurately, maintain experimental integrity, and eliminate unnecessary biomechanical stresses. In short, the individual will respond to his operating enviroment more effectively. Figure 7-1 summarizes these human factors design objectives and the particular laboratory issues they address.

The discussion that follows has been structured around the following issues:

1.   Some of the key human variables that contribute to the handling of toxic chemicals in the laboratory

121

2.   A description of some of the types of facilities where toxic chemicals are used
3.   A characterization of chemical containment
4.   Design recommendations for laboratory operating environments, based on these topics

For discussion purposes, the major human variables are sometimes classified as follows:

- Physical parameters
- Psychophysical tasks
- Psychological issues

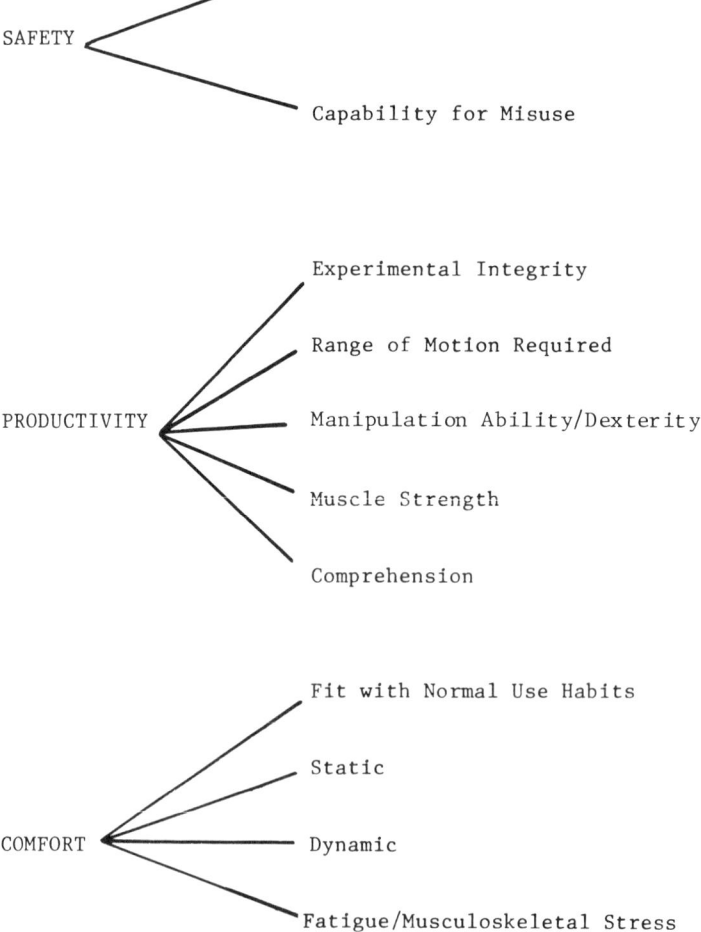

Figure 7-1.   Human factors design objectives in the laboratory.

However, the current treatise is limited to: the physical parameters of anthropometry, biomechanics and certain environmental conditions, and psychophysical tasks containing nonseparable elements of cognitive and motor skills.

PHYSICAL PARAMETERS

Anthropometry

Anthropometry, the science of measuring the human body, includes a variety of static and dynamic anatomic and strength measurements. (The discussion of human strength is deferred to the section on biomechanics.) Anthropometric data have been collected for both men and women of various races, sizes, and physical abilities. These data are given in terms of percentiles, each representing that percentage of the population which is as small or smaller. Specifically, percentile 1 is the smallest possible physical dimension and percentile 100 is the largest. Figure 7–2 typifies the range and detail of the data collected for standing adult males[1]. The data are presented for percentiles 2.5 to 97.5 because designers will usually design for 95% of the population. (It should be noted that the first and last few percentiles represent rare individuals.) If women are to be included in the workforce, then the range from 2.5 percentile female to 97.5 percentile male will then include 95% of the total population, as illustrated in Figure 7–3.

One might ask, "Why not simply design for the *average* user?" The reasons are twofold. First, consider locating a visual barrier such that it can be used by the average chemist or technician. Since the average is the 50th percentile, 50 percent of the population would find the barrier unusable or inconvenient, possibly to the point of danger. Secondly, there is no such thing as an "average" person. Although the average for each measurement is the 50th percentile, the probability of any individual having every measurement in this single percentile is so low as to be virtually nonexistent. For example, someone with 50th percentile height may have no other dimension at that percentile. This fact was illustrated in a study performed by Hertzberg[2] where more than 4,000 men were measured to establish if they were average. After ten measurements were completed, all the study subjects were eliminated.

The above discussion is applicable to the creation of a normal work area. The reach envelope shown in Figure 7–4 represents the windshield wiper pattern developed by Squires in 1956 and studied further by Konz[3]. As these diagrams suggest, the inner and outer boundaries to the work area can be set by combining the envelopes for the 5th percentile female and the 95th percentile male to accommodate the widest range of users.

In the laboratory, anthropometric characteristics can determine whether equipment will be within reach, whether workers will bump elbows with adjacent colleagues, or even whether objects can be seen from their visual angle. Equipment intended for use with one hand may be too large for the 5th percentile female to hold in a stable position or too small for the 95th percentile male to grasp in a usable orientation.

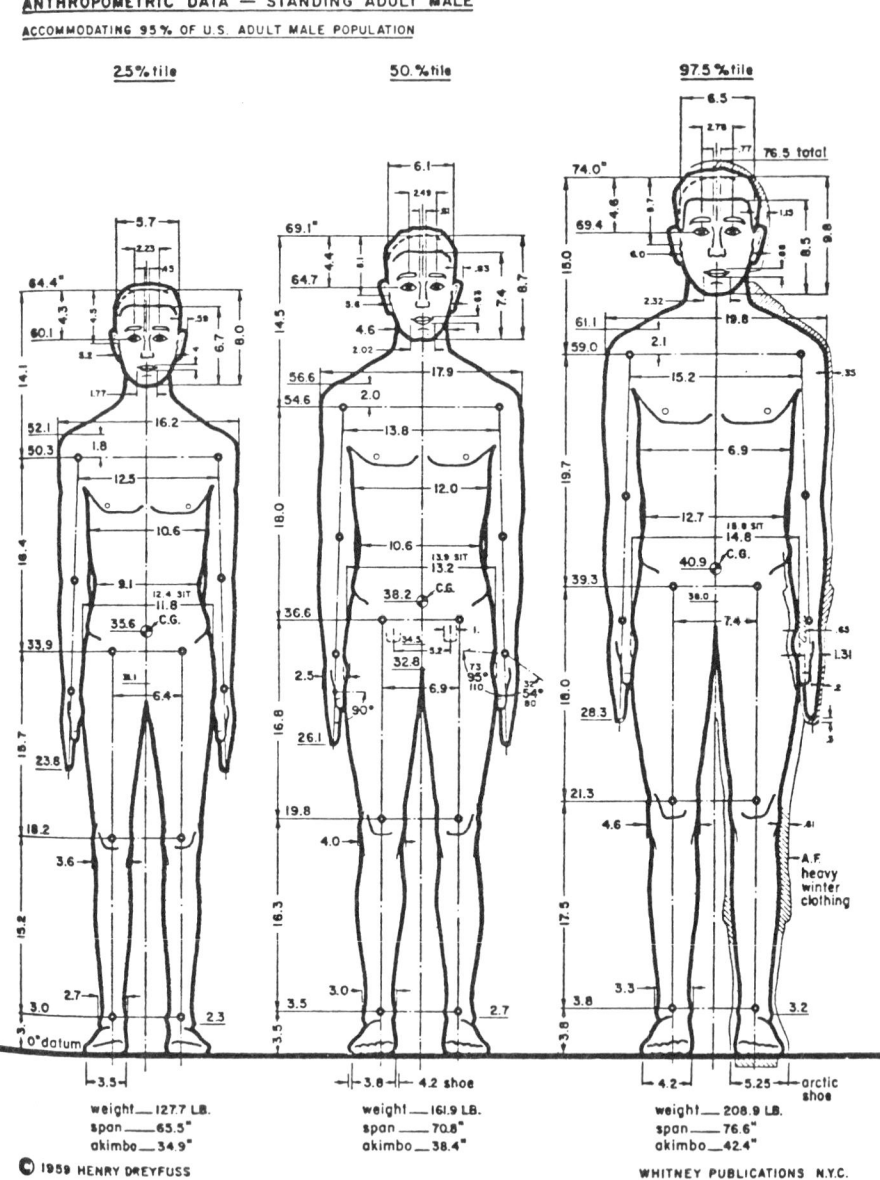

Figure 7-2.   Size differences in the adult male.

Finally, it should be noted that laboratory design and layout should be performed to accommodate "most" of the user population. Identifying the population which will be excluded depends on the associated consequences (i.e., productivity gains or losses, additional costs). Therefore, the challenge is in defining "most of the user population."

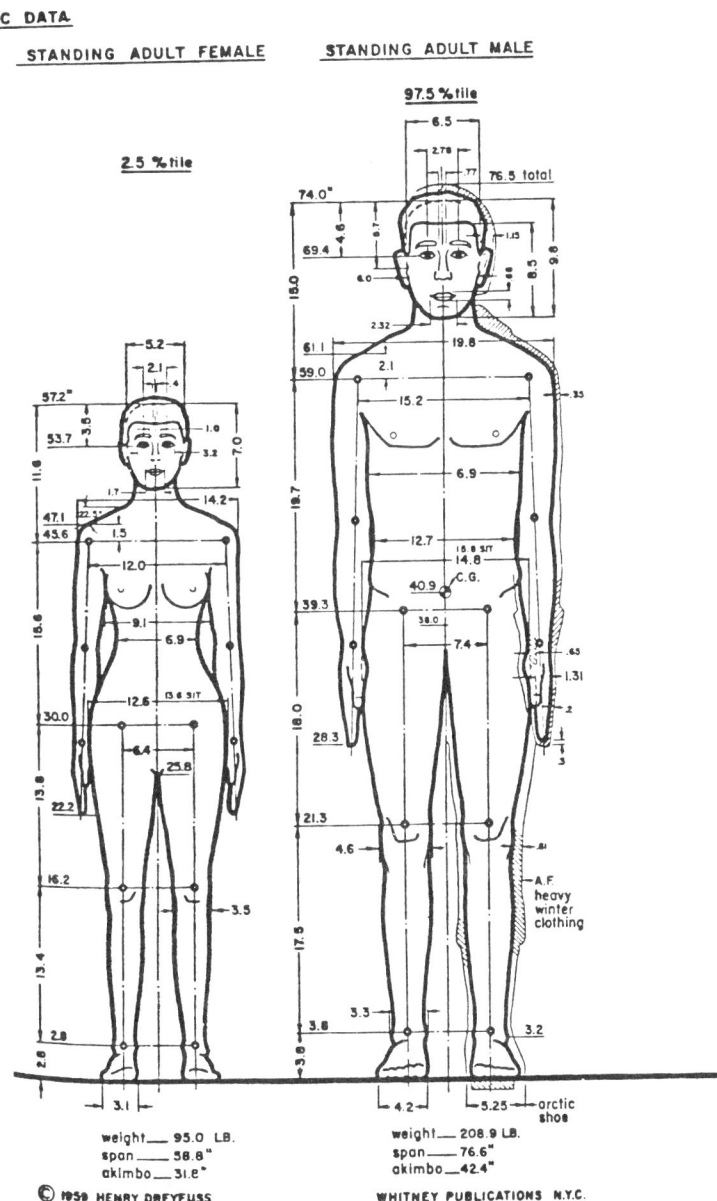

Figure 7-3. Size ranges for males and females.

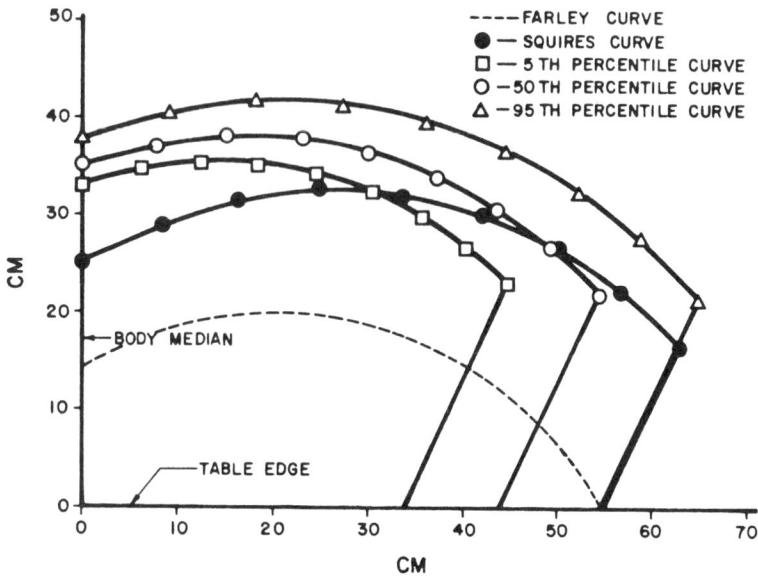

Normal male work area (Konz and Goel, 1969) differs from recommendations by Farley and Squires in that Farley did not consider movement of the elbow and Squires did not adjust for human variability.

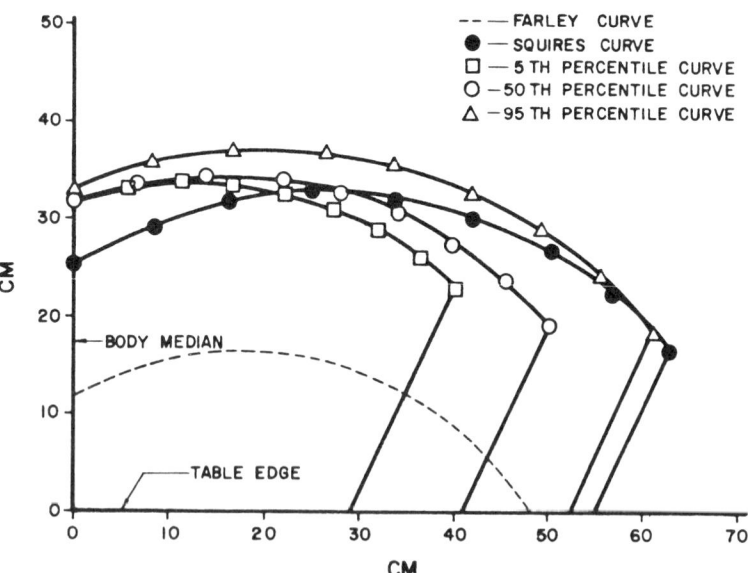

Normal female work area (Konz and Goel, 1969) is slightly smaller than for males.

Figure 7-4. Normal work areas for men and women. Reprinted with permission from *Work Design* by Stephen A. Konz, Grid, Inc., Columbus, Ohio, 1969, p. 29.

Biomechanics

Biomechanics considers the human body as a mechanical system, composed of levers and forces. The anthropometric strength measurements are arranged in percentiles, as previously described. Some estimates exist for the time interval over which a given percentile of maximum strength can be used; past this point the human becomes too fatigued to perform the task efficiently, safely, or at all. As in classical physics, biomechanics is divided into static and dynamic systems. Approximate loads are relatively easy to calculate, even though they are based on physiological as well as mechanical factors.

The motionless human body, due to its mass and configuration, has a static load. One such illustration is an extended arm. An arm held in an unsupported extended position can maintain motor control for only a short time, due to the force of its own weight and gravity acting on it. Another illustration often found in the laboratory is bending of the trunk from a standing position. Figure 7–5 illustrates the load due to the weight of the upper body. This static load greatly increases oxygen consumption and is very fatiguing [4]. It can be seen that the load is concentrated on only one or a few vertebra, providing an obvious explanation of localized back pain, especially in tall workers.

Environmental Factors

Appropriate lighting in a work area greatly contributes to the health and safety of the workers. Poor visibility, due to the small size of the details or low level of contrast or illumination, causes the rate of eye assimilation to decrease and the related task to be more time-consuming. Additionally, if lighting in the normal field of vision is exces-

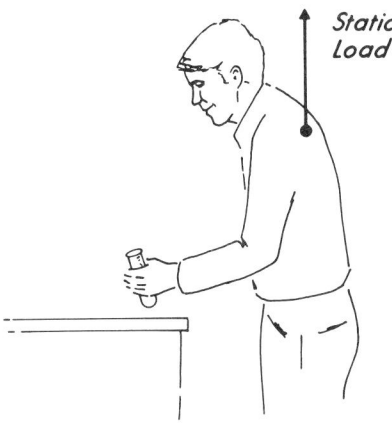

Figure 7–5.   Sample static load.

sive, an individual can experience discomfort due to the stress created in the eye muscle responsible for the relative size of the pupil. Some of the factors affecting the optimal level of lighting are:

- The number and visual acuity of the people using a particular area
- The tasks performed in the area
- The relative contrast of the items being illuminated
- Size of the task area
- Viewing angle of the user
- Quality of illumination (absence of glare, color of light)
- Amount of available daylight

Finally, in using lights as signals, they must be detectable and conform to population stereotypes without cluttering the visual fields.

Noise resembles lighting in that for many tasks there is an optimal range above or below which performance degrades. Although noise is generally thought of as an annoyance or a hazard, a low level can be of value in either masking unpleasant sounds or aiding a vigilance task. As with lights, noises are often used as signals. Care should be taken that signals are audible and distinguishable, without producing "sensory overload."

PSYCHOPHYSICAL PARAMETERS

Population Stereotypes

Population stereotypes are those compatibility relationships in such general use that "everyone knows" them. Some examples are:

- Hot is on the left.
- Green means go ahead.
- Turning a knob clockwise increases whatever the knob controls.

In designing for human use, it is necessary to know which stereotypes apply. Some relationships are intrinsic to a situation, or obvious in terms of spatial images, whereas others are cultural (and care must be taken to ensure that the user population is from the appropriate culture). McCormick [5] notes: "When the most compatible relationships are not obvious, it is necessary to identify them on the basis of empirical experiments."

Cognizance of these compatibility relationships increases the efficiency of task performance, and strongly impacts safety. For example, if one were to place the hot water faucet on the right, there is a reasonably high probability that someone would be burned. The same kind of mistake is easily made for other types of equipment, causing injury, and more insidiously, causing incorrect experimental results.

Negative Transfer

Frequently, a response is learned which is at least partially intrinsic, as contrasted with the preceding discussion. Transfer occurs when a person who has learned to use a piece of equipment applies this knowledge to similar pieces of equipment. Transfer positive when the tasks are truly similar and negative when one or more elements of the new task are reversed. Negative transfer is often encountered when using ordinary kitchen stove burners, due to the diversity and creativity of control knob arrangements. The rate at which a new skill is learned is frequently affected by negative transfer. Fitts and Posner[6] state: "It is not the learning of an opposite response per se which leads to negative transfer, but it is the necessity of making an opposite response to the same or similar stimulus cues."

In addition, those who have apparently successfully learned the new skill and can perform without error may still revert to the original pattern when under stress, such as that encountered in an emergency situation. This fact has implications in standardization of laboratory equipment and procedures, at least for critical controls or elements.

Coding

The purpose of coding is to provide identification. With controls, coding can be provided using shape, color, size, labeling, and location, taking advantage of population stereotypes and previous operator training[7]. Shape and size coding provides tactile identification. However, if the operator must wear gloves, the effectiveness of this type of coding can be significantly reduced. Labeling should be brief, visible, obvious, and located in a consistent relative position to controls. Where color coding is used, the effect of population stereotypes is more obvious (e.g., emergency stop buttons should be red). Since location coding is strongly dependent on previous training, the effects of negative transfer should be carefully considered.

When possible, coding redundancy should be used, thus identifying a control by more than one method. For example, label, location, and color can all be used for the same control. Color coding should not be used as the only identification method, since its reliability clearly depends on whether workers are screened for color blindness.

Although most of the literature on coding is concerned with controls, coding can be used to identify areas, equipment, and personal protection articles.

FACILITY CHARACTERISTICS

There are three types of facilities where toxic chemicals are used, which, for discussion purposes, can be categorized as follows: in vivo, in vitro, and basic chemistry facilities, each with its own hazards due to the nature of the experimental work.

Animal studies are conducted at in vivo facilities. Typically in NTP studies, only one group of animals is housed in a particular area, and all studies are conducted in a barrier facility, with separation of clean and dirty areas. Air pressure differences are used to ensure that air flow goes from clean to dirty corridors through each area. Additionally, there are 10 to 15 air changes per hour, with temperature controlled at 72–76° F and humidity maintained at 40–60%.

Chemicals are sometimes mixed in a special dose preparation lab within this area; if they are mixed elsewhere they can contaminate other areas. Although hoods and glove boxes are used, often chemicals must be mixed with animal feed—a particularly hazardous activity. Workers are required to change clothes in a shower area upon entering and shower-out after potential exposure to a toxic agent.

The second type of facility uses bacteria, fruit flies, and cell cultures for "in vitro" toxicity testing. The facility, noticeably smaller than the "in vivo" type, typically does not use barriers; hoods and glove boxes are typically used for control purposes.

In a basic chemistry facility workers rarely wear personal protection suits. Separate corridors are not used, but often air pressure differences control flow. Special glove boxes, hoods, ventilation, and basic climate control are important features in this type of facility.

CONTAINMENT CHARACTERIZATION

System Concepts

Any potentially hazardous system can be characterized as containing three elements: source, path, and receiver. A hazard emanates from the source, is conducted along the path, and affects the receiver.

Containment of the hazard at its source is the best method of protection. This approach is not always possible since detailed knowledge of the nature of the hazard and the physical handling operation is required in order to determine all the characteristics which must be contained. Blockage of the path provides the next line of defense. Again, it is necessary to know the chemical characteristics and means of use so that all possible paths are considered. Finally, the receiver can be protected. This technique is the least desirable, since it restricts the functionality of the receiver, and these restrictions can themselves decrease safety.

Source Containment

Containment of a hazard at its source is done through engineering controls. For the aforementioned facilities, the engineering controls used are barriers, glove boxes, and hoods, thus physically containing toxic agents. Temperature and humidity controls contain the source at a more basic level by providing conditions under which diffusion of a chemical is less likely to occur.

Path Blockage

Blocking the path of a hazard is generally done through work practices. Any action which prevents a toxic agent from actually reaching the receiver falls in this category. The usual methods are handling practices and showering to wash away chemicals before they can reach the skin. Separate geographic locations for chemicals not totally contained also provide path blockage. For intrinsically hazardous activities, such as cage washing, mixing of chemicals with feed or with other chemicals, obtaining small amounts of a chemical from a large storage vat, or cleaning up spills, path blockage requires careful planning.

Receiver Protection

Receiver protection, or personal protection, is the last line of defense. If a toxic agent surmounts this final barrier, it will have hazardous effects. If personal protection is required for a task, the obvious inference is that the first two barriers cannot be relied upon. Therefore, workers are understandably reluctant to perform tasks requiring these devices.

The usual types of personal protection are a jump suit and booties made of synthetic material with very low permeability. In addition, gloves, respirator, and safety glasses are worn. These devices impose restriction on the wearer by inhibiting vision, movement, touch sensitivity, or other functions.

DESIGN FOR THE HUMAN

Basic Considerations

All design is toward a goal. If a safe environment is to be provided, then safety must be the primary goal, thus giving the adage "safety first" a new and important meaning. Safe practices must be made more convenient than unsafe ones. Therefore, operating practices should follow population stereotypes, take previous training into consideration, and use coding when possible. If the range of workers is not to be restricted, designs must consider 95% of the total population.

For laboratory tasks, hazards should be stopped at the earliest line of defense possible. Therefore, one must determine which lines of defense are possible and the human engineering needed to maintain them.

Physical Separation

Initially, a determination must be made as to which hazards can be physically contained. For these cases, the usual engineering controls of barriers, air pressure differences, ventilation, and climate control can be supplemented with human engineering barriers. If a piece of equipment or an undiluted supply of a chemical is not to be removed from an area, it should be made biomechanically immovable by 95% of the laboratory population. Those items which are not to be touched by humans should be placed out of reach.

Where feasible, automation or robotics should be considered for tasks which are hazardous to humans. If tasks are automated, care should be taken to provide maximum information and emergency training to the observer, including visibility, audio input, and monitoring devices with warning signals.

Work Practices

When toxic agents must be handled by humans, training assumes paramount importance. Standard methods and procedures must be developed that consider both the person and the task in worst-case situations.

For personnel, education and experience vary. Using the worst-case baseline, the least education and experience for any worker hired determines the extent of training. Skill-level certification ensures compliance with training requirements.

Since laboratory methods are usually task- and chemical-specific, they should be written and available for reference. When the method varies with the chemical for a given task, the chemicals can be classed and containers for each class color coded. The written reference method for each chemical class is then coded with the same color.

Once a method has been written, it should be analyzed for strength requirements. The static workload should be examined. Comparison with population stereotypes and previous training should be made, to detect potentially unsafe differences. The method should then be physically demonstrated using nontoxic agents to determine any hazards still existing. The method or the physical equipment can then be adjusted to eliminate the hazard. For example, a worker will not breathe effluent which is lighter than air if the effluent is ejected at a point higher than his nose.

Emergency procedures also require training. As noted earlier, previous training often takes precedence under emergency conditions. Simulated emergencies can be used to fixate a learned response. When emergency procedures vary with type of emergency, alarms should have distinctly different sounds or visual signals. The broadcasting of voice instructions in emergency situations may prevent confusion.

Supervision must be adequate to maintain compliance with methods and procedures. If a method is not being followed, either the method should be changed or the alternate unsafe method made impossible by arrangement of other physical characteristics.

Protective Clothing

If a worker must wear protective clothing, the hazard, the person, and the task are each considered. Clothing can be divided by type of protection afforded rather than by amount of standard clothing worn. For example, for cage washing, it may be more reasonable to provide a special cooled suit which completely encloses the worker rather than to add a full-face respirator to a standard jump suit.

Provision for anthropometric and physical characteristics should be made. Presence of facial hair, wearing of eyeglasses, and physical sex differences all change mobility and sensory input. The clothing changes the temperature and humidity to the worker, possibly increasing or decreasing his susceptibility to a hazard and affecting his productivity.

Design Procedures

If a new facility is to be designed, the first step is a thorough analysis of hazards, tasks, and required human characteristics. Classification into areas allows simultaneous and modular development of each area. Tasks can be simulated, as can hazards. The entire plan can thus be addressed for human engineering before construction begins.

When the facility already exists, the same procedure can be followed to upgrade safety characteristics. When upgrading is to be only partial, analysis of the entire affected facility should be performed. Since data exists for accidents, critical incidents, and "near misses" in existing facilities, various areas can be identified for improvement.

Many hazards are correctable through human engineering. If equipment is designed for the human user, if new methods are written so that tasks can be performed in a safe manner, and if training is personalized and thorough, a gradual adaptation of the task to humans can be accomplished.

REFERENCES

1. Dreyfuss, H. *Measure of man,* (New York: Whitney Library of Design, 1955).
2. Hertzberg, H.T. *Some contributions of applied physical anthropology in human engineering,* (USAF, WADD, TR 60–19, January 1960).
3. Konz, S. *Work design.* (Columbia, OH: Grid Publishing Inc., 1979).
4. Grandjean, E. *Fitting the task to the man,* 3rd ed. (Taylor & Francis Ltd., 1980).
5. McCormick, E.J. *Human factors in engineering and design,* 4th ed. (New York: McGraw-Hill, 1976).
6. Fitts, M.P. and M.I. Posner, *Human performance.* (Brooks/Cole, May 1969).
7. Chapanis, A., and R.G. Kinkade. "Design of controls," in *Human engineering guide to equipment design* (rev). H.P. Van Cott and R.G. Kinkade, Ed. (Washington, D.C.: Government Printing Office, 1972).

PART II

Establishment of a Safety Program

CHAPTER 8

Preparation of Chemical-Specific Health and Safety Documents

Andrew T. Prokopetz and Douglas B. Walters
National Toxicology Program, National Institute of Environmental Health Sciences, P.O. Box 12233, Research Triangle Park, North Carolina 27709

William S. Baillargeon
Hazardous Materials Group, Radian Corporation, 8501 Mo-Pac Boulevard, P.O. Box 9948, Austin, Texas 78766-0948

Elizabeth M. Prescott and R. Scott Stricoff
Arthur D. Little, Inc., Acorn Park, Cambridge, Massachusetts 02140

INTRODUCTION

The National Toxicology Program (NTP) performs the majority of its toxicological testing by contract due to limited on-site laboratory capabilities. As a result, the NTP must provide health and safety information on chemicals tested in this fashion to help safeguard all personnel who come in contact with these materials. Documents such as the National Institute for Occupational Safety and Health (NIOSH) Health Hazard Alerts [1], Current Intelligence Bulletins [2], NIOSH Criteria Documents [3,4], NIOSH/OSHA (Occupational Safety and Health Administration) Occupational Health Guidelines [5], the National Institutes of Health (NIH) Safety Data Sheets [6], the Royal Society of Chemistry's Laboratory Hazards Data Sheets [7], and General Electric's Material Safety Data Sheets [8] provide information for industrial chemicals. This chapter deals with the information requirements and preparation of workable health and safety documents for chemicals which are used largely for research.

Guidelines and criteria for the preparation of health and safety documents are limited in the literature [9,10,11]; however, it is generally recognized that chemical health and safety information should be presented in a precise and concise manner, using a format with key-worded headings to indicate categories of concern. Such a formatted document should be easily readable in emergency situations where specific information needs to be quickly discerned. The information must be easily understood by personnel from all disciplines who may be using the document (e.g., toxicology, pathology, animal care, occupational medicine, chemistry, engineering, and health and safety).

In the NTP, formatted chemical health and safety documents are varied according to two major testing requirements. *In vivo* (live animal) studies usually test large quantities of chemicals whose identity is known to the investigator. *In vitro* (microbial or tissue culture) studies use smaller quantities with testing often performed "blind" (i.e., the chemical identity is unknown). The time period for which a health and safety document is needed is also dependent upon the type of test. NTP studies vary in duration from short-term (one-month) studies (i.e., typically *in vitro*) to extended long-term bioassays (*in vivo*) where a chemical may be tested for a five-year period. Therefore, the documents must provide information on storage and stability to help ensure the integrity of a chemical for the duration of a testing protocol. These testing constraints on the content of the health and safety documents are illustrated in a workable formatting scheme in the next section.

Approximately 50% of the chemicals tested by the NTP's carcinogenesis testing program in the last three years have been found to be carcinogenic in at least one test species. Hence, it is felt that there is a high toxicological risk associated with the chemicals selected for NTP test. This toxicological risk, coupled with the dangerous properties often present in the test chemicals (e.g., flammability or explosivity), is of major concern. One purpose of health and safety documents is to help describe handling, storage, use, and emergency response.

CONTENTS OF A HEALTH AND SAFETY DOCUMENT

There are two basic formats for health and safety documents employed by the NTP in toxicity studies. The first type is a Chemical-Specific Health and Safety Guideline (CSG) which was developed for use in studies with known test chemicals. The second format requires a combination of two documents, a Safety and Handling Document (SHD) and an Emergency Procedures Document (EPD), which are used in testing "blind" compounds. The contents of each format are described below.

Chemical-Specific Health and Safety Guideline

The general requirements listed above for Chemical-Specific Health and Safety Guidelines for known chemicals necessitate that information relevant to the four categories of concern listed in Table 8-1 be searched for in the literature and key worded into the document. These four categories should be arranged as in Table 8-1 according to their importance in an emergency situation. This ordering allows first for a brief summary highlighting important areas of concern and then for proper identification of the chemical. Next are cautionary information based upon known toxicological properties of the chemical and emergency procedures. This information should be in a prominent and accessible location in the document. This should be followed by the physical-chemical properties which can be used for structure-activity correlations in emergency situations and for better understanding of the handling of the chemical in day-to-day operations. Finally, the list of the references used in the preparation of the document should be included, along with copies of the important articles. These four categories can be broken down into 13 sections which make up the key words highlighted in the document and which are used in the search scheme for its preparation. These sections are listed in Table 8–2, and the purpose of each is explained below.

A summary on the first page of the document allows the reader a quick overview of the hazards associated with the particular chemical and the protection equipment needed. Use of key words and phrases, such as highly flammable, reacts violently with water, explosive, are important in this section. The summary leads the reader to the sections of importance which follow in the document.

Identification numbers and synonyms allow positive verification of the compound of concern. NIOSH's Registry of Toxic Effects of Chemical Substances (RTECS) number permits the reader quick access to this valuable listing. The Wiswesser Line Notation (WLN) number allows cross-checking with other compounds of similar structure and permits elementary structure-activity analogies. The Chemical Abstract Service (CAS) number, as well as other identification numbers, firmly identifies one specific chemical, but often may be misleading. A slight variation in hydration or optical activity of a chemical may lead to a different CAS number, even though the same basic chemical-physical properties pertain. This is one of the reasons for double identification with both test name (or synonym) and CAS number. A CAS number matchup may not be obtained, but a synonym may match the test chemical. Redundancy is important in this section to minimize problems such as transposition of digits in individual identity numbers.

The section on health hazard information first lists the allowable limits of exposure, including (where data are available) both OSHA's permissible exposure limit (PEL) and American Conference of Governmental Industrial Hygienists (ACGIH's) Threshold Limit Value (TLV) and indicates the routes of exposure applicable for this chemical. It is important to list all relevant requirements (i.e., OSHA standards for general industry [12]), recommendations (i.e., TLV's adopted by the

Table 8–1. Chemical-Specific Health and Safety Guideline (CSG): Major Categories

---

I. Summary and identification of chemical
II. Health hazard information and emergency procedures
III. Chemical-physical properties
IV. References

Table 8-2. Chemical-Specific Health and Safety Guideline (CSG): Key Words

I. Summary of major concerns
II. Identification numbers and synonyms
   A. Numbers
      1. Chemical Abstract Service (CAS) number
      2. Registry of Toxic Effects of Chemical Substances (RTECS) number
      3. Wiswesser Line Notation (WLN) number
   B. Synonyms
III. Health hazard information
   A. Permissible exposure limit (PEL)/threshold limit valve   (TLV)/time-weighted average (TWA)
   B. Route of exposure
   C. Effects of overexposure
      1. Acute hazard
      2. Chronic hazard
IV. Emergency first aid procedures
   A. Eye
   B. Skin
   C. Inhalation
   D. Ingestion
V. Protective equipment and monitoring procedures
   A. Eye
   B. Gloves
   C. Clothing
   D. Ventilation
   E. Analytical method for monitoring workroom air
   F. Respiratory
VI. Spill, leak, and disposal procedures
   A. Stability
   B. Waste disposal recommendations
VII. Chemical hazards
   A. Stability
   B. Incompatibility
   C. Handling and storage
   D. Special precautions
VIII. Fire hazards
   A. Flash point
   B. Autoignition temperature
   C. Explosive limits in air
   D. Extinguishant
   E. Special precautions
IX. Physical properties
   A. Molecular formula
   B. Molecular weight
   C. Molecular structure
   D. Appearance/odor
   E. Physical state
   F. Melting point
   G. Boiling point

H. Specific gravity (water = 1)
I. Vapor density (air = 1)
J. Vapor pressure (@ 20° C or 68° F)
K. Solubility
    1. Water
    2. Organic solvents
    3. Acids and bases
    4. Vegetable oils/miscellaneous solvents
X. Toxicity data
  A. Route of exposure
  B. Species
  C. Dose/result
XI. Additional toxicity/metabolism data
XII. References
XIII. Copies of pertinent articles in reference list

ACGIH [13], limits recommended by NIOSH [1,2,3,4], or guidelines (state, local, internal policy) for the various routes of exposure to this chemical. The section on the effects of overexposure details the acute and chronic hazards as well as important notes for the medical response team (e.g., CNS depression, irritant to mucous membranes, central stimulant).

The emergency first aid procedures are written to assist personnel in the proper care of exposed individuals. These statements range from routine procedures such as washing exposed areas with soap and water to more specific recommendations such as whether or not to induce vomiting for ingested exposure. This last recommendation may not be readily apparent to the emergency response teams due to their lack of information concerning the physical-chemical and toxicological properties of most research chemicals. Generally, vomiting is not recommended if: (1) the chemical is corrosive (i.e., either highly acidic or alkaline), (2) toxicity is greater via inhalation than ingestion and the victim may inhale the vomited material, or (3) convulsions may occur [14].

It is important that protective equipment recommendations be chemical specific. In the absence of literature information, recommendations are based on the physical-chemical and toxicological properties of the test chemical as well as the experimental protocol. Next, consideration is given to various methods of containment and protection. (The first and most important protection that should be afforded the worker is through engineering controls. Personal protection should always serve as a backup.) Finally the quantities handled also determine the protective equipment needed. If the quantity tested is small (milligram to gram range) and can be safely handled in a properly functioning hood, the respirator requirement may be unnecessary, but if the quantity is larger and must be handled outside a hood, more stringent respirator requirements are necessary, and an analytical method of monitoring workroom air is recommended. Based on these analytical results and previous considerations listed above, the protective equipment needed for varying ranges of chemical contamination of the air is listed, similar to the NIOSH Health Hazard Alert Bulletins [1].

Similarly, monitoring is also valuable in determining the effectiveness of clean-up procedures after occurrence of a spill. The spill and leak procedures are worded toward avoidance of dry sweeping for cleanup to reduce formation of aerosols. If a solvent is used for cleanup, consideration must be given to the chemical and toxicological properties of the chemical and the solvent (e.g., solubility, volatility, flammability, incompatibility, and toxicity). Waste disposal recommendations are also based on the physical-chemical properties as well as on local, state, and federal regulations for this particular chemical. Generally speaking incineration is the method of choice [15] (see Chapter 19).

The chemical hazards specified in the next section assist in the proper handling, storage, and use. For example, it may be necessary to store a chemical for five years or longer during a chronic bioassay. Thus, assurance of chemical integrity and minimization of dangerous situations developing from decomposition products is achieved.

Fire hazard data include information on the chemical's flashpoint or its combustibility, the autoignition temperature, the explosive limits in air (both upper and lower limits), degradation products, the preferred extinguishant, and any other special fire precautions. This information is crucial in emergency situations and may assist in the development of experimental protocols (e.g., for inhalation studies where the dose levels may border on the explosive limits).

The physical property information given in the safety and health document can assist in compound identification (e.g., appearance, odor, and physical state), provide more in-depth storage and handling data (e.g., melting and boiling points, vapor pressure, and density), and permit some flexibility in spill cleanup (e.g., solubility in various solvents). These data may also assist in structure-activity correlations when further information is lacking. Changes in some of the more obvious physical properties, such as physical state or appearance, may provide an initial clue that decomposition of the test chemical is occurring.

The toxicity and additional toxicity/metabolism data can assist medical staff, trained in occupational medicine and toxicology, in treating exposed individuals. It also serves to alert contract personnel to the severity of the acute and chronic hazards and again may assist in the development of experimental protocols (e.g., in establishing exposure levels).

The key information in the preceding sections should be footnoted with the references, which are then listed in the last part of the document. Important references should be included for further in-depth review.

Safety and Handling and Emergency Procedures Documents

The information included in the health and safety documents for known test chemicals is rearranged when testing unknown compounds. In the NTP, this is accomplished by supplying two documents with each test chemical. The first, a Safety and Handling Document (SHD), explains the hazards associated with the particular chemical and the personal protection needed, while not disclosing its identity. The second, an Emergency Procedures Document (EPD), is a sealed document to be opened only in the event of an emergency. Breaking the seal decodes the chemical's identity and details the procedures recommended for an emergency situation. The basic components of both the SHD and the EPD are listed in Tables 8-3 and 8-4. The information included in each of these components is basically the same as that in the Chemical-Specific Health and Safety Guideline, and the previous discussion of the contents of this document pertains for the SHD and EPD as well. A complete discussion can be found elsewhere[9,10,11].

Table 8-3. Elements of a Safety and Handling Document (SHD)

   I. Aliquot number
  II. Personal protection equipment
     A. Dependent on type of lab and test protocol
 III. Acute hazards
 IV. Spills and leakage
  V. Storage precautions
 VI. Chemical and physical properties
     A. Physical description
     B. Melting point
     C. Boiling point
     D. Solubility
        1. Water
        2. Dimethyl sulfoxide
        3. Ethanol and other organic solvents
     E. Flammability
     F. Stability
     G. Toxicity

Table 8-4. Elements of an Emergency Procedures Document (EPD)

   I. Aliquot number
  II. Primary name
 III. Identification numbers and synonyms
     A. Numbers
        1. CAS number
        2. RTECS number
        3. WLN number
     B. Synonyms
 IV. Acute hazards
  V. Symptoms
 VI. First aid
     A. Skin contact
     B. Inhalation
     C. Eye contact
     D. Ingestion
 VII. Spills and leakage

PREPARATION OF HEALTH AND SAFETY DOCUMENTS

Once the type of document and the data needed for its preparation have been identified, the next critical step is the formation of a proper literature search scheme. Figure 8–1 illustrates a versatile flow diagram with numerous cross-checks utilizing most of the available pertinent literature. This cross-checking prevents obtaining misinformation from compounds with similar names or structures. Redundancy at this point is better than accidents in the laboratory arising from omissions or errors in the safety document.

This search scheme first checks in-house literature, as listed in Appendix A, which can and should be extensive and continually updated. Appendix A is the current list of comprehensive chemical data reference sources, routinely searched when compounds are selected for NTP testing. Some references, such as the *Colour Index* or the *Food Chemicals Codex,* are useful for certain classes of compounds (e.g., dyes or food products, respectively); while other references, such as the *Merck Index* or Sax's *Dangerous Properties of Industrial Materials,* may be referred to for thousands of chemicals. The in-house literature search should set the groundwork for more extensive data base searching. Appendix B tabulates data bases that are accessible to the National Toxicology Program through such vendors as Lockheed, Systems Development Corporation, the National Library of Medicine, and other similar sources. Several of these vendors are adding two new data bases per month, many of which are pertinent to the preparation of a health and safety document. Thus updating is crucial.

Upon completion of the literature review and compilation of the information, there may still be some missing data. For example, solubility, vapor pressure, and other physical-chemical properties may be needed and can be experimentally determined at the NTP chemical respository or analytical resources laboratories, if necessary.

Once the above information is accumulated, the data is reviewed by a panel of experts. This is the final step in the preparation, and one of the most critical in the process. Numerous gaps may occur that need to be filled by input from a chemist, industrial hygienist, toxicologist, or an individual with a medical background. Supplementation of missing information is prepared using structure-activity relationships in which known data from closely analogous compounds are analyzed and extrapolated or interpolated to areas where this information is missing. Numerous problems can occur if this process is not critically evaluated. For example, a disposal method in the literature for benzidine-based dyes called for a reduction step that could have transformed a potential carcinogen into a known carcinogen—benzidine. Common sense is of the essence.

CONCLUSION

Health and safety documents should be geared toward the needs of the personnel who will use them. These documents should be adaptable to the changing needs of the

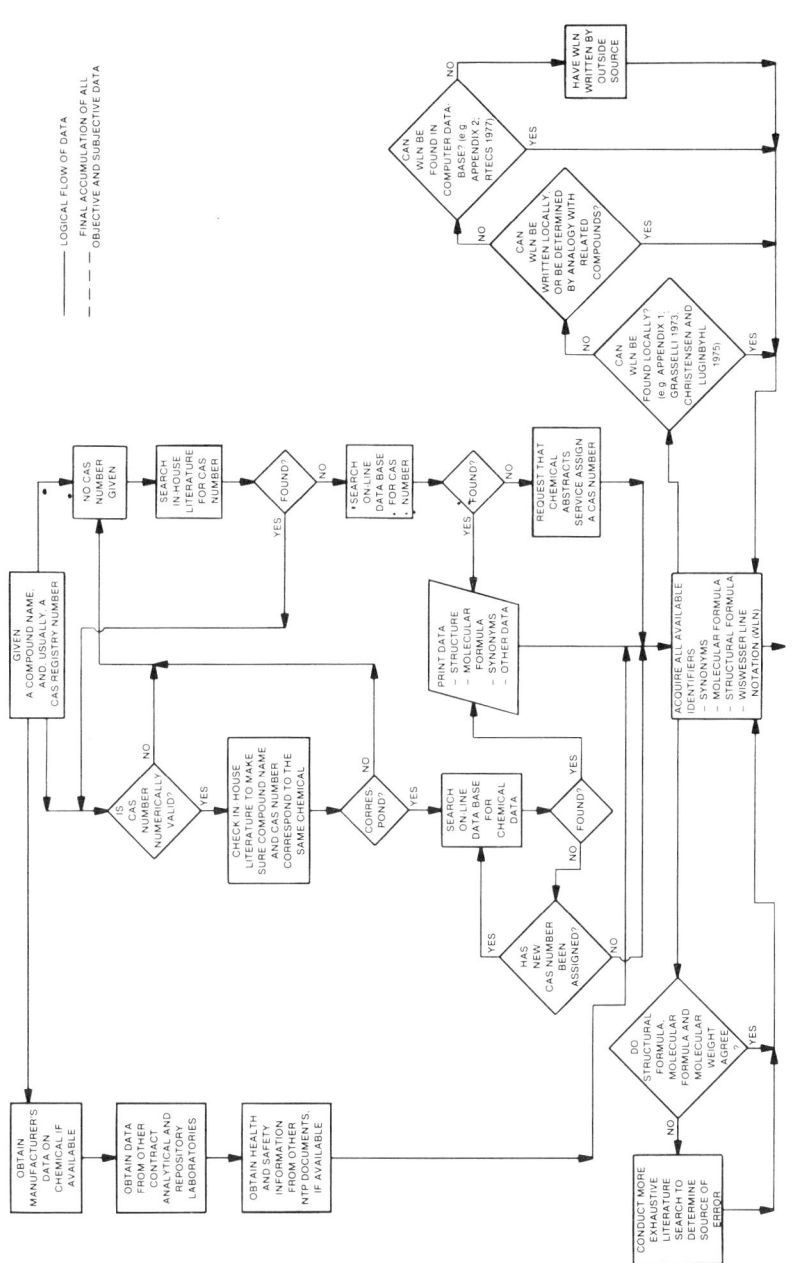

Figure 8-1. Flow chart of literature search scheme for hazardous materials research and evaluation.

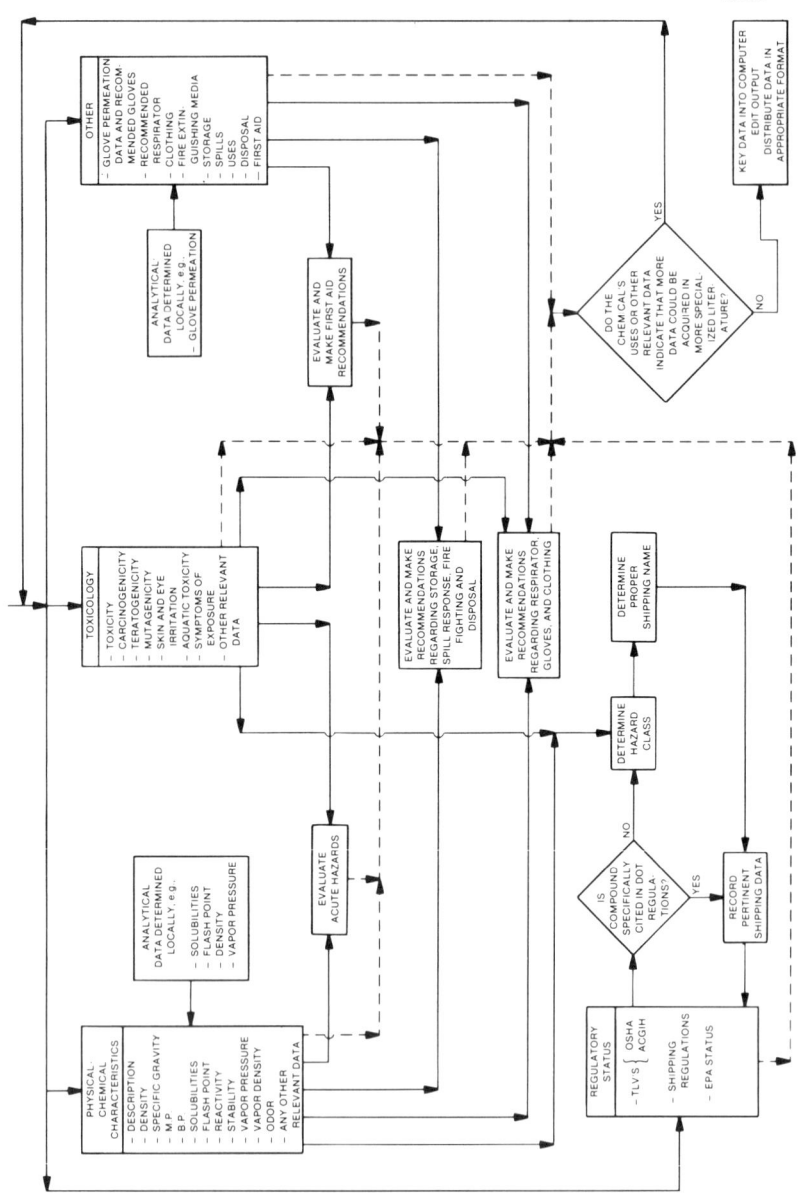

Figure 8-1. *(continued).*

laboratory staff; conveniently packaged to allow storage directly in the laboratory for quick access; and as informative and concise as possible.

REFERENCES

1. "Health Hazard Alert," DHHS (NIOSH) Publication.
2. "Current Intelligence Bulletin," DHHS (NIOSH) Publication.
3. "NIOSH Criteria Document," DHHS (NIOSH) Publication.
4. Bahlman, L.J. "NIOSH Current Intelligence System: An Occupational Safety and Health 'Hazard Alerting System'," *Am. Indust. Hyg. Assoc. J.* 41 (1): A30–A37, 1980.
5. Mackison, F., R.S. Stricoff, and L.J. Partridge, Eds. *NIOSH/OSHA Occupational Health Guidelines for Chemical Hazards*, DHHS (NIOSH) Publication No. 81–123 (1981).
6. "Safety Data Sheets," Division of Safety, National Institutes of Health (1982).
7. "Laboratory Hazards Data Sheet." Royal Society of Chemistry (University of Nottingham, England).
8. Nielsen, J.M., Ed. *Material Safety Data Sheets* (General Electric Co., 1980).
9. Meiners, Alford F. "Preparation of Carcinogen Monographs," in *Safe Handling of Chemical Carcinogens, Mutagens, Teratogens and Highly Toxic Substances, Vol. 1,* D.B. Walters, Ed. (Ann Arbor, MI: Ann Arbor Science, 1980), pp. 291–311.
10. Walters, D.B., L.H. Keith, and J.M. Harless. "Chemical Selection and Handling Aspects of the National Toxicology Program," in *Environmental Health Chemistry,* J.D. McKinney, Ed. (Ann Arbor, MI: Ann Arbor Science, 1981), pp. 580–585.
11. Keith, L.H., J.M. Harless, and D.B. Walters. "Analysis and Storage of Hazardous Environmental Chemicals for Toxicological Testing," in *Environmental Health Chemistry,* J.D. McKinney, Ed. (Ann Arbor, MI: Ann Arbor Science, 1981), pp. 608–613.
12. *Code of Federal Regulations,* Title 29, Part 1910, Subpart Z, "Occupational Health and Environmental Control."
13. "TLVs, Threshold Limit Values for Chemical Substances and Physical Agents in the Work Environment with Intended Change for 1982," ACGIH Report ISBN: 0–936712–39–2, 1982.
14. Dreisbach, R.H. *Handbook of Poisoning* (Los Altos, CA: Lange Medical Publications, 1980), p. 19.
15. Wilkinson, T.K. and H.W. Rogers. "Disposal of Chemical Carcinogens, Mutagens and Teratogens from Research Facilities," in *Safe Handling of Chemical Carcinogens, Mutagens, Teratogens and Highly Toxic Substances, Vol. 2,* D.B. Walters, Ed. (Ann Arbor, MI: Ann Arbor Science, 1980), pp. 575–593.

APPENDIX A

Comprehensive Chemical Data Source List

Advisory Committee on Pesticides. Further Review of the Safety for Use in the U.K. of the Herbicide 2,4,5-T. Advisory Committee on Pesticides. 1980.

Airline Tariff Publishing Co. Official Air Transport Restricted Articles Tariff No. 6-D Governing the Transportation of Restricted Articles by Air. Airline Tariff Publishing Co. Washington, DC. 19 April 1980 Revision.

Aldrich Chemical Company. Aldrich Catalog/ Handbook of Fine Chemicals. Aldrich Chemical Co., Inc. Milwaukee, WI. 1982.

Alliance of American Insurers. Handbook of Organic Industrial Solvents. 5th Ed. Alliance of American Insurers. Chicago. 1980.

American Conference of Governmental Industrial Hygienists. Documentation of the Threshold Limit Values. 4th ed. American Conference of Governmental Industrial Hygienists. Cincinnati, OH. 1980.

American Conference of Governmental Industrial Hygienists. Threshold Limit Values for Chemical Substances and Physical Agents in the Work Environment with Intended Changes for 1982. American Conference of Governmental Industrial Hygienists. Cincinnati, OH. 1982.

Block, J.B. The Signs and Symptoms of Chemical Exposure. Charles H. Thomas. Springfield, IL. 1980.

Buckingham, J., Ed. Dictionary of Organic Compounds. 5th ed. Chapman and Hall. New York. 1982.

Bureau of Explosives, Association of American Railroads. Hazardous Materials Regulations of the Department of Transportation by Air, Rail, Highway, Water and Military Explosives by Water, Including Specifications for Shipping Containers. Bureau of Explosives Tariff No. BOE–6000–A. Bureau of Explosives. Washington, DC. 1981.

Christensen, H.E. and T.T. Luginbyhl, Eds. Registry of Toxic Effects of Chemical Substances. National Institute for Occupational Safety and Health. Rockville, MD. 1975.

Clayton, G.D. and F.E. Clayton, Eds. Patty's Industrial Hygiene and Toxicology. Vol. 2. Third Revised Edition. John Wiley and Sons. New York. 1981.

Commission of the European Communities. Constructing EINECS: Basic Documents. Official Journal of the European Communities. Office for Official Publications of the European Communities. Luxembourg. 1981.

Commission of the European Communities. Constructing EINECS: Basic Documents, Compendium of Known Substances. Vols. 1–3. Office for Official Publications of the European Communities. Luxembourg. 1981.

Commission of the European Communities. Constructing EINECS: Basic Documents, European Core Inventory. Vols. 1–4. Office for Official Publications of the European Communities. Luxembourg. 1981.

Cone, M.V., M.F. Baldauf, F.M. Martin and J.T. Ensminger, Eds. Chemicals Identified in Human Biological Media, A Data Base, First Annual Report, Vol. I, Parts 1 and 2, Records 1–1580. Interagency Collaborative Group on Environmental Carcinogenesis, National Cancer Institute, National Institutes of Health Bethesda, MD. 1980.

Cone, M.V., M.F. Baldauf, F.M. Martin and J.T. Ensminger, Eds. Chemicals Identified in Human Biological Media, A Data Base, Second Annual Report, Vol. II, Parts 1 and 2, Records 1581–3500. Interagency Collaborative Group on Environmental Carcinogenesis, National Cancer Institute, National Institutes of Health. Bethesda, MD. 1981.

Council for Agricultural Science and Technology. The Phenoxy Herbicides. 2nd ed. CAST Report No. 77. Council for Agricultural Science and Technology. Iowa State University, Ames, Iowa. 1978.

Deichmann, W.B. and H.W. Gerarde. Toxicology of Drugs and Chemicals. Academic Press. New York. 1969.

Dreisbach, R.H. Handbook of Poisoning: Prevention, Diagnosis and Treatment. 10th ed. Lange Medical Publications. Los Altos, CA. 1980.

Estrin, F.E., P.A. Crosley and C.R. Haynes, Eds. CFTA Cosmetic Ingredient Dictionary. 3rd ed. The Cosmetic, Toiletry and Fragrance Assn. Inc. Washington. 1982.

Fletcher, J.H., O.C. Dermer and R.B. Fox, Eds. Nomenclature of Organic Compounds, Principles and Practice. American Chemical Society. Washington, DC. 1974.

Furia, T.E. and N. Bellanca. Teneroli's Handbook of Flavor Ingredients. The Chemical Rubber Co. Cleveland, OH. 1971.

Goodman, L.S. and A. Gilman. The Pharmacological Basis of Therapeutics. 5th ed. Macmillan Publishing Co. New York. 1975.

Gosselin, R.E., H.C. Hodge, R.P. Smith and M.N. Gleason. Clinical Toxicology of Commercial Products. 4th ed. Williams and Wilkins Co. Baltimore. 1976.

Grant, W.M. Toxicology of the Eye. 2nd ed. Charles H. Thomas. Springfield, IL. 1974.

Grasselli, J.G., Ed. CRC Atlas of Spectral Data and Physical Constants for Organic Compounds. CRC Press, Inc. Cleveland, OH. 1973.

Haque, R., Ed. Dynamics, Exposure and Hazard Assessment of Toxic Chemicals. Ann Arbor Science Publishers. Ann Arbor, MI. Undated.

Hartwell, J.L. Survey of Compounds Which Have Been Tested for Carcinogenic Activity. 2nd ed. Public Health Service Publication No. 149. National Cancer Institute, National Institutes of Health. Bethesda, MD. 1963.

Hawley, G.G., Ed. The Condensed Chemical Dictionary. 10th ed. Van Nostrand Reinhold. New York. 1981.

Hayes, W.J., Jr. Pesticides Studied in Man. Williams and Wilkins. Baltimore. 1982.

Huff, B.B., Ed. Physicians' Desk Reference. 36th ed. Medical Economics Co. Oradell, NJ. 1982.

International Agency for Research on Cancer, World Health Organization. IARC Monographs on the Evaluation of Carcinogenic Risk of Chemicals to Man. Vols. 2–20. International Agency for Research on Cancer. Geneva. 1973–1979.

International Air Transport Association. Restricted Articles Regulations. 23rd ed. International Air Transport Assn. Geneva. 1980.

International Technical Information Institute. Toxic and Hazardous Industrial Chemicals Safety Manual for Handling and Disposal with Toxicity and Hazard Data. International Technical Information Institute. 1978.

Lewis, R.J., Sr. and R.L. Tatken, Eds. Registry of Toxic Effects of Chemical Substances. DHEW (NIOSH) Publication No. 81–116. National Institute for Occupational Safety and Health. Cincinnati, OH. 1980.

Lewis, R.J., Sr. and R.L. Tatken, Eds. Registry of Toxic Effects of Chemical Substances. Microfiche Ed. National Institute for Occupational Safety and Health. Cincinnati, OH. Quarterly Updates.

Lyman, W.J., W.F. Reehl and D.H. Rosenblatt. Handbook of Chemical Property Estimation Methods, Environmental Behavior of Organic Compounds. McGraw-Hill. New York. 1982.

Mackison, F.W., R.S. Stricoff and L.J. Partridge, Eds. Occupational Health Guidelines for Chemical Hazards. DHHS (NIOSH) Publication No. 81-123. National Institute for Occupational Safety and Health. Cincinnati, OH. 1981.

Manufacturing Chemists Association. Guide for Safety in the Chemical Laboratory. 2nd ed. Van Nostrand Reinhold. New York. 1982.

Meidl, J.H. Explosive and Toxic Hazardous Materials. Glencoe Publishing Co. Encino, CA. 1970.

Meyer, E. Chemistry of Hazardous Materials. Prentice-Hall. Englewood Cliffs, NJ. 1977.

National Cancer Institute, National Institutes of Health, Public Health Service, U.S. Department of Health, Education and Welfare. Survey of Compounds Which Have Been Tested for Carcinogenic Activity. 1961-1967 Vol. Sections I and II. DHEW (NIH) Publication No. 73-35. Public Health Service Publication No. 149. National Cancer Institute. Bethesda, MD. 1973.

National Cancer Institute, National Institutes of Health, Public Health Service, U.S. Department of Health, Education and Welfare. Survey of Compounds Which Have Been Tested for Carcinogenic Activity. 1968-1969 Vol. DHEW (NIH) Publication No. 72-35, Public Health Service Publication No. 149. National Cancer Institute. Bethesda, MD. 1972.

National Cancer Institute, National Institutes of Health, Public Health Service, U.S. Department of Health, Education and Welfare. Survey of Compounds Which Have Been Tested for Carcinogenic Activity. 1970-1971 Vol. DHEW (NIH) Publication No. 73-453, Public Health Service Publication No. 149. National Cancer Institute. Bethesda, MD. 1973.

National Cancer Institute, National Institutes of Health, Public Health Service, U.S. Department of Health, Education and Welfare. Survey of Compounds Which Have Been Tested for Carcinogenic Activity. 1978 Vol. DHEW (NIH) Publication No. 80-453 (Formerly Public Health Service Publication No. 149). National Cancer Institute. Bethesda, MD. 1980.

National Fire Protection Association. Hazardous Chemicals Data. National Fire Protection Association. Boston. 1975.

National Fire Protection Association. Fire Protection Guide on Hazardous Chemicals. 7th ed. National Fire Protection Association. Boston. 1978.

National Fire Protection Association. Flash Point Index of Trade Name Liquids. 9th ed. National Fire Protection Association. Boston, MA. 1978.

National Institute for Occupational Health and Safety. NIOSH Manual of Sampling Data Sheets, 1977 Ed. DHEW (NIOSH) Publication No. 77-159. National Institute for Occupational Safety and Health. Washington, DC 1977.

National Institute for Occupational Health and Safety. Occupational Safety and Health Administration. Pocket Guide to Chemical Hazards. DHEW (NIOSH) Publication No. 78-210. National Institute for Occupational Safety and Health. Washington, DC 1978.

National Research Council, Committee on Codex Specifications. Food Chemicals Codex. 3rd Ed. National Academy Press. Washington, DC 1981.

National Toxicology Program. Chemical Registry Handbook, Parts I and II. National Toxicology Program. Research Triangle Park, NC. 1981.

Occupational Safety and Health Administration. Tentative OSHA Listing of Confirmed and Suspected Carcinogens by Category. Occupational Safety and Health Administration. Washington, DC. 1979.

Office of the Federal Register, National Archives and Records Service, General Services Administration. Code of Federal Regulations, Title 40, Protection of Environment, Parts 100 to 399 (Revised as of July 1, 1980). Government Printing Office. Washington, DC. 1979.

Packer, K., Ed. Nanogen Index, A Dictionary of Pesticides and Chemical Pollutants. Nanogens International. Freedom, CA. 1975 (Updated 1979).

Plunkett, E.R. Handbook of Industrial Toxicology. Chemical Publishing Co. New York, NY. 1976.

Proctor, N.H. and J.P. Hughes. Chemical Hazards of the Workplace. J.B. Lippincott. Philadelphia. 1978.

Rappoport, Z.V.I., Ed. CRC Handbook of Organic Compound Identification. 3rd ed. CRC Press, Inc. Cleveland, OH. 1975.

Rigaudy, J. and S.P. Klesney. Nomenclature of Organic Chemistry, Sections A, B, C, D, E, F and H. Pergamon Press. New York. 1979.

Ross, S.S., Ed. Toxic Substances Sourcebook. Series 1. Environmental Information Center, Inc., Toxic Substances Reference Department. New York. 1978.

Sax, N.I., Ed. Industrial Pollution. Van Nostrand Reinhold. New York. 1974.

Sax, N.I. Dangerous Properties of Industrial Materials. 5th ed. Van Nostrand Reinhold. New York. 1979.

Shepard, T.H. Catalog of Teratogenic Agents. 3rd ed. The Johns Hopkins University Press. Baltimore. 1980.

Shubik, P. and J.L. Hartwell. Survey of Compounds Which Have Been Tested for Carcinogenic Activity. Supplement 2. Public Health Service Publication No. 149. National Cancer Institute, National Institutes of Health. Bethesda, MD. 1969.

Sittig, M. Hazardous and Toxic Effects of Industrial Chemicals. Noyes Data Corporation. Park Ridge, NJ. 1979.

Sittig, M., Ed. Priority Toxic Pollutants, Health Impacts and Allowable Limits. Noyes Data Corporation. Park Ridge, NJ. 1980.

Sittig, M. Handbook of Toxic and Hazardous Chemicals. Noyes Publications. Park Ridge, NJ. 1981.

Slein, M.W. and E.B. Sansome. Degradation of Chemical Carcinogens. Van Nostrand Reinhold. New York. 1980.

Society of Dyers and Colourists. Colour Index. Vols. 1–7. The Society of Dyers and Colourists. Yorkshire, England. American Association of Textile Chemists and Colorists. Research Triangle Park, NC. 1971–1982.

Steere, N.V., Ed. Handbook of Laboratory Safety. 2nd ed. CRC Press, Inc. Cleveland, OH. 1971.

Strauss, H.J. Handbook for Chemical Technicians. McGraw-Hill. New York. 1979.

Sunshine, I., Ed. CRC Handbook Series in Analytical Toxicology, Section A: General Data, Vol. 1. CRC Press, Inc. Boca Raton, FL. 1969.

Thienes, C.H. and T.J. Haley. Clinical Toxicology. 5th ed. Lea and Febiger. Philadelphia, PA. 1972.

Thomas, C.L., Ed. Taber's Cyclopedic Medical Dictionary. 14th ed. F.A. Davis Co. Philadelphia. 1981.

Thompson, J.F., Ed. Analytical Reference Standards and Supplemental Data for Pesticides and Other Organic Compounds. EPA Publ. No. 600/9-76-012. U.S. Environmental Protection Agency, Office of Research and Development, Health Effects Research Laboratory. Research Triangle Park, NC. 1976.

Trease, G.E. and W.C. Evans. Pharmacognosy. 11th ed. Balliere Trindall. London, England. 1978.

U.S. Coast Guard, Department of Transportation. Chemical Hazards Response Information System (CHRIS), A Condensed Guide to Chemical Hazards. U.S. Coast Guard Publication No. CG-446-1. U.S. Coast Guard. Washington, DC. 1974.

U.S. Coast Guard, Department of Transportation. Chemical Data Guide for Bulk Shipment by Water. 5th ed. U.S. Coast Guard Publication No. CG 388. U.S. Coast Guard. Washington, D.C. 1976.

U.S. Coast Guard, Department of Transportation. Chemical Hazards Response Information System (CHRIS), Hazardous Chemical Data. U.S. Coast Guard Publication No. CG 446 2. U.S. Coast Guard. Washington, DC. 1978.

U.S. Department of Transportation, Materials Transportation Bureau, Office of Hazardous Materials Operations. An Index to the Hazardous Materials Regulations, Title 49, Code of Federal Regulations, Parts 100-199 (January 3, 1977 Revision). U.S. Department of Transportation. Washington, DC. 1977.

U.S. Environmental Protection Agency, Office of Toxic Substances. Toxic Substances Control Act Chemical Substances Inventory, Initial Inventory. 6 Vols. U.S. Environmental Protection Agency. Washington, DC 1979.

U.S. Environmental Protection Agency, Office of Pesticides and Toxic Substances. TSCA Chemical Assessment Series, Chemical Hazard Information Profiles (CHIPs), August 1976-August 1978. U.S. EPA Publication No. EPA-560/11-80-011. U.S. Environmental Protection Agency. Washington, DC. 1980.

U.S. Environmental Protection Agency, Office of Pesticides and Toxic Substances. TSCA Chemical Assessment Series, Chemical Screening: Initial Evaluations of Substantial Risk Notices, Section 8(e), January 1, 1977-June 30, 1979. U.S. EPA Publication No. EPA-560/11-80-008. U.S. Environmental Protection Agency. Washington, DC. 1980.

U.S. Environmental Protection Agency, Office of Toxic Substances. Toxic Substances Control Act Chemical Substances Inventory, Cumulative Supplement II to the Initial Inventory. U.S. Environmental Protection Agency. Washington, DC. 1982.

Verschueren, K. Handbook of Environmental Data on Organic Compounds. Van Nostrand Reinhold. New York, NY. 1977.

Wade, A. and J.E.F. Reynolds, Eds. Martindale; The Extra Pharmacopoeia. 27th ed. The Pharmaceutical Press. London, England. 1977.

Weast, R.C. and M.A. Astle, Eds. CRC Handbook of Chemistry and Physics. 63rd ed. CRC Press, Inc. Boca Raton, FL. 1982.

Weiss, G., Ed. Hazardous Chemicals Data Book. Noyes Data Corporation. Park Ridge, NJ. 1980.

Williams, L.R., E. Calliga and R. Thomas. Hazardous Materials Spill Monitoring: Safety Handbook and Chemical Hazard Guide, Part A. U.S. EPA Report No. EPA-600/4-79-008a. U.S. Environmental Protection Agency. Washington, DC. 1979.

Williams, L.R., E. Calliga and R. Thomas. Hazardous Materials Spill Monitoring: Safety Handbook and Chemical Hazard Guide, Part B—Chemical Data. U.S. EPA Report No. EPA-600/4-79-008b. U.S. Environmental Protection Agency. Washington, DC. 1979.

Windholz, M., Ed. The Merck Index. 9th ed. Merck and Co. Rahway, NJ. 1976.

Wiswesser, W.J., Ed. Pesticide Index. Entomological Society of America. College Park, MD. 1976.

Worthing, C.R., Ed. The Pesticide Manual, A World Compendium. 6th ed. British Crop Protection Council. London, England. 1979.

APPENDIX B

List of Databases and Databanks Accessible to the NTP

Name of Database/ Databank	Dates	Subject Description
ACS Primary Journal Database (CFTX)	1980– (1976– J. Med. Chem.)	Full-text coverage of American Chemical Society journals.
AGLINE (Previously was DOANE)	1977–	Agricultural practice, production, products, and marketing including agribusiness news, farm chemicals and fuels, livestock production, government policies and programs, and legis/regs.
AVLINE	Current	Nonprint materials in the health sciences.
BIOSIS (Biological Abstracts)	L: 1972– S: 1980–	Comprehensive worldwide coverage of the life sciences.
BIOSIS (earlier files)	L: 1969–1971 S: 1969–1979	Comprehensive worldwide coverage of the life sciences.
CA Search (Chemical Abstracts; CAS)	1967–	Comprehensive worldwide coverage of chemistry and related subjects.
CANCERLIT	1963–	Cancer.
CANCERPROJ	Current	Summaries of ongoing research projects in cancer.
CAS Online	1967–	Provides access to substances sharing desired structural features or meeting specific requirements such as CAS RN, molecular formula, etc.
CASSI (Chemical Abstracts Source Index)	1907– (limited coverage 1830–)	Bibliographic and library holdings information for primary literature relevant to the chemical sciences.
CATLINE	1871–	Catalog of all serials and monographs cataloged by the National Library of Medicine.
CDI (Comprehensive Dissertation Index; Dissertation Abstracts)	1861–	U.S. and some non-U.S. doctoral dissertations.

154

Name of Database/ Databank	Dates	Subject Description
CHEMDEX/ CHEMDEX2	1972	Similar to CHEMNAME, but like CHEMLINE, ring structure is included.
Chemical Regulations and Guidelines System (CRGS)	May 1981–	Guide to U.S. federal government regulatory material relating to the control of chemical substances. Covers aspects of regulations such as tariffs and registration requirements and health and safety regulations.
CHEMLAW	Current	U.S. chemical regulations including full text as published in CFR and *Federal Register*. Includes drug, chemical process, food container, chemical testing, hazardous waste disposal regulations, and other regulations.
CHEMLINE	Current	Chemical dictionary.
CHEMNAME	Current (1967–)	Chemical dictionary of substances cited two or more times in CA Search.
CHEMSDI	Latest 6 wks.	Current awareness file for CA Search.
CHEMSEARCH	Latest 6 wks.	Dictionary listing of the most recently cited chemical substances in CA Search. Companion to CHEMNAME and CHEMSIS.
CHEMSIS	1967–	Chemical substance dictionary for singly indexed substances cited during the 8th, 9th, 10th, and 11th Collective Index periods of CA Search.
CHEMZERO	1965–	Chemical substance records for which there are no citations in CA Search 67+.
CLINPROT	Current	Summaries of clinical investigations of new anticancer agents and treatment.
Conference Papers Index	1973–	Coverage of papers presented at life science, engineering, and physical science meetings.
CRDS (Chemical Reactions Documentation Service)	1944–	Based on *Journal of Synthetic Methods*, provides up-to-date information on new developments in the field of synthetic organic chemistry. Access limited to CRDS subscribers.
CTCP (Clinical and Toxicology of Commercial Products)	Current	*Clinical Toxicology of Commercial Products* on-line.
ENVIROLINE (ESI)	1971–	Environmental sciences.

Name of Database/ Databank	Dates	Subject Description
Environmental Bibliography (EPB; ENVIROBIB)	1974–	Coverage of periodical literature on air and water pollution, ecology, energy, nutrition, health, and land use.
Environmental Mutagens (EMI; EMIC)	1969–	Chemical mutagens. Also subfile of Toxline.
Environmental Tetratology (ETI, ETIC)	1912– (1975– present—most complete)	Testing and evaluation of teratogenic activity of chemical, biological, and physical agents and dietary deficiencies of warm-blooded animals. Also subfile of Toxline.
Excerpta Medica	June 1974–	Human medicine, toxicology, occupational health, environmental health, forensic science, etc.
FRSS (Federal Register Search System	1978–	All citations to chemicals, substances and materials published in the *Federal Register*.
FSTA	1969–	Food sciences and technology.
Hazardline (Occupational Health Services)	1982–	State Laws, Regulations, Safety Data Sheet information.
IPA (International Pharmaceutical Abstracts)	1970–	Pharmacy practice and education.
Life Sciences Collection	1978–	Major areas of biology, medicine, biochemistry, ecology, and microbiology, and some aspects of agriculture and veterinary science.
MEDLINE (MEDLARS-ON-LINE)	1966–	Biomedical journal literature.
MEDOC (Medical Documents)		Government documents in health sciences.
MIDAS (Metals Information Designations and Specifications)	Current	Provides access to designation and specification numbers for ferrous and nonferrous metals and alloys, element concentrations, physical properties, uses, forms, etc.
Non-Ferrous Metals Abstracts	1961–	All aspects of nonferrous metallurgy and technology.
NTIS (National Technical Information Services/ Government Reports Announcements)	1964–	Government-sponsored research, development, and engineering reports and analysis prepared by Federal agencies, their contractors or grantees.

Name of Database/ Databank	Dates	Subject Description
OHM-TADS (Oil and Hazardous Materials–Technical Data System)	Current	Information pertinent to emergency spill response efforts including physical, chemical, biological, toxicological, and commercial data for these materials.
PESTDOC/ PESTDOC-II	1968–	Pesticides, herbicides, and plant protection designed specifically for information requirements of agricultural chemical manufacturers exclusive of fertilizers.
Research in Progress (RIP)	Current	Inventory of energy-related research, development and demonstration projects in the areas of energy, environment, mineral, or fuel resources.
RINGDOC/ RING6475	1964–	Pharmaceutical literature for pharmaceutical manufacturers.
RTECS	1977 with quarterly updates.	*Registry of Toxic Effects of Chemical Substances.*
Safety Science Abstracts	1975–	Safety.
SANSS (Structure and Nomenclature Search System)	Current	Chemical structure and nomenclature data linked with the other CIS databases and more than 66 non-CIS information sources.
SCISEARCH	1965–	Multidisciplinary index to scientific and technical literature.
SUPERINDEX	Current	Back-of-the-book index entries of about 600 of the most-used scientific, technical, and medical reference books.
TDB (Toxicology Data Bank)	Current	Data on WLN, synonyms, toxicity, manufacture, chemical-physical properties, disposal methods, etc., of chemical substances.
TOXLINE/ TOXBACK	1965–	Toxicology, adverse effects of drugs and chemicals, environmental pollution, and industrial health and safety.
TSCA	June 1979–	Contains dictionary listing of chemical substances in the *Initial Inventory* and *Cumulative Supplement II* of the *Toxic Substance Control Act (TSCA) Chemical Substances Inventory* and their non-confidential plant and product information.

Name of Database/ Databank	Dates	Subject Description
TSCA Initial Inventory	June 1979–	Nonbibliographic dictionary listing of chemical substances in the *Initial Inventory* and *1st Supplement* of the *Toxic Substance Control Act (TSCA) Chemical Substances Inventory.*
TSCAPP (TSCA Plant and Production)	Current	Nonconfidential plant and production information for the chemicals on the *Toxic Substances Control Act (TSCA) Inventory.*
WDROP (WaterDROP)	1970–	Identification of organic water pollutants published since 1970.

CHAPTER 9

The Requirements and Pitfalls of Laboratory Worker Medical Surveillance

G. Stewart Young
Arthur D. Little, Inc., Acorn Park,
Cambridge, Massachusetts 02140

INTRODUCTION

Occupational Safety and Health in Carcinogenesis Laboratories

In the last three decades, our awareness of problems associated with the handling of carcinogens in the laboratory has increased. Despite the small quantities of toxic agents used in laboratories, epidemiological studies of chemists and laboratory workers have shown an increased incidence of mortality from various types of cancers in comparison with the general population. Some of these studies have tentatively associated exposures to organic chemicals[1] and aromatic amines[2,3] as causes for the increased mortality and morbidity. In an isolated example, two out of three laboratory workers who were exposed to N-nitrosodimethylamine showed signs of liver damage[4]. Subsequent animal research verified the hepatotoxicity and carcinogenicity of this chemical. A major problem that has been recognized in recent years is the dissemination of potentially carcinogenic material throughout the laboratory even when control technology perceived as state of the art is employed. This first controlled study which indicated the widespread movement of potentially carcinogenic material around a laboratory facility using a spore model was reported by Darlow et al. [5]. Later Sansone et al. [6] used sodium fluorescein as a tracer and produced similar results showing contamination problems. Both researchers concentrated on laboratory procedures resulting in the generation of aerosols, such as weighing and mixing of feed in animal bioassays. Sansone's results showed 2–470 ng of fluorescein in the weighing room when the feed was prepared in an acceptable laboratory hood, and 7 ng of fluorescein on a cotton noseplug of a technician who was using an approved respirator.

Not until the early 1970s were safety regulations and formal guidelines applied to carcinogen laboratories. Earlier good laboratory practices for carcinogen handling were adopted from the techniques used to protect the integrity of experimental material in microbiological studies [7–9]. In addition, formal guidelines from the American National Standards Institute (ANSI Z33. 1–1961) for exhausted ventilation systems and from the American Conference of Governmental Industrial Hygienists (*Threshold Limit Values for Chemical Substances and Physical Agents in the Workroom Environment*, and *Industrial Ventilation Manual)* were also available for reference and use.

Currently, the Occupational Safety and Health Administration (OSHA) has compound-specific regulations for a small group of carcinogens including asbestos, coal tar pitch volatiles, 4-nitrobiphenyl, alpha-naphthalamine, methyl chloromethyl ether, 3,3′-dichlorobenzidine (and its salts), *bis*-chloromethyl ether, beta-naphthylamine, benzidine, 4-aminodiphenyl, beta-propiolactone, 2-acetylaminofluorene, 4-dimethylaminoazobenzene, ethyleneimine, N-nitrosodimethylamine, vinyl chloride, inorganic arsenic, benzene, coke oven emissions, 1,2-dibromo-3-chloropropane, and acrylonitrile [10]. In general, these standards apply to industrial workplace exposures and specifically exclude from regulation some laboratory uses of the chemicals when in solutions at concentrations of 0.1–1.0%. However, several of OSHA's other regulations do apply to laboratory operations, including 29 CFR 1910.134 (respiratory protection), and subpart G (occupational health and environmental control, which includes ventilation and ionizing and nonionizing radiation regulations). In order to fill the gaps in regulations which cover carcinogen handling in laboratories, the Department of Health, Education and Welfare (DHEW) Laboratory Chemical Carcinogen Safety Standards Subcommittee issued guidelines [11]. These guidelines cover medical surveillance, worker education, work practice and engineering controls, and specific responsibilities for program management for carcinogen handling in the laboratory. In turn, these general guidelines have been adapted to specific laboratory procedures for the National Institute of Environmental Health Sciences (NIEHS) research efforts in evaluating carcinogens, mutagens, and various toxic chemicals [12]. Specific layouts for chemical containment laboratories are detailed in the protocol, which also includes sections on custom-designed glove boxes, decontamination sinks, and waste water treatment facilities.

Similarly, the National Cancer Institute (NCI) has implemented DHEW's guidelines for animal handling during carcinogen bioassays [13]. These carcinogen safety standards cover personal protective equipment and operating practices for animal care personnel. Both the NCI and NIEHS guidelines call for further tailoring of health and safety procedures for carcinogens to each laboratory which actually performs the bioassay work [12,14].

The efficacy of the commonly employed control techniques has been the subject of much recent work. Some of the current research focuses upon permeability of various types of protective equipment [15,16], the efficiency and effectiveness of laboratory hoods [17,18], clean and dirty corridor systems for animal handling facilities [19], and monitoring techniques to ensure reduced exposures to laboratory personnel from carcinogens [20–22]. Initial results of the above studies indicate that accepted or standard protective equipment and work practice techniques are not always achieving the intended goal of providing protection to laboratory personnel in carcinogen laboratories. In order to provide a greater degree of protection for laboratory personnel, laboratory occupational safety and health programs are being improved.

Occupational Safety and Health in the National Toxicology Program

The National Toxicology Program (NTP) was established in November 1978 as a Department of Health and Human Services (DHHS) interagency cooperative effort to develop the scientific information necessary to protect the health of the American public from exposure to hazardous chemicals. In addition to testing chemicals for toxic properties, the program also develops more efficient test methods.

The NTP coordinates the testing of chemicals for carcinogenicity and provides an organizational focus through which such testing can be given greater emphasis within the National Cancer Institute. Evolving from NCI's long history of research into chemical carcinogenesis, the NTP incorporates a variety of program elements, including the testing of chemicals in lifetime experiments in animals, the testing of chemicals in short-term batteries, and continuing research into improved (i.e., in terms of sensitivity, speed, and cost) test methods.

The scope of activities under NTP is necessarily broad. Hundreds of individual chemicals have been and are currently being tested *in vivo* and *in vitro* to identify their carcinogenic and other toxicologic properties. This testing involves administration of substances in the solid, liquid, and gaseous phases via ingestion, gavage, skin painting, implantation, injection, and inhalation.

Many independent laboratories, ranging from universities and hospitals to national laboratories and professional testing laboratories, conduct NTP testing under contract. Because a thorough understanding of the potential toxicity/carcinogenicity of a bioassay subject is always lacking when the test is in progress, it is important that a safety program be implemented to protect against excessive exposure of laboratory personnel and the surrounding environment to the test agent, its metabolites, and its degradation products. While each participating laboratory is required to develop and implement its own safety program, the NTP retains responsibility for evaluating these programs.

To assist in the evaluation of health and safety practices of the NTP and its contract laboratories, NTP has issued a task order contract with the Occupational Safety and Health Unit at Arthur D. Little, Inc., for comprehensive health and safety/industrial hygiene services. Recognizing that the health and safety problems of NTP laboratories differ from those of an industrial production facility, the NTP required support services in basic industrial hygiene (recognition, evaluation, and control of hazards) as well as specialized experience in nonroutine analytical chemistry applications, engineering control and personal protective equipment evaluation and development, biological testing procedures and protocols, and statistical design of sampling strategies. This chapter resulted from a preliminary study of biological monitoring which was conducted to assist the NTP in the development of biological monitoring for laboratory workers in the bioassay program and to explore potential techniques and procedures for monitoring exposure to a limited number of chemicals on test.

APPROACHES FOR BIOLOGICAL MONITORING

A comprehensive occupational safety and health program should include three distinct monitoring activities: environmental monitoring, biological monitoring, and medical monitoring. Biological and medical monitoring are often referred to as medical surveillance. This chapter includes definitions and descriptions of biological and medical monitoring, discussion of some of the problems associated with these monitoring activities, and a discussion of some of the requirements and recommendations developed by agencies such as the Occupational Safety and Health Administration. There are several general references which provide recommendations for the design and management of biological and medical monitoring programs [12, 23-27].

Monitoring in Occupational Safety and Health Programs

Environmental monitoring involves monitoring of chemicals in the working environment. These chemicals may be airborne or they may be deposited on surfaces in the workplace. Biological monitoring involves monitoring of chemicals which have passed from the working environment into the biological or internal environment of the worker. Medical monitoring involves the monitoring of the health status of employees, particularly adverse health effects or pathological events that may be due to exposure to chemicals in the workplace. Monitoring can also be defined in terms of the degree of prevention that it provides. For example, primary preventive measures are intended to prevent the occurrence of disease; secondary preventive measures are intended to identify disease in its early stages and to prevent its progression. Environmental and biological monitoring are primary preventive measures intended to control exposure to toxic substances; medical monitoring is a secondary preventive measure intended to identify disease or preferably to identify the precursors to disease and initiate therapy as well as to assist in the identification of toxic exposures.

Environmental monitoring is a fundamental aspect of the practice of industrial hygiene and is an essential part of any occupational safety and health program; however, environmental monitoring has some significant limitations. First, environmental monitoring is useful for identifying and evaluating the levels of airborne chemicals or chemicals deposited on surfaces, but it cannot fully evaluate exposures that may occur from skin absorption or ingestion of chemicals. Environmental monitoring standards and sampling procedures have been developed to assess chemical exposures which occur with some regular frequency such as on a daily basis for most of an 8- to 10-hour work shift. Exposures that occur infrequently or last for a short time are difficult to assess with standard environmental monitoring procedures. Another limitation is the focus on occupational exposures, which ignores the potential adverse health effects of nonoccupational exposures. Finally, environmental monitoring cannot account for the effect of habits such as smoking or drinking and metabolic factors such as variations in breathing rate, lung volume, or individual sensitivities. Because of these limitations, an occupational safety and health program should not rely solely upon environmental monitoring but should supplement environmental monitoring with biological and medical monitoring.

Medical Surveillance: Biological and Medical Monitoring

Waritz defines biological monitoring as: "Analysis of exhaled air, analysis of some biological fluid, such as urine, blood, tears, or perspiration, or analysis of some body component, such as hair or nails, to evaluate past exposure to a chemical" [28: p. 258]. The time perspective of biological monitoring entails evaluating past exposure. Also, distinctions can be made between direct and indirect monitoring. Direct monitoring involves analysis of the chemical or its immediate metabolites; indirect monitoring, analysis of the effects that result from the action of the chemical or its metabolites on some body system. (There is certainly some overlap between the indirect biological monitoring of the secondary effects of a chemical and medical monitoring of adverse health effects or pathological events. This overlap is due to the lack of information concerning the association between the secondary effects or physiological changes and the subsequent development of functional disorders. In practice, the distinction is mostly a problem of semantics.)

In general, direct biological monitoring is preferable to indirect biological monitoring because it allows analysis of an exposure. With indirect monitoring damage may have already occurred by the time data can be interpreted, and the time lag required for indirect monitoring obscures the relationship between effects and specific exposures.

Medical monitoring also involves the analysis of body fluids or other components, but the purpose is to evaluate the pathological effects of past exposure. In the most general sense, medical monitoring can be defined in terms of cancer screening as follows: "The application of a relatively simple, inexpensive test to a large number of persons in order to classify them as likely, or unlikely, to have the cancer which is the object of the screen" [29]. The objective of such an activity is to reduce the level of morbidity and mortality due to the development of the subject disease in the population being monitored. It should be noted that the focus of medical monitoring is on the probability of disease being present, rather than the confirmed diagnosis of disease. Thus, the tests which are conducted in a medical monitoring program tend to be simpler, less expensive, less invasive, and more comfortable than diagnostic test procedures.

Biological and medical monitoring are part of a continuum which begins with environmental monitoring and which, as a whole, coincides with the progression from exposure to a toxic substance to the ultimate development of disease. Figure

9-1 describes this progression and the relationship between exposure, disease, and monitoring activities. Environmental monitoring focuses on the chemical in the occupational environment prior to or during the actual exposure by inhalation, ingestion, or absorption of the chemical. After the chemical enters the body, biological monitoring is concerned with detecting the substance or its metabolites in various biological media. Finally, after the chemical of interest is metabolized, deposited, accumulated, excreted, or otherwise processed, medical monitoring focuses on identifying physiological or pathological changes which are attributable to the exposure.

Uses for Biological Monitoring

The following uses of biological monitoring correspond, to some extent, with the problems associated with environmental monitoring.

- identification of unsuspected exposures
- guidance for therapy
- documentation of level of exposure
- identification of unusual sensitivity
- evaluation of multiple exposures
- validation of area monitoring

Periodic biological monitoring can help to identify unsuspected exposures. In other words, it serves as a quality control measure for engineering and administrative control programs or personal protective measures. For example, an employee may be inhaling chemical vapors because of a poorly fitted respirator, and biological monitoring of a urine sample could detect abnormal levels of the chemical. In addition, biological monitoring can be used to confirm exposure and quantify the exposure level. This may be crucial when an antidote such as atropine, which may be toxic in the absence of organophosphate exposure, is being considered. Finally, biological monitoring can be useful for documenting levels of exposure, evaluating nonoccupational, mixed, or intermittent exposures, and as a validation of personal or area environmental monitoring[28].

Pitfalls of Biological Monitoring

There are many uses for biological monitoring and also many problems or pitfalls which must be considered when planning and conducting monitoring programs. Some of these problem areas are:

- logistics
- sampling and analysis
- professional jurisdictions
- interpretation of data
- legal and ethical issues

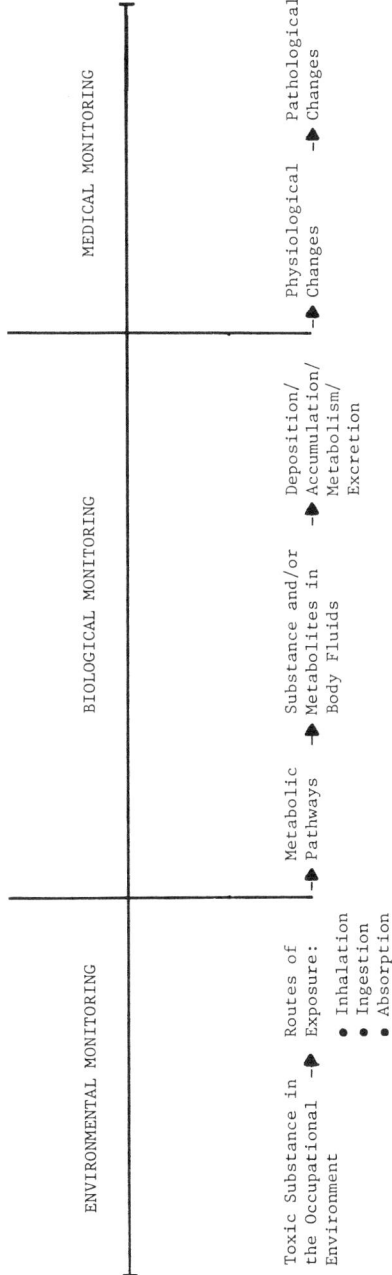

Figure 9-1.   The relationship between exposure, disease, and monitoring.

There are numerous logistical problems which must be resolved such as selecting employees for monitoring, working up a schedule which minimizes interference with the work schedule, ordering, stocking, and handling materials and supplies, shipping samples to analytical laboratories, and ensuring the cooperation of labor and management. Sampling and analysis of samples can be a problem because widely accepted procedures are limited and, for the more exotic compounds, biological monitoring methods may be nonexistent.

Even if the sampling and analysis are successfully completed, someone must interpret the results and decide whether or not they are acceptable. Problems associated with interpretation are discussed in the following section. Finally, biological monitoring is complicated by a variety of legal and ethical issues such as compulsory versus voluntary testing, obligations to report results, confidentiality of records, and the jurisdictions of various professional groups.

Biological monitoring is considered by some to be a medical procedure; others consider it to be more akin to industrial hygiene. To the extent that biological monitoring involves an assessment of exposure, it is, in fact, a part of industrial hygiene, although medical expertise or certification is required for any invasive procedures.

Interpretation of Monitoring Results

The ability to sample a biological medium and to analyze it for toxic chemicals is relatively straightforward; however, interpretation of the analytical data is a complex problem and is the most serious pitfall for successful biological and medical monitoring[30,31]. A few of the problems associated with interpreting monitoring data are:

- several sources of variation
- false negative and false positive results
- additional data requirements
- need for coordination with industrial hygienists
- need for cooperation of labor
- unintentional discrimination

For example, the results of monitoring may vary because of some underlying biological or temporal cycle such as menstruation or circadian rhythms. The results may also vary because of measurement error either on the part of the observer or the instruments. Few tests are 100% accurate, and a small percentage of the results are either false negatives or false positives. Either case presents a problem—the employee with a false negative result is given a false sense of security and the employee with a false positive result may be subjected to unnecessary and sometimes painful or hazardous diagnostic or therapeutic procedures.

Often interpretation requires the collection and review of additional data which may include comprehensive personal and medical histories and the results of previous environmental and biological monitoring. For example, habits such as smoking or hobbies involving chemical exposures may interfere with biological monitoring while physiological differences may interfere with medical monitoring.

Finally, interpretation requires coordination with industrial hygienists so that whenever problems are identified, the source of exposure will also be identified and controlled. The cooperation of labor groups is also essential and sometimes a problem, especially if labor fears that adverse monitoring results will lead to dismissal or undesirable job transfer. Interpretation can also be discriminatory because most standards do not recognize the physiological differences between racial, ethnic, and age groups. Reproductive effects have not been studied intensively, and the effects on men have received much less attention than the effects on women, although there is every reason to believe that men can be at substantial risk.

Genetic Monitoring

In recent years interest has focused on genetic monitoring as a particular form of medical monitoring which can be used to identify the effects of chemical exposures [32,33]. In part, genetic monitoring developed as a result of concern about the mutagenic effects of chemicals. It also developed because damage to genetic material, even if it is minor and innocuous in terms of health, may be a useful early warning of potential physiological and pathological changes. A variety of tests have been developed including cytogenetic tests which analyze chromosomal structure and tests of body fluids such as urine for mutagenic activity *in vitro*. Theoretically, genetic monitoring could be used to detect hypersusceptible workers and thus prevent exposure to potentially toxic substances by placing such employees in jobs with less chance of exposure. In reality, genetic monitoring involves complex legal, ethical, and emotional issues. Ultimately, we must decide whether the workplace should be safe for everybody, even the most sensitive members of the population, or whether we should adopt a policy which accepts some finite level of exposure and risk or which discriminates against some people during job placement because of their metabolic variations or genetic inheritance. Such questions are the subject of current debate and will not be easily or quickly resolved.

OSHA Requirements for Biological and Medical Monitoring

The requirements currently promulgated by the Occupational Safety and Health Administration (OSHA) for biological and medical monitoring are limited and consist mainly of the following general medical examinations and tests [34,35]:

physical exam	hematology
special exams	hormone assay
chest x-ray	sperm counts
pulmonary function	respiratory questionnaire
sputum cytology	blood lead
urinalysis	zinc protoporphyrin
blood chemistry	exit exam

Vinyl chloride is an example of a chemical which has received considerable attention because of its carcinogenic properties, and yet OSHA requirements for medical monitoring are limited to a general physical, a medical history, and a series of biochemical tests (total bilirubin, alkaline phosphatase, SGOT, SGPT, gamma glutamyl transpeptidase) to assess liver function. In addition, OSHA recommends several other tests including pulmonary function tests, chest x-ray, urinanalysis, serum enzyme and protein assay, hepatitis antigen assay, and liver scanning.

Requirements for Respirator Users

OSHA has more specific medical monitoring requirements for workers who wear respirators (see Code of Federal Regulations, CFR, 1910.134 Respiratory Protection, and chemical-specific regulations such as CFR 1910.1001 Asbestos). These regulations require periodic review of the medical status of respirator users to assure that they are physically able to work while wearing the equipment. CFR 1910.1001 also addresses issues such as seniority status and pay rates which cannot be jeopardized if the employee is not able to wear a respirator.

Requirements for Recordkeeping

OSHA has also issued requirements for recordkeeping (CFR 1910.20) which specifically distinguish between "exposure" and "medical" records. These distinctions are particularly important for preserving the confidentiality of medical records. OSHA has proposed regulatory reforms which include several changes in the requirements for recordkeeping including certain exemptions, limitations, and reductions.

The Development of Biological Monitoring Programs

The organizational structure and scope of activity of occupational safety and health programs are highly variable both at the corporate level and at the individual facility. In any case there are certain disciplines and activities which can be identified as being potential elements in a comprehensive program. Some elements are common to most programs (e.g., fire protection or first aid) while other elements are only found in the more sophisticated facilities (e.g., epidemiology and biostatistics). The various disciplines which may contribute to an occupational safety and health program include the following:

industrial hygienist	physician
chemical engineer	nurse
ventilation engineer	first-aider
safety engineer	benefits/personnel officer
firefighter	toxicologist
biohazard officer	epidemiologist
radiation control officer	biostatistician

These disciplines should work in a coordinated fashion. Many organizational relationships exist, and Figure 9–2 depicts one simple arrangement which separates the program into industrial hygiene, occupational medicine, and safety components.

Biological monitoring requires coordination between the industrial hygiene component of the program and the medical component. Table 9–1 describes a scenario consisting of a sequence of events which lead to the biological monitoring of a laboratory employee. This hypothetical presentation illustrates the interplay which occurs between industrial hygiene and medicine.

While it is clear that biological monitoring focuses on the evaluation of exposure and medical monitoring on the evaluation of pathological changes resulting from exposure, there is a considerable overlap or "gray area" between the two activities. For example, do we consider monitoring of carboxyhemoglobin formation or cholinesterase inhibition to be monitoring of exposure or response? If we correlate environmental carbon monoxide levels with levels of carboxyhemoglobin in the blood, then we can argue that it is a form of biological monitoring. On the other hand, carboxyhemoglobin results in reduced oxygen transfer and subsequent asphyxiation and so its formation can be considered to be an adverse health effect resulting from carbon monoxide exposure, making this type of monitoring a medical activity. While the distinction between biological and medical monitoring may seem to be simply a problem of semantics, it also involves serious issues such as confidentiality of records and the jurisdiction of various professional groups.

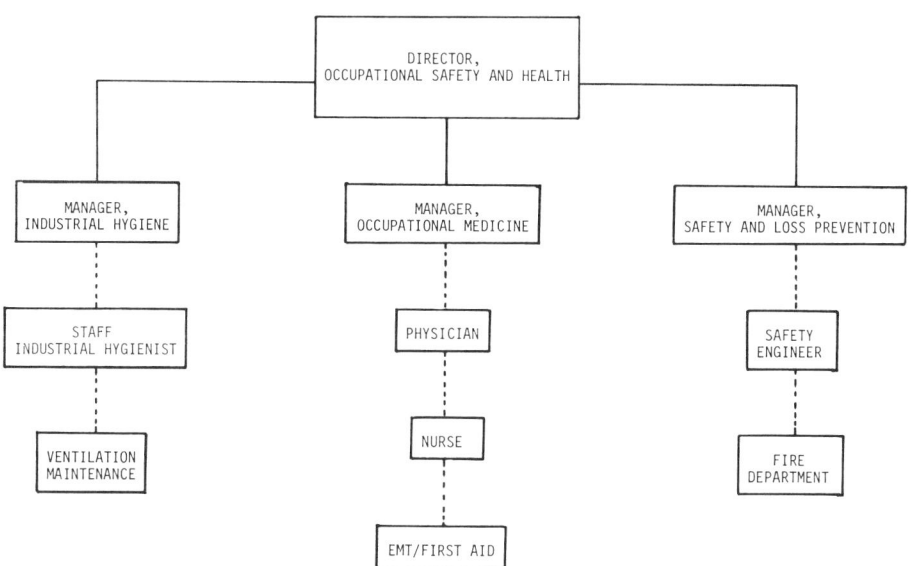

Figure 9–2. Hypothetical organization of an occupational safety and health program.

Table 9-1.   Hypothetical Series of Events Leading to Biological Monitoring
of a Laboratory Employee

- *Employee hired.*
- *Preplacement physical exam.*
  Physician reviews job/hazard description and decides that employee health is not at risk from employment.
- *Employee works.*
- *Periodic air samples.*
  Industrial hygienist takes periodic personal air samples to evaluate employee exposure. No airborne chemicals are detected during the periodic sampling.
- *Periodic biological monitoring.*
  Industrial hygienist takes periodic noninvasive biological samples (invasive samples are taken by nurse or physician). Analysis reveals abnormal levels of chemical in the sample.
- *Industrial hygienist identifies exposure source.*
  Industrial hygienist controls exposure by removing employee from work or providing protective equipment.
- *Industrial hygiene/medical consultation.*
  Industrial hygienist informs medical staff about biological monitoring results.
- *Medical staff monitors employee health status.*
- *Industrial hygienist controls source of exposure.*
- *Industrial hygienist monitors other employees.*
- *Industrial hygiene/medical consultation.*
  Reevaluate employee and consider replacement in original position or elsewhere.

Issues for Program Implementation

In order to implement a program of biological monitoring, a number of issues must be resolved, including the basic problem of definitions. Some of these issues are relatively simple, such as organizational and administrative issues, while others, such as some of the legal and ethical issues or the selection of analytical techniques, are complex and may not be satisfactorily resolved with the current state of knowledge. The following section discusses some issues related to the implementation of biological monitoring programs. The discussion is presented in terms of the general questions which arise when one considers implementing a program of biological monitoring. Subsequent sections discuss existing programs at selected facilities and the feasibility of implementing biological monitoring in NTP-sponsored research laboratories.

The initial question which must be answered is: Do we need a biological monitoring program? If we know that there are no exposures or that environmental monitoring is providing sufficient data for evaluating exposure, then biological monitoring may not be necessary. On the other hand, biological monitoring data have many uses. For example, periodic biological monitoring may identify unsuspected exposures from intermittent sources or exposure routes such as absorption or ingestion which are not detected by traditional air monitoring. Since biological monitoring is a more direct measure of exposure than environmental monitoring, it can be used to confirm and document levels of exposure estimated from area or personal sampling. Medical personnel can use biological monitoring data to confirm exposure and to guide the choice of therapeutics. Such data could also be used to identify unusual sensitivities or metabolic abnormalities.

If we decide that biological monitoring is a worthwhile activity, we must decide whom to sample as well as when and where the samples will be taken. If cost is not a concern, we could monitor all employees; however, even environmental monitoring is limited to a subset of the total workforce and so it is likely that we would select employees whose exposure is representative of the overall workforce exposure.

The next question which must be resolved is to decide what to monitor. Should we monitor the chemical itself or some metabolite? For example, if we are monitoring employees exposed to styrene, we should note that almost all of the styrene is metabolized and that the principal metabolite is mandelic acid [27]. In experimental animals, however, there are considerable interspecies differences such as metabolism of styrene to hippuric acid rather than mandelic acid. Such differences complicate biological monitoring for chemicals which have not been well studied because human data are often lacking and animal data may not provide a valid method.

Once we have determined the substance to be monitored, we must decide what kind of sample to take (e.g., blood, urine, breath, hair, nails) and what kind of analysis to conduct (e.g., colorimetric, chromatographic, spectrophotometric). While blood is probably the most relevant sampling medium in terms of the exposure of vital organs, the sampling process is painful and requires special skill and procedures both for sampling and processing the sample. Other media such as urine or breath are relatively easy to collect because they do not require invasive techniques, but since they are excretory samples, they are less accurate as a quantitative estimate of internal exposure [28]. The choice of analytical techniques varies from simple colorimetric dipstick tests to tests that require sophisticated equipment. Selection of a method depends in part on determining which methods have been evaluated and are considered to be acceptable and in part on the availability of resources for in-house or commercial analysis.

After a sample is taken and analyzed, the result must be interpreted. It must be determined whether or not the worker is exposed to the substance in question and, if exposed, whether or not the level of exposure is within acceptable bounds. Unfortunately, even under laboratory conditions, the precision of biological monitoring is generally less than $\pm 20\%$. Phenol is an exceptional case with a precision below $\pm 10\%$ because of relatively simple metabolism and a high excretion rate, while nitrobenzene tends to accumulate in adipose tissue and, because of complex metabolic pathways, cannot be measured with a precision less than $\pm 20\%$ [27]. Under real working conditions interpretation of results is much more difficult than in the laboratory because individuals vary widely in their metabolic functions, dietary habits, work and other exposures, and other factors which confound the results of biological monitoring.

Future Developments

There appears to be a resurgence of interest in biological and medical monitoring. Research on indoor air quality, particularly pollutants in residential or other nonindustrial environments, has led to the realization that pollutant exposure occurs throughout the day and night and that environmental monitoring gives a limited perspective on the 24-hour spectrum of exposure. Also, in recent years there has been increasing dissatisfaction with current permissible exposure limits which are based, to a large extent, on limited toxicological and epidemiological data. In fact, more than three decades ago, Elkins recommended biological monitoring as a more accurate measure of exposure than environmental monitoring [36].

Interest in biological and medical monitoring is evident in the activities of regulatory agencies, industry, and labor organizations. Professional societies such as the American Industrial Hygiene Association (AIHA) have renewed their interest and have formed an Ad Hoc Committee for Biological Monitoring. Despite the increasing activity, new methods will take time to develop, and regulations or requirements will require not only new methods but also considerable peer review and commentary before promulgation. The following section reviews selected biological monitoring programs at NTP contract laboratories and shows that the existing programs are extremely limited in scope.

REVIEW OF SELECTED BIOLOGICAL MONITORING PROGRAMS

Biological Monitoring at NTP Contract Laboratories

Tracor Jitco, Inc., is one of the prime contractors for the NTP carcinogenesis bioassay program and, in order to fulfill a requirement of contract no. N01-CP-43350, "Bioassay Operations Program," they provided health and safety guidance for all operations, both prime and subcontract, connected with the test program. Accordingly, Tracor Jitco has developed a carcinogenesis bioassay health and safety plan which includes a recommended medical surveillance program for contract laboratories [37]. It is a general program which does not provide any chemical-specific recommendations nor does it distinguish between medical surveillance and biological monitoring.

Tracor Jitco also conducted surveys of the medical programs at the various laboratories working under contract for the NCI/NTP carcinogenesis bioassay program [38]. A physician at Tracor Jitco, and several colleagues visited Gulf South Research Institute, Physiological Research Laboratory, Midwest Research Institute, Battelle Northwest, Bioassay Systems, Litton Bionetics, Mason Research Institute, Microbiological Associates, Papanicolaou Cancer Research Institute, and Battelle Columbus Laboratory. The site visit reports suggest that these laboratories have developed comprehensive medical monitoring programs; however, the physician did recommend that the laboratories should include the acid phosphatase test in the blood profile as a specific test for prostatic carcinoma and he also recommended proctosigmoidoscopy every other year for employees over 40 years of age. He also reminded several laboratories of the OSHA requirements for cardiovascular and respiratory examination of prospective respirator users. There were no indications that any of the laboratories had established biological monitoring programs and the medical programs seemed to focus on general health status rather than the relationship between potential job hazards and adverse health effects.

Safety and health personnel at Litton Industries, EGG, and SRI International indicated that biological monitoring programs at their laboratories were limited to a few pilot programs. For example, at the EGG facility in Maryland, new laboratory employees are given a physical examination, a blood screen, and a serum sample for future baseline comparisons. Physical examinations are given every six months for laboratory personnel. EGG personnel are currently unsure about their needs for a biological monitoring program, particularly for employees involved in commercial testing because the identity of the test compound is often unknown.

Litton conducts similar baseline and periodic physical examinations and has conducted some chemical-specific examinations (i.e., blood cholinesterase, urinary selenium, and metabolites of trichloroethylene). Since many of the tests which they conduct are short-term (about two days), they do not feel that biological monitoring will have any value. They also test many coded materials or unknowns and so cannot determine the appropriate monitoring procedures and analytical techniques.

Biological Monitoring at U.S. Government Laboratories

Federal agencies operate a wide variety of laboratories. For example, the United States Department of Agriculture (USDA) has approximately 400 laboratories conducting research with toxic substances. Several agencies within the USDA, notably the Science and Education Administration and the Food Safety and Quality Service, have health monitoring programs which are designed to protect laboratory employees whose work regularly poses the possibility of exposure to toxic materials. General guidelines for medical surveillance have been developed and recommended by the USDA medical director[39].

The Laboratory Chemical Carcinogen Safety Standards Subcommittee of the Department of Health, Education and Welfare Committee to Coordinate Toxicology and Related Programs has proposed guidelines for the laboratory use of chemical substances posing a potential occupational carcinogenic risk[11]. These guidelines are less specific than the USDA guidelines, but they include a more comprehensive discussion of the rationale for medical and biological monitoring in periodic health assessments. An excerpt from the guidelines follows:

> The nature of a program for providing periodic health assessments is complicated by several factors. Among these are (1) many laboratory workers handle a variety of toxic chemicals so that the medical surveillance should ideally seek evidence of adverse effects from all these substances, (2) some cancer-causing chemicals have little or no toxicity

other than the production of neoplasms, and (3) most tumors do not become evident until many years (often 20–30) after the initiating events.

Medical monitoring will, therefore, sometimes for necessity and more often for efficiency, usually concentrate on events likely to precede overt evidence of tumorigenesis. For example, some carcinogens, such as dimethylnitrosamine, have high acute toxicity, especially to the liver, and evidence of such acute toxicity can be obtained within a few hours or days following exposure. Some tumors, such as those induced by carbon tetrachloride, are normally preceded by marked changes in liver cells, usually detectable by clinical tests. Others, e.g., angiosarcomas induced by such substances as vinyl chloride, will often cause detectable cell changes in nearby tissue as the probable result of space occupation. It should be noted that detection of such toxic changes does not necessarily presage tumor development, but should, nevertheless, precipitate the institution of corrective work practices and improved engineering controls. For the medical department to be effective, it must have relevant information, such as mode and mechanism of toxic action, frequency and severity of exposure, and exposure concentrations, if known. Some of this information will be available in individual Safety Data Sheets. However, this information should be supplemented by the principal investigator when appropriate.

Biological monitoring will sometimes be a useful method of detecting exposure and perhaps of estimating the degree of exposure. Biological monitoring usually involves the analysis of body fluids or excreta (usually urine, sometimes blood, rarely expired air) for the toxic substance or a biotransformation product. An example is the detection of acetyl derivatives in the urine of persons absorbing benzidine [27]. Even if exposure cannot be quantified, as is sometimes the case, the mere detection of the metabolite, if its presence is specific to the individual carcinogen or its chemical class, is sufficient to indicate the need for corrective action.

In some cases, especially with less well known carcinogens, those in the research laboratory will be better informed on possible biological monitoring procedures than will the medical department. In such cases, the investigators should discuss the possibilities with the medical department. Specialized analytical procedures and equipment may be needed for some of this monitoring, procedures and equipment that may not be available to the dispensary but which are available in the research laboratory. The investigators should undertake such monitoring procedures themselves only with prior approval by and participation of the medical department. This is to ensure that appropriate precautions will be taken such as (1) precautions related to data interpretation, e.g., standard corrections for dilution of urine, (2) precautions for the individual, such as assurance that invasive procedures will not be used, and (3) precautions for the individual's privacy, such as maintenance of appropriate security for individual records.

Agencies and institutes within the Department of Health and Human Services have developed safety and health programs which provide general information regarding medical and biological monitoring. A typical example is the Safety and Health Manual of the National Institute for Environmental Health Sciences (NIEHS) which requires that all laboratory personnel be examined on at least a 12-

to 18-month schedule [12]. The examination recommended by NIEHS consists of the following:

- comprehensive medical history
- complete physical examination
- necessary inoculations
- any special diagnostic tests (e.g., urinary or sputum cytology, skin exam, slit lamp exam) as dictated by the nature of the individual's work
- other examinations deemed necessary by the examining physician

No information of a chemical-specific nature is provided in this type of general safety and health manual. This is due to the large number of potential exposures and the lack of more specific information for monitoring procedures.

Many of the research laboratories of the U.S. Fish and Wildlife Service have developed health monitoring programs. For example, the Fish Control Laboratory at LaCrosse, Wisconsin; the Pesticide Laboratory at Columbia, Missouri; and the Wildlife Research Center at Patuxent, Maryland, all have adopted programs based upon the USDA program [40-43]. These programs involve blood chemistry profiles, electrolyte profiles, enzyme assays, urinalysis, and other common tests. They do not include chemical-specific biological or medical monitoring. Finally, the U.S. Navy Occupational Health program acknowledges that periodic evaluation of workers exposed to toxic substances is necessary, but it only cites a few examples of chemicals and their target organs [44].

Biological Monitoring at Other Selected Private Sector Organizations

Most industrial facilities are subject to OSHA regulations, which include specific requirements for biological monitoring and medical surveillance [10]. Also, NIOSH has published criteria documents or proposed regulations which recommend such testing. OSHA regulations currently adopted or pending are limited to a few chemicals such as asbestos, carcinogens, vinyl chloride, coke oven emissions, benzene, inorganic arsenic, cotton dust, acrylonitrile, and inorganic lead. These standards all require medical monitoring, but only the lead standard specifically requires the inclusion of biological monitoring results in the medical record [35].

Some private sector organizations have developed comprehensive programs. For example, Kaiser Aluminum and Chemical Corporation has developed occupational health surveillance charts which summarize medical and industrial hygiene considerations for all airborne contaminants and physical stresses in its industrial operations [45]. Biological monitoring is recommended for the contaminants which are listed in Table 9-2. A footnote to the charts specifies that the selection of testing laboratory and analytical method is to be approved by the medical director and that specimens are to be collected only by an approved physician or under the direct supervision of one.

Table 9–2.   Typical Corporate Recommendations for Biological
Monitoring[45]

Contaminant	Recommendations for Biological Monitoring
Cadmium oxide	urinary cadmium
Carbon monoxide	carboxyhemglobin
Carbon tetrachloride	urinalysis[a]
Chloroform	urinalysis
Fluorides	urinary fluorides (both preshift and postshift)
Lead	blood lead and urinary lead
Manganese	urinalysis
Mercury	blood mercury and urinary mercury
Particulate polycyclic organic matter	urinalysis
Toluene	urinary hippuric acid
Vinyl chloride	urinalysis
Xylene	urinalysis

[a]Recommendations for urinalysis do not specify chemicals or their metabolites
for monitoring.

BIOLOGICAL MONITORING AT NTP LABORATORIES

In previous sections biological monitoring has been described as an important aspect of a comprehensive occupational safety and health program and as an activity which provides a unique perspective for the evaluation of chemical exposures. If we focus our attention on the specific attributes of the NTP laboratory work environment, however, we find that the theoretical value of biological monitoring cannot be fully translated into a practical program. The following sections address the role of biological monitoring at NTP laboratories and show where such an activity may be useful. Finally, some recommendations for work which will promote the implementation of limited biological monitoring are provided.

Biological Monitoring for NTP Test Compounds

The initial premise of the NTP investigation was that literature search would identify valid biological monitoring methods for a host of NTP test compounds. Subsequent searching proved that this premise was too optimistic and that the data base was quite limited. In fact, the limited data base is one important reason for including a compound with possible carcinogenic properties in the NTP program in the first place. With the exception of several analgesic compounds such as 4-hydroxyacetanilide, methdilazine, and methylphenidate which have been extensively investigated, the relevant literature is limited to a few reports on analytical methods. However, there are no reports of practical methods for biological monitoring, even for the more widely studied compounds. (Note that "practical methods" means more than a sensitive analytical method. It requires an understanding of the dose-response relationship, the precision and accuracy of the data, and the meaning of the data as a measure of exposure.) Since the initial literature search was limited to human studies, an additional search was conducted for studies of nonhuman subjects but no useful information was discovered. In any case, information derived from laboratory animal experimentation may not be particularly useful because the metabolic pathways and kinetics of metabolism vary widely from species to species and so it is difficult to extrapolate animal data to develop biological monitoring procedures for humans.

Biological Monitoring for Common NTP Compounds

While the initial focus of this task was the compounds being tested for carcinogenic and other toxic properties, we realized after conducting several unproductive literature searches that practical methods for biological monitoring were not available for these compounds. Concurrently, we realized that, in terms of both duration and concentration, exposures to the test compounds were much less significant than exposures to the solvents and reagents which are routinely used in NTP laboratories. Examination of industrial hygiene data on formaldehyde exposures (see Figure 9–3) demonstrates that there is a wide range of exposure from undetectable levels to a maximum, in this case, of 15 ppm in the breathing zone of a necropsy technician. While the median exposure is between 0.19 ppm and 0.25 ppm, more than 40% of 31 samples are greater than 0.50 ppm and about 16% of the samples are greater than 1 ppm.

Formaldehyde has been the subject of considerable research in recent years because of speculation about carcinogenic properties. Reported methods for biological monitoring, which initially involved direct measurement of formaldehyde in blood and urine, commonly involve measurement of formic acid, a rapidly formed metabolite of formaldehyde. Makar and Tephly [46] have described an improved analytical procedure specific for formate in blook, urine, or tissue extract. Using spectrophotofluorometry, formate concentrations as low as 6 mg/liter of blood can be measured. Tephly has indicated that his group at the University of Iowa has developed a rapid colorimetric test for formate which might be a convenient procedure for large-scale or repetitive biological monitoring programs, but he is uncertain about the relationship between the biological measurement of formate at low levels and subsequent adverse health effects.

On the other hand, investigators at Colorado State University have reported the results of a pilot study which shows that airborne levels of formaldehyde on the order of 0.1 ppm are too low for meaningful biological monitoring of formic acid

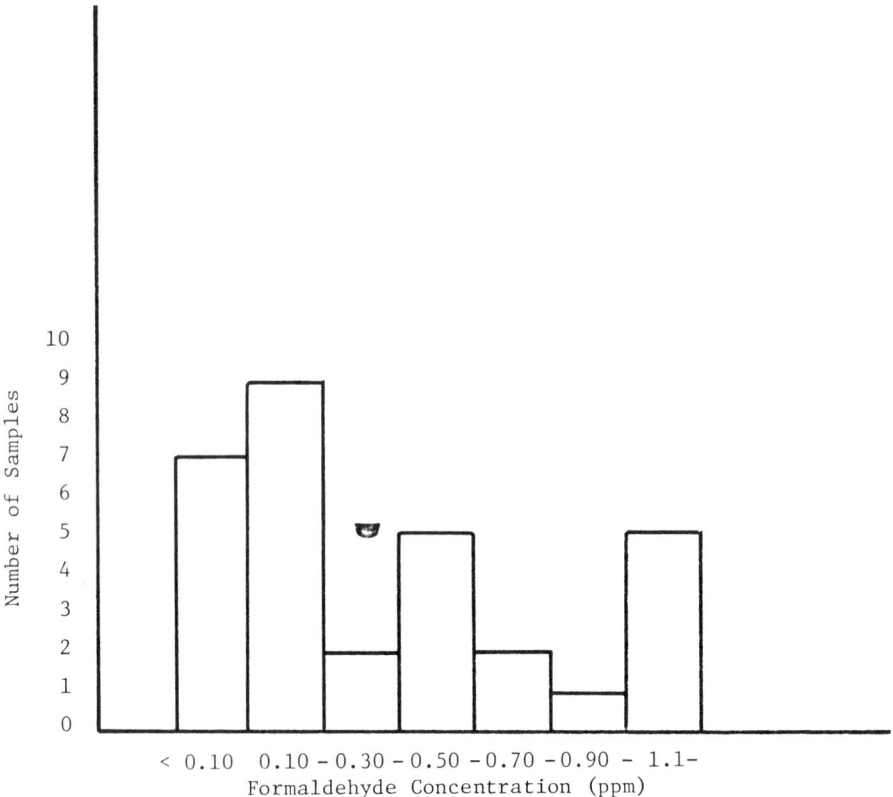

Figure 9-3.   Bioassay laboratory formaldehyde sampling.

[47]. Using gas chromatography-mass spectrophotometry, these investigators found no significant shifts in urinary formic acid before and after low-level exposures to formaldehyde in a veterinary laboratory environment. Beaulieu, the principal investigator, has indicated that his group is abandoning biological monitoring for formaldehyde and is focusing on changes in pulmonary function which they reported as having a potential dose-response relationship. Beaulieu also reported that some veterinary students continued to exhibit abnormal decrements in pulmonary function after several months (i.e., summer vacation) without formaldehyde exposure and that additional studies are under way.

Obviously, biological monitoring is a complex activity even for a common chemical such as formaldehyde. The work by Beaulieu et al. [47] suggests that the airborne levels found in the laboratory environment are too low for meaningful monitoring, while Makar and Tephly [46] are developing analytical techniques which may be useful, at least for monitoring, if not for risk assessment.

RECOMMENDATIONS

An important goal of this chapter is to provide guidance and recommendations regarding the development of biological monitoring programs at NTP contractors' laboratories. While initially we focused on the chemicals currently on test, we have broadened our perspective to include not only test chemicals but also reagents, solvents, and other chemicals used routinely in NTP laboratories (e.g., formaldehyde).

Regarding NTP test chemicals, routine biological monitoring is not recommended at this time because the exposures, if they occur, are for short durations at low concentrations, practical methods are not available, and data interpretation is difficult because of a lack of field experience. Biological monitoring may be useful occasionally when there is reason to believe (e.g., from air monitoring or personal reports) that an exposure has occurred. In such a situation, one would compare a postexposure sample with a stored baseline sample to confirm that environmental contaminants were taken into the body. Confirmation could then trigger certain types of periodic biological or medical monitoring.

Routine biological monitoring may eventually be feasible for those chemicals such as formaldehyde which are commonly used in NTP laboratories. The problem, in this case, is that exposures are frequent but low in concentration. If the chemical is rapidly converted to a common metabolite, it may be difficult to distinguish between preexposure and postexposure levels. In fact, interpretation of biological monitoring data is much more complicated than this simple example suggests. For example, during this task we examined the literature regarding formaldehyde and identified two research groups which have adopted widely divergent approaches to the problem of biological monitoring.

REFERENCES

1. Olin, G.R. "The Hazards of a Chemical Laboratory Environment—A Study of the Mortality in Two Cohorts of Swedish Chemists," *Am. Indust. Hyg. J.* 39: 557, July 1978.
2. Case, R.A.M., J.M. Davis, and G.M. Edwards. "Some Environmental Carcinogens," *Ann. Repr. Br. Empire Cancer Camp.* 44: 55, 1966.
3. Case, R.A.M. *Proc. R. Soc. Med.* Volume 62: 1061, 1969.
4. Barnes, J.M. and P.N. Magee. "Some Toxic Properties of Dimethylnitrosamines," *Br. J. Indust. Med.* 11: 167, 1954.
5. Darlow, H.M., et al. "Hazards from Experimental Skin Painting of Carcinogens," *Arch. Envir. Health* 18: 881, July 1968.
6. Sansone, E.B., et al. "Sources and Dissemination of Contamination in Material Handling Operations," *Am. Indust. Hyg. J.* 38: 433, September 1977.
7. Wedum, A.G. and G.B. Phillips. "Criteria for Design of a Microbiological Research Laboratory," *ASHRAE J.* 6: 46, 1964.
8. Morris, E.J. "A Survey of Safety Precautions in the Microbiological Laboratory," *J. Med. Lab. Tech.* 17: 70, 1960.

9. Anderson, R.E., et al. "Potential Infectious Hazards of Common Bacteriological Techniques," *J. Bacteriol.* 64: 473, 1952.

10. U.S. Department of Labor, Occupational Safety and Health Administration. Subpart Z: Toxic and Hazardous Substances 1910.1001–1910.1045, *General Industry* (rev.) (Washington, D.C.: U.S. Government Printing Office, November 7, 1978).

11. U.S. Department of Health, Education and Welfare, Laboratory Chemical Carcinogen Safety Standards Subcommittee. Guidelines for the Laboratory Use of Chemical Substances Posing a Potential Occupational Carcinogenic Risk (rev. draft), June 5, 1979.

12. Walters, D.B., Ed. *NIEHS Safety and Health Manual,* DHEW (NIH) 79–1848, 1979.

13. Sontag, J.M., et al. *Guidelines for Carcinogen Bioassay in Small Rodents.* U.S. Department of Health, Education and Welfare. National Cancer Institute (Bethesda: DHEW (NIH) 76–801, February 1976).

14. NIH(RG)30. Safety and Health Clause. HEWPR 3–7.5002. August 1979.

15. Sansone, E.G. "The Effect of Environmental Factors on Protective Clothing Material Permeability." Paper presented at the American Industrial Hygiene Association Conference, Houston, May 18–23, 1980.

16. Johnson, T.C. and W.D. Merciez. *Permeation of Halogenated Solvents Through Drybox Gloves* (U.S. Atomic Energy Commission, RFP-1608, 1971).

17. Caplan, K.J. and G.W. Knutson. "Development of Criteria for Design, Selection, and In-Place Testing of Laboratory Fume Hoods and Laboratory Room Ventilation Air Supply," Final Report ASHRAE RP-70, March 1, 1978.

18. Sansone, E.G. and A.M. Losikoff. "A Note on the Chemical Contamination Resulting from the Transfer of Solid and Liquid Materials in Hoods," *Am. Indust. Hyg. J.* 38: 489, September 1977.

19. Henke, C.B. "Design Criteria for Animal Facilities," in *Laboratory Animal Housing* Proceedings of a symposium held at Hunt Valley, Md., September 22–23, 1976 (Washington, D.C.: National Academy of Sciences, 1978), p. 142.

20. Melcher, R.G. "Monitoring Trace Amounts of Organic Chemicals in the Laboratory Atmosphere," in *Safe Handling of Chemical Carcinogens, Mutagens, and Teratogens, and Highly Toxic Substances,* Vol. I (Ann Arbor, MI: Ann Arbor Science, 1980), p. 169.

21. Pellizzari, E.D. "State-of-the-Art Techniques for Monitoring Environmental Carcinogens, Mutagens, and Teratogens," in *Safe Handling of Chemical Carcinogens, Mutagens, Teratogens, and Highly Toxic Substances,* Vol. I (Ann Arbor, MI: Ann Arbor Science, 1980), p. 185.

22. Segal, A., and G. Loewengart. "Development of a Personal Monitoring Device for the Detection of Direct-Acting Alkalating Agents," in *Safe Handling of Chemical Carcinogens, Mutagens, Teratogens, and Highly Toxic Substances,* Vol. I (Ann Arbor, MI: Ann Arbor Science, 1980), p. 197.

23. Anderson, J.H. "Medical Aspects of Occupational Health in a Laboratory Setting," in *Laboratory Safety: Theory and Practice,* A.A. Fuscaldo, F.J. Erlick, and B. Hindman, Eds. (New York: Academic Press, 1980).

24. Baselt, R.D. *Biological Monitoring Methods for Industrial Chemicals* (Davis, CA: Biomedical Publications, 1980).

25. Haegele, L. "Selected Medical Problems Often Associated with Laboratory Personnel," in *Laboratory Safety: Theory and Practice,* A.A. Fuscaldo, F.J. Erlick, and B. Hindman, Eds. (New York: Academic Press, 1980).

26. Linch, A.L. *Biological Monitoring for Industrial Chemical Exposure Control* (West Palm Beach: CRC Press, 1974).

27. Piotrowski, J.K. "Exposure Tests for Organic Compounds in Industrial Toxicology," National Institute for Occupational Safety and Health (NIOSH), DHEW (NIOSH) Publication No. 77–144, 1977.

28. Waritz, R.S. "Biological Indicators of Chemical Dosage and Burden," in *Patty's Industrial Hygiene and Toxicology,* Volume III, L.J. Cralley and L.V. Cralley, Eds. (New York: John Wiley and Sons, 1979).

29. Cole, P. and A.S. Morrison. "Basic Issues in Cancer Screening," paper presented at the UICC Workshop on Screening, Toronto, April 24, 1978.

30. Frankenburg, W.K. "To Screen or Not to Screen: Congenital Dislocation of the Hip," *AJPH* 71: 1311–1313, 1981.

31. Lilienfeld, A.M. "Some Limitations and Problems of Screening for Cancer," *Cancer* 33: 1720–1724, 1974.

32. Fuscaldo, K.E. "Genetic Monitoring," in *Laboratory Safety: Theory and Practice,* A.A. Fuscaldo, B.J. Erlick, and B. Hindman, Eds. (New York: Academic Press, 1980).

33. Kilian, D.J. "Use of Human Biological Monitoring for Risk Assessment of Mutagenesis and Carcinogenic Effect," in *Safe Handling of Chemical Carcinogens, Mutagens, Teratogens, and Highly Toxic Substances,* Vol. I (Ann Arbor, MI: Ann Arbor Science, 1980) pp. 247–258.

34. Biotechnology, Inc. OSHA Medical Surveillance Requirements and NIOSH Recommendations, prepared for the National Aeronautics and Space Administration, January 1980.

35. Messinger, H.B., R. Clappo, P. Nolan, and L. Stagner. "An Analysis of Medical Monitoring Data Required by OSHA Health Regulations," U.S. Department of Labor, Report No. ASPER/CON–78/0167/A, 1979.

36. Elkins, H.B. *The Chemistry of Industrial Toxicology* (New York: John Wiley and Sons, 1950).

37. Tracor Jitco, Inc., carcinogenesis bioassay health and safety plan.

38. Tracor Jitco, Inc., site visit reports.

39. Jacykewycz, O. USDA Medical Guidelines for Employees Exposed to Toxic Substances, transcript of a seminar presented March 28, 1978.

40. U.S. Fish and Wildlife Service. Region G. Guidelines for Establishing Laboratory Employees Health Monitoring Programs, no date available.

41. U.S. Fish and Wildlife Service, Columbia National Fisheries Research Laboratory. Laboratory Safety Plan, no date available.

42. U.S. Fish and Wildlife Service, Patuxent Wildlife Research Center. Safety and Health Plan, no date available.

43. U.S. Fish and Wildlife Services, Fish Control Laboratories. Health monitoring program, staff memorandum, September 6, 1977.

44. Naval Medical Training Institute. *Occupational Health Manual,* 1972.

45. Hughes, J.P. "Overview of Medical Surveillance Procedures," American Occupational Medicine Association Postgraduate Seminar 8, April 10, 1978.

46. Makar, A.B. and T.R. Tephly. "Improved Estimation of Formate in Body Fluids and Tissues," *Clin. Chem.* 28: 385, 1982.

47. Beaulieu, H.J., et al. "Formaldehyde: Chronic, Low-Level Exposures—Effects on Formic Acid in Human Urine," abstract of a presentation to the American Industrial Hygiene Association, 1982 (submitted for publication).

CHAPTER 10

Safety Training Programs for Toxicity Testing Laboratories

J. David Sakura
Arthur D. Little, Inc., Acorn Park,
Cambridge, MA 02140

INTRODUCTION

Laboratory personnel involved with toxicology testing may be exposed to numerous chemical and biological hazards that pose serious risks to worker health. A key element in a total health and safety program designed to minimize worker exposure to test materials is a comprehensive safety training program. A well-conceived and properly executed laboratory training program provides the laboratory worker with sufficient practical experience and technical information so that the worker can operate safely within a hazardous work environment.

This chapter deals with the development, objectives, and characteristics of a successful safety training program for laboratory personnel who work with or come into contact with toxic and genotoxic materials. Suggested modules for a model safety training program are presented along with a listing of resource materials that can be used to enhance a training program.

DEVELOPMENT OF A LABORATORY SAFETY TRAINING PROGRAM

Requirements and Needs for Training

The handling of hazardous materials such as chemical carcinogens in a toxicology testing laboratory must be performed in such a manner as to minimize worker exposure to these chemicals. This important health and safety objective can be achieved by establishing a program of laboratory work practices and using selected engineering controls. Additionally, in order to meet these objectives, a laboratory safety training program must be organized and presented since training has long been recognized as the fundamental method for effecting self-protection in the workplace[1].

For most laboratory personnel this training includes several years of informal instruction in the safe handling of chemicals while enrolled in undergraduate and graduate science courses. Besides informal training, courses in laboratory safety are becoming increasingly more common in the undergraduate curriculum [2, 3]. Thus, new laboratory employees are likely to have received fairly extensive general training in the proper handling of chemicals in the laboratory. However, additional instruction and training in the proper handling of specific test chemicals will be necessary to provide workers with an adequate degree of protection.

Besides voluntarily offering employee training, laboratories are often required by federal, state, and local regulations to provide employee training in steps necessary to reduce the risk associated with handling hazardous materials. The National Cancer Institute safety standards [4] and the National Institutes of Health laboratory safety guidelines [5] encourage training of all employees who are working with or may potentially come into contact with chemical carcinogens. In keeping with these guidelines, health and safety minimum requirements for the National Toxicology Program (NTP) call for NTP laboratories to provide documentation of an employee training program.

Objectives of a Laboratory Training Program

Because of the uniqueness of many of the chemicals under investigation, a training program must be responsive to the special needs of a worker involved with toxicity testing. Thus the objectives of a laboratory training program should be to enable laboratory personnel to work safely and to understand the potential hazards in the workplace. The following are some specific objectives for a laboratory training program:

- To provide information and instruction regarding the personal hazards associated with the activities in a laboratory. Information regarding the potential hazards associated with areas where toxic and genotoxic materials are used is especially important for new employees. Often these individuals may have had limited experience working with these hazardous materials, and thus may be unfamiliar with or unaware of the degree of hazards involved. In addition, a new employee training program should also clearly articulate the safety policies of the laboratory, and the shared responsibilities of the supervisor and staff should be clearly understood.
- To provide specific instruction in the necessary personal precautions that must be taken while working in a high-hazard laboratory. Each laboratory should have a well-defined set of standard operating practices (SOPs) that must be conveyed in an understandable fashion. Included in the SOPs are details on recommended laboratory practices and engineering controls that are designed to limit worker exposure.
- To overcome and correct deficiencies in improper laboratory practices. Proper use of protective clothing and equipment should be reviewed on a regular basis.

Personal hygiene including laboratory policies regarding eating, smoking, and drinking in the laboratory should be addressed.

- To increase safety awareness among all laboratory personnel. In order to prevent accidents or injury in the laboratory, a training program must encourage the person to act in a safe manner at all times. This behavior requires both heightened safety awareness by the individual and a positive attitude regarding safety among all laboratory personnel[6].
- To provide laboratory personnel with updated health and safety information. Regular training sessions offer the opportunity to disseminate new information on laboratory safety and health hazards in a timely manner. This information, if properly presented, can convey to the employee the sense that individual awareness of laboratory safety is a dynamic, ongoing process, and that safety in the laboratory has been given a position of importance in the overall objectives of the laboratory.

The objectives of a laboratory health and safety training program should be tailored to meet the requirements of a particular laboratory. A needs assessment by persons responsible for health and safety in the laboratory may indicate additional training objectives. For example, local conditions such as a number of relatively new, inexperienced workers may initially require special emphasis on one or more training objectives.

Implementation of a Successful Laboratory Safety Training Program

Several recent studies describe the elements of successful safety training programs for the workplace [7, 8]. Because of the nature of the hazards present and the variability in the level of prior training in laboratory safety and health, laboratory personnel present special training problems that must be addressed in order to effect a successful program. The following is a discussion of some of the elements of a training program for laboratory personnel that take into account some of these problem areas.

1. The training program must be tailored to provide baseline information necessary for the worker to perform the assigned tasks. New techniques and procedures must be learned (or relearned) along with instruction in the principles and proper use of special equipment such as glove boxes, blenders, and laminar flow biological safety cabinets. A thorough understanding of the operation of all laboratory equipment is important, since malfunction of equipment, such as hoods or biological safety cabinets, designed to protect the worker is generally first recognized by personnel directly affected.

2. The instruction material should be presented at the highest technical level possible. Because of the high educational level of most laboratory personnel, all training materials (audiovisuals, etc.) must be carefully screened as to their appropriateness of subject matter and level of presentation.

3.   The pedagogical approach should be appropriately geared to the adult level and employee participation should be conducted at a similar level.
4.   Instructions should be given by a senior member of the staff, who is familiar with laboratory procedures, and preferably by one who has had additional training in health and safety.

In a survey of training programs, Heath [9] identified the amount of student participation as an important characteristic in a successful training program. Thus, in planning a laboratory safety training program, considerable attention should be given to the degree and type (active or passive) of student participation. In many learning situations, instruction should follow a three-step process—information, demonstration, and practice. Thus, after instructional material is initially conveyed by lecture, audiovisual or written material, some type of hands-on demonstration should follow, where students would practice the exercise under supervision. Instruction in the proper use of personal protective equipment, e.g., respirators, protective clothing, and fire and emergency response, lends itself well to this approach. Training sessions conducted with the highest level of realism are most effective especially when demonstrating to new employees laboratory procedures and practices.

In general, while audiovisual materials should be an integral part of any training module, the use of audiovisuals should not supersede personal instruction. As a precautionary measure, audiovisual materials should be carefully screened in order to assure that the instructional materials are not presented either too simplistically or condescendingly.

Resource Material for Laboratory Training

Technical information useful as course material for laboratory training programs is readily available from a number of government sources [10–13]. Resource guides and annotated bibliographies are also available for course development [14, 15]. Private organizations like the National Safety Council [16] and the National Fire Protection Association [17] are also ready sources of laboratory health and safety information.

For laboratory supervisory personnel and other key individuals responsible for training, several intensive day-long courses are available. For example, a course entitled "The Safe Handling of Chemical Carcinogens in the Research Laboratory" has been presented on a regular basis by the Illinois Institute of Technology Research. Day-long training courses in the hazards associated with the handling of chemical carcinogens have been developed by the National Institutes of Health and by the National Cancer Institute, Office of Research Safety, Division of Safety. A series of symposia conducted by the Division of Safety at the National Institutes of Health are held annually with each symposium focusing on a specific topic that relates to health and safety in biomedical research facilities [18, 19]. Finally, private organizations such as the American Chemical Society and the National Safety Council annually sponsor training programs in laboratory safety and health.

Audiovisual materials should be an integral part of any training session. A listing of government and special audiovisual materials in occupational safety and health is available [20], and many of these films can be obtained from the National Audio-visual Center, Washington, D.C. [21]. Private sources of audiovisual material include the National Safety Council, manufacturers of safety equipment, chemical supply houses, and commercial audiovisual supply houses.

A Modular Approach to Laboratory
Safety Training Programs

A modular approach offers considerable flexibility in developing a laboratory safety training program that meets the particular training needs of a laboratory. This method involves: (1) selection of modules based upon factors such as the nature of the chemical, biological and physical hazards, the profile of the employee, past health and safety injury and illness data; (2) a teaching approach that uses appropriate materials and teaching methods; and (3) evaluation of the effectiveness of the training program. Evaluation could include the degree of compliance of government regulations, scores in laboratory safety inspections, or a decrease in laboratory-related injury and illnesses.

A MODEL LABORATORY SAFETY TRAINING
PROGRAM

The following is an example of a modular approach to training, adopted from a program developed by the National Institute of Environmental Health Sciences (NIEHS) Office of Health and Safety. Course objectives, suggested topics, and related audiovisual material are given for each module.

- *Module I: Introduction to Laboratory Health and Safety*
  Objective: To introduce new employees to the policies of the laboratory and outline the responsibilities of employer and employee.
  Topics: Safety awareness; employer/employee responsibilities.
  Suggested audiovisual: "Safety. Isn't It Worth It?" (Film Communicators, North Hollywood, California).
- *Module II: Personal Protection*
  Objective: To train employees in the proper use of personal protective equipment.
  Topics: Protective clothing including gloves; proper fit and use of respirators; eye protection; and personal hygiene.
  Suggested audiovisual: "Face and Eye Protection in the Chemical Laboratory" (National Society for the Prevention of Blindness); "MSA Air Purifying Respirator" (Mine Safety Appliance Co., Pittsburgh, Pennsylvania).
- *Module III: Operational Practices*
  Objective: To acquaint the employee with the proper use of laboratory hoods, biological safety cabinets, and other work practices.

Topics: Laboratory ventilation; clean and dirty work areas; housekeeping; and good laboratory work practices.

Suggested audiovisual: "Nobody's Perfect" (National Audio-visual Film Center); "Effective Use of Laminar Flow Biological Safety Cabinets" (National Audio-visual Film Center).

- *Module IV: Emergency Response*
  Objective: To train employees in the proper response to fires and chemical emergencies.
  Topics: Decontamination and cleanup of chemical spills; fire extinguishers; and safety showers.
  Suggested audiovisual: "28 Grams of Prevention" (Film Communicators, North Hollywood, California); "Using Fire Extinguishers the Right Way" (National Fire Protection Association, Quincy, Massachusetts); "The First Two Minutes—Firefighting with a Hand Portable Extinguisher" (The Ansul Company, Marinette, Wisconsin); "Seconds Count" (BNA Communications Inc., Rockville, Maryland).

- *Module V: Principles of Toxicology and Risk Assessment*
  Objective: To discuss basic principles of toxicology and risk assessment.
  Topics: Classification of chemical agents; routes of exposure; consequences of exposure; and evaluation of risk.
  Suggested audiovisual: "Assessment of Risk in Cancer Virus Laboratory" (National Audio-visual Center).

- *Module VI: Hazards Found in Bioassay Laboratories*
  Objective: To instruct in the proper handling of laboratory test animals.
  Topics: Hazards and risks associated with animal handling; proper laboratory procedures in dose preparation and administration; animal facility maintenance.
  Suggested audiovisual: "Hazard Control in the Animal Laboratory" (National Audio-visual Center).

RESEARCH NEEDS IN LABORATORY SAFETY TRAINING

Measures of Effectiveness of Training

A long-standing premise of training programs has been that by providing information and instruction in job safety and health, hazards in the workplace can be reduced. However, most recent studies on the effectiveness of training do not indicate a direct or clear-cut effect of training on reducing injury and illnesses in the workplace [9, 22]. Surry [23] concluded that training apparently reduces accident liability during the first few months of employment, but that training does not have a long-term effect on accident rates. Safety training apparently speeds up the "rate of acquisition of skills, which also occurs during on-the-job experience."

New attention should therefore be given to devising better methods for evaluating the effectiveness of laboratory training programs. In general the evaluation process should enhance existing programs by: (1) identifying the strengths and weaknesses of a training module: (2) measuring how closely the training module fulfilled the stated objectives; and (3) documenting the short and long-term effects on changes in employee attitude and behavior. Based upon these evaluation criteria, new training modules can be developed or existing programs changed. Interactive computer-based learning modules offer a partial solution to the need for more suitable measures of training effectiveness. Thus the self-pacing feature of an interactive learning system allows trainees to proceed based upon an immediate evaluation of their learning progress. Other attractive features of a computer-based training program are: presentation of subject matter that can be tailored to meet the user's information requirements, and instructional strategies that can be varied and presented in a manner that holds the trainee's attention.

Custom-made Training Modules on Video Tape

Besides individualized computer-based instruction programs, custom-made video tapes offer the potential for adding a personalized dimension to the instructional material used for laboratory safety training [24]. By developing training modules and presenting them on video tapes, the format and content of the training session can be tailored to the needs of the viewer audience. In the case of those aspects of laboratory training which involve highly specialized work practices, video taping of the actual work procedure adds a level of realism not possible with other audiovisuals. This feature is especially important for new employees, since they can readily access the video tape and can repeatedly review the training material, until the procedure is thoroughly understood.

SUMMARY

A laboratory safety training program is an important element in the health and safety program for toxicity testing laboratories. A well-conceived and properly executed training program requires a clear understanding of the interrelationships between program objectives, course content, and approaches to learning. Because of the wide variety of potential course materials currently available from governmental and private sources, special attention must be given to selection of training materials that are appropriate for highly trained laboratory personnel. To meet the informational shortcomings found in existing training materials, custom-made training video tapes and computer-based instruction programs can be used to convey to the trainee specialized and up-to-date safety information.

REFERENCES

1 . Cohen, A., M.J. Smith, and W.K. Anger. "Self-protective Measures against Workplace Hazards," *J. Safety Res.* 11:121-131, 1979.

2. Nicholls, L.J. "An Undergraduate Chemical Laboratory Safety Course," *J. Chem. Ed.* 59(10):A301-A304, 1982.

3. Renfrew, M.M., Ed. *Safety in the Chemical Laboratory*, Volume 4 (Easton, PA: J. Chemical Education, 1981).

4. "National Cancer Institute Safety Standards for Research Involving Chemical Carcinogens," DHEW Publication No. (NIH) 77-900, 1975.

5. "National Institutes of Health Guidelines for the Laboratory Use of Chemical Carcinogens," DHHS NIH Publication No. 81-2385.

6. Martin, J.C. "Behavioral Factors in Laboratory Safety: Personnel Characteristics and the Modification of Unsafe Acts," in *Laboratory Safety—Theory and Practice*, A.A. Fuscaldo, B.J. Erlick, and B. Hindman, Eds. (New York: Academic Press, 1980), p. 322.

7. Heath, E.D. "Worker Training and Education in Occupational Safety and Health: A Report on Practice in Six Industrialized Western Nations, Part III," *J. Safety Res.* 13:121-131, 1982.

8. Smith, M.J., H.H. Cohen, A. Cohen, and R.J. Cleveland. "Characteristics of Successful Safety Programs," *J. Safety Res.* 10:5-15, 1978.

9. Heath, E.D. "Worker Training and Education in Occupational Safety and Health: A Report on Practice in Six Industrialized Western Nations, Part III," *J. Safety Res.* 13:73-87, 1982.

10. "Laboratory Safety Monography. A Supplement to the NIH Guidelines for Recombinant DNA Research," DHEW (NIH), 1979.

11. DHEW. *National Institute of Health Biohazards Safety Guide* (Washington, D.C.: U.S. Government Printing Office, 1974).

12. "Working Safely with Flammables and Combustible Liquids," DHEW (NIOSH) 78-206, 1975.

13. "Carcinogens—Regulation and Control: Working with Carcinogens—A Guide to Good Health Practices," DHEW (NIOSH) 77-206, 1977.

14. "Laboratory Safety Publications and Training Aids: An Annotated Bibliography," DHHS (NIH) Administrative Document, 1981.

15. "A Resource Guide to Worker Education Materials in Occupational Safety and Health," U.S. Department of Labor (OSHA), 1982.

16. Gatwood, G. and L. Oldendorf, Eds. "Research and Development Safety Notebook," (Chicago: National Safety Council, 1976).

17. National Fire Protection Association, Inc. "Fire Protection for Laboratories Using Chemicals," Batterymarch Park, Quincy, MA, NFPA 45-1982.

18. "Laboratory Ventilation for Hazard Control," proceedings of a Cancer Research Safety Symposium, October 21-22, 1976, NIH Publication No. 82-1293, 1982.

19. "Management of Hazardous Chemical Wastes in Research Institutions," proceedings of the 1981 NIH Research Safety Symposium, May 20-21, 1981, NIH Publication No. 82-2459.

20. "Audio-visual Resources in Occupational Safety and Health: An Evaluative Guide," DHHS (NIOSH) Publication No. 82-102, 1981.

21. "A Reference List of Audio-visual Materials Produced by the United States Government, Supplement 1980," General Services Administration, National Audio-visual Center (Washington, D.C.: U.S. Government Printing Office, 1980).

22. Pfeifer, C.M. "An Evaluation of Policy Related Research on Effectiveness of Alternative Methods to Reduce Occupational Illnesses and Accidents," a study prepared with the support of the National Science Foundation, 1974.
23. Surry, J. "Industrial Accident Research: A Human Engineering Appraisal," Department of Industrial Engineering, University of Toronto, June, 1969.
24. Cohen, K.S. "The Video tape Revolution," *Occupation. Health Safety* 51 (7): 9-12, 1982.

CHAPTER 11

A Respirator Protection Program for Toxicology Laboratories

Joseph A. Coco
Office of Occupational Safety and Health,
Litton Bionetics, Inc.,
5516 Nicholson Lane, Kensington, Maryland 20895

INTRODUCTION

The purpose of this chapter is to provide information and guidance to the reader who may need to develop, implement, and administer a respiratory protection program in an industrial toxicology laboratory. Translating Occupational Safety and Health Administration (OSHA) regulations into practice is never an easy task; this may be especially true for the professional whose specialty is not occupational health and safety. At present, there are no OSHA industry standards for laboratories per se; therefore, many of the health and safety regulations need to be adapted from applicable general industry or specific industry standards. The OSHA standard for respiratory protection is an example of a general industry standard. This chapter seeks to highlight the key elements of a respiratory protection program and discuss the specific problem areas that arise from the nature of toxicology research. At times these specific problems make compliance with some of the elements of an OSHA-acceptable respiratory protection program difficult.

The toxicology laboratory has recently emerged as a significant "industry" in its own right. As a result, increasing numbers of people are employed in an occupation which health and safety professionals consider a unique working environment. That is, no other industry offers to the worker an environment in which there is a risk of exposure to such a wide variety of chemical substances. Some types of chemicals tested include: solvents, intermediates, pesticides, pharmaceuticals, fuels (both natural and synthetic), plasticizers, food additives, cosmetics, biocides, explosives, and pigments.

The safe conduct of toxicology studies therefore requires the consideration of many factors, one of the most important being the quality of air in the work environment. Airborne contaminants found in the workplace constitute perhaps the single greatest job-related hazard to laboratory workers, especially in regard to potential long-term consequences. Thus, major efforts must be made to recognize, evaluate, and control this hazard.

Many activities, routine operations, and emergency situations can generate airborne contaminants which can present health risks to researchers, technicians, animal care staff, and other support personnel. Various types of routine operations which can produce significant airborne contamination include: weighing, transferring, grinding, and blending of neat chemicals; dispensing of dosed feed[1]; dumping of contaminated bedding and dosed feed. Other activities which can pose an inhalation hazard are the removal of dosed animals from inhalation chambers, skin painting or gavaging animals with volatile test materials, and handling freshly dosed animals and contaminated caging materials. Emergencies must also be considered. These contingencies include chemical spills, leaks, and fires. The hazard may be in the form of a gas, vapor, aerosol, or any combination of these. Accordingly, several recognized methods for controlling and minimizing employee exposure to hazardous materials have been developed.

Methods for controlling airborne hazards include engineering controls such as general dilution ventilation, local exhaust ventilation, chemical fume hoods, and carcinogen hoods (class II type B biological safety cabinets). Other methods of control include isolation by means of special containment devices such as glove boxes. The approaches to controlling airborne hazards are not limited to engineering systems; other supplementary approaches involve proper work practices, procedures, and techniques. Quite often respirators are employed to supplement other control methods, especially when operational conditions cannot be totally controlled by engineering and administrative methods. Respiratory protection is also employed when these methods are not readily applicable or practicable[2]. In addition, it is not always economically feasible to create and maintain engineering controls[3]. Respiratory protection, however, should not be considered a substitute for engineering control methods. Respirators are primary protective devices for normal operations only when no other method of control is possible[4]. Therefore, the use of respirators is an acceptable method of control only after consideration of all factors involved, and when current engineering and administrative control methodology cannot completely eliminate hazards. Such is the case for some aspects of toxicology research.

RESPIRATORY PROTECTIVE EQUIPMENT

Respiratory protective devices vary in design, application, and protective capability. Therefore, the user must assess the respiratory hazard and understand the specific uses and limitations of available equipment to ensure proper selection[3]. A discussion of some of the major types of respirators currently available will be beneficial to those not totally familiar with this approach to hazard control.

Respirators may be broadly classified as either negative-pressure or positive-pressure devices, each class having various types and configurations[5]. As the terminology implies, a negative-pressure respirator creates negative pressure inside the facepiece when the wearer draws air into the lungs through air-purifying elements or certain types of clean-air supplying valves or tubing. Because the pressure inside the facepiece is negative with respect to the user's environment, it is very important that the face-to-facepiece seal be "tight" to prevent inward leakage of contaminated air [5]. A positive-pressure respirator maintains a positive pressure inside the facepiece through a valve system from a source of compressed air that forces air into the respirator under pressure. Because the pressure differential is positive, the face-to-facepiece seal is less critical. Any leakage that might occur will usually be outward, thereby maintaining an uncontaminated atmosphere in the respirator. However, inward leakage can occur even with positive-pressure devices[5].

In general, respiratory protective equipment falls into two basic categories, according to the method of operation[4]:

1.   air-purifying devices: (a) particulate-removing (mechanical filter) type; (b) gas- and vapor-removing (chemical media) type; and (c) combination particulate-removing and gas/vapor-removing type
2.   supplied-air devices: (a) air-line respirators (using a source of filtered, compressed air or compressed oxygen) of continous flow, demand flow, or pressure demand type; and (b) self-contained breathing apparatus (using a portable source of air worn by the user) of closed-circuit (recirculating) or open-circuit (demand or pressure-demand) type.

Air-Purifying Respirators

An air-purifying respirator is one that removes contaminants from the ambient air. The purification of the air is accomplished by mechanically filtering out particulate contaminants with fibrous media or by removing contaminating gases or vapors by chemical means [6]. Cartridges, canisters, and other filters are employed for this purpose.

Air-purifying respirators generally operate in the negative-pressure mode. Although the device is used in conjunction with a tight-fitting facepiece seal, the negative pressure results in various degrees of penetration of contaminants into the respirator. Full-facepiece respirators generally allow less penetration through the seal than half-facepiece respirators. Properly fitted half-face respirators may leak up to 10%; properly fitted full-facepiece respirators, up to 1%. Therefore, since an inherent characteristic of the design of this category of respirator is that the facepiece is under negative pressure during inhalation, some leakage is expected. The limitations placed upon the several types of air-purifying respirators are based primarily upon the ability to obtain an initial fit of the respirator, maintain the quality of fit during wearing, and not exceed the use limitations of the facepiece and air-purifying media.[7]

Air-purifying media consist of fibrous filters or sorbents contained in suitable protective housings (filter holders, cartridges, or canisters). A filter is a fibrous medium used for the removal of aerosols, that is, airborne solid or liquid particulates. There are many classes of mechanical filters specifically designed for various classes of airborne particulate matter. However, none of these filters provides protection against gases, vapors, or oxygen deficiency [7]. It should be noted that attempts to protect the worker by means of a surgical mask are inadequate because such a mask provides poor protection against inhaled aerosols [8] and no protection against vapors and gases. The service life of a particulate filter is limited by the amount of material that can be retained before the resistance to inhalation increases significantly [6]. Sorbents of various types are used for removing gases and vapors from the air stream [9]. Generally activated charcoal or impregnated charcoal is used as the adsorbent for organic compounds, but for some compounds, especially those of low molecular weight and high volatility, charcoal provides little protection to the user [10]. It has been shown that not all organic vapors behave the same when adsorbed on activated charcoal. Variations in concentration, amount of carbon, relative humidity, temperature, and breathing rate all influence the rate at which these vapors are adsorbed [6, 11-16]. Efficiency also varies with vapor pressure, boiling point, molecular weight and structure, and polarizability of the air contaminant [13, 17].

The evaluation of respirator cartridges and canisters for their efficiency to adsorb organic vapors has become increasingly important. As new exposure guidelines are established by toxicity testing, concern about the protective capacity of air-purifying respirators against these vapors in the work environment arises [18]. All cartridges and canisters are labeled for respiratory protection against specific gases and vapors and their maximum use concentration. Each is also color-coded to indicate the type of protection afforded. The OSHA regulation on respiratory protection requires that approved or accepted respiratory protective devices be used where respiratory protection is required [19]. The National Institute for Occupational Safety and Health (NIOSH) is responsible for approving and listing respiratory protective devices [20, 21]. The most frequently used respirators in the toxicology laboratory are those approved for "organic vapors" which may be also rated for other contaminants such as acid gases or pesticides. Many users feel that such devices guarantee effectiveness against all organic vapors [16]. This is not necessarily true, especially when one discovers that cartridges and canisters stamped "NIOSH/MESA Approved" (MESA, Mine Enforcement Safety Administration) for organic vapors have passed a test that is based on performance against only one air contaminant—carbon tetrachloride. The ability of a respirator cartridge or canister to adsorb other chemicals may be greater or less than that of carbon tetrachloride [22]. Respirator cartridge evaluations have been performed for many different organic vapors [11, 13, 17, 18, 23]. The breakthrough time which is the basis for these evaluations is a complex function of the chemical vapor or gas, the activated carbon, and the prevailing experimental conditions [16]. Equations have been developed which can be used to calculate breakthrough time for cartridges and canisters [11, 14, 16]. Although it has been suggested that the industrial hygienist use experimentally derived breakthrough times to establish the service life of an air-purifying device [11], this may not be practical in the toxicology laboratory because of time constraints. Even if breakthrough times were experimentally determined or calculated, such information would be of limited value for this type of work environment for the following reasons: (1) airborne levels can vary between operations and within operations; (2) personnel typically wear the same cartridges (or canister) in a variety of different chemically contaminated atmospheres; and (3) humidity levels (which significantly affect adsorption capacity) can vary greatly in different operations. In addition, breakthrough times can vary significantly for an air contaminant with the same kind of cartridge but made by different manufacturers [18]. Because of the many variables involved with accurately predicting the service life of these devices in the field, the prevailing rule of thumb indicates that a cartridge or canister can be used until the contaminant vapor is detected inside the mask [16, 22]. At times this may not be adequate because olfactory sensitivities can vary widely among individuals. Even those individuals with good olfactory senses may experience olfactory fatigue [22]. Because of the sensory limitations of the wearer, air-purifying respirators are usually not recommended for protection against vapors and gases that have poor warning properties as it is possible for the user to be exposed to excessive concentrations without knowing it [2]. If the odor threshold (or other sensory information such as taste or irritation) is greater than its threshold limit value (TLV), then the chemical is said to have poor warning properties. Use practices are recommended for chemical cartridge respirators for various groupings of compounds, based on their odor-threshold-to-TLV ratio [2]. Because of the many limitations [6, 7] on the use of air-purifying devices, these types of respirators must be used in strict accordance with the manufacturer's instructions and warnings.

Supplied-Air Respirators

An atmosphere-supplied respirator is one that furnishes respirable air or oxygen to the wearer from an uncontaminated supply such as a compressed breathing air or oxygen cylinder, an oxygen-generating canister, or a breathing air compressor that draws its supply from an uncontaminated ambient atmosphere. This type includes air-line respirators and self-contained breathing apparatus.

Air-line respirators provide protection against contaminants by providing an adequate supply of respirable air by any of the following modes of operation: continuous flow, demand flow, and pressure demand flow [6]. Continuous flow and pressure demand flow are positive-pressure devices whereas demand flow is a negative-pressure device. Air is supplied in an air-line respirator through a hose to a half facepiece, full facepiece, hood, helmet, or suit. The quality [24] and quantity [6] of air going to the facepiece must meet prescribed specifications. Special precautions must be taken to prevent extraneous air contaminants, especially carbon monoxide, from entering the air supply [6]. Other precautions, such as proper air pressures and the use of ancillary equipment, must be taken to ensure safe use of these devices [7].

Air-line respirators can be used in atmospheres not immediately dangerous to life or health, especially where working conditions demand continuous use of a respirator [6, 7]. Although most atmosphere-supplying respirators are capable of providing protection against high concentrations of many toxicants, no device is 100% effective [6, 25]. Some leakage into the facepiece may occur. Many of the air-line devices employing a tight-fitting facepiece use the same basic facepiece as many of the air-purifying respirators, and thus have some of the same limitations. Two additional limitations are (1) there is no respiratory protection if the air supply fails unless there is an auxiliary supply available; and (2) the air hose limits travel distance.

These limitations preclude their use as emergency and rescue devices [6]. As is the case with all safety equipment, these devices must be used within the limits set by the manufacturer.

A self-contained breathing apparatus (SCBA) consists of a respirator with the supply of air, oxygen, or oxygen-generating material carried by the wearer. These devices can be either open-circuit, such that exhaled air passes to the ambient atmosphere through the facepiece exhaust valve, or closed-circuit (recirculating) wherein the carbon dioxide is removed from the exhaled air, oxygen is added, and the recycled air is rebreathed. An open-circuit SCBA uses compressed air, compressed oxygen, liquid air, or liquid oxygen. A closed-circuit SCBA uses compressed, liquid, or chemically generated oxygen. Compressed oxygen is never to be used in an open-circuit SCBA in which compressed air has previously been used. Compressed air might contain slight amounts of oil that would coat orifice housings; oxygen passing through such an orifice under high pressure could cause an explosion or fire [6].

SCBAs generally provide the highest level of respiratory protection currently available. They can be either negative- or positive-pressure devices, but most are positive-pressure. The demand open-circuit SCBA, like the demand air-line respirator, is under negative pressure during initial inspiration by the wearer until the demand valve opens and pressurizes the facepiece with supplied air. The possibility of facepiece leakage with this type of unit places serious limitations on its use [6]. Because of the low protection provided by the demand SCBA and the availability of adequate substitutes, it has been recommended that they may not be used and further, that NIOSH delete the approval schedule for them [26]. The basic limitation of SCBAs is the length of time that each of these devices can be used. This is limited by the air or oxygen supply that the wearer can carry. In order to use this type of respiratory protection safely, the manufacturer's instructions must be followed. Units are assigned nominal ratings for the length of time they would protect the average person doing moderately heavy work. It must be emphasized that these ratings serve only as a guide and that the air supply can be consumed more rapidly in a stress situation. Therefore, these units are provided with a warning device (e.g., a bell) that indicates when the remaining service life has been reduced to the point that the wearer should return to an uncontaminated atmosphere. Further limitations on the use of SCBAs may be attributed to their size and weight, especially for work in confined spaces. They are, however, the respirator of choice for emergencies and high-hazard work.

It must be remembered that all respirators have limitations; no respirator is capable of providing absolute protection. There is one limitation applicable to all respiratory equipment—certain gaseous contaminants can enter the body by means other than the respiratory tract [7]. For those materials that can penetrate skin special "impermeable" protective clothing must be worn to prevent systemic poisoning. However, this clothing is incapable of providing complete protection. As with all safety equipment, effective use begins with an understanding of the uses and limitations of the equipment. Above all, the equipment must be selected in a manner which ensures the proper level of protection for a given level of hazard.

NEED AND SELECTION

OSHA regulations [19] obligate the employer to provide employees with respiratory protective devices when they are needed. These regulations also obligate the employee to use the provided respiratory protective equipment in accordance with instructions and training. OSHA permissible practices and requirements for a minimally acceptable respiratory protection program are summarized as follows:

1. written standard operating procedures governing the selection and use of respirators
2. respirator selection based on the hazard to which the worker is exposed
3. instruction and training in the use and limitations of the respirator
4. assignment of respirators to individuals for their exclusive use, where practicable
5. regular cleaning and disinfection of respirators
6. storage of respirators in a convenient, clean, and sanitary location
7. inspection of routinely used respirators during cleaning; replacement of worn or deteriorated parts; inspection of emergency respirators at least once a month and after each use
8. maintenance of appropriate surveillance of work area conditions and degree of employee exposure and stress
9. regular inspection and evaluation to determine the continued effectiveness of the program
10. assignment of tasks requiring respirators exclusively to persons who are physically able to perform the work and use the equipment; a physician's screening of problematic health conditions
11. use of NIOSH/MESA-approved respirators

Each of these criteria must be met to have a respiratory protection program that is acceptable to OSHA. Most of these requirements are fairly straightforward and present little difficulty for implementation. However, in the toxicology laboratory, two major difficulties emerge: (1) the selection of the respirator on the basis of hazard to which the worker is exposed, and (2) the maintenance of appropriate surveillance of the degree of exposure. The major reason for these problems is that many chemicals received for toxicity testing have incomplete chemical identification and little or no physical, chemical, safety, or health data. This is especially true for chemicals received for genotoxicity studies. The majority of commercial test materials submitted by clients for these types of studies are identified only by a code designation. Few material safety data sheets submitted by clients identify chemical class or family, much less the identity of the test material. As such, many of the entries on these material safety data sheets are left blank by the client. The words "proprietary," "confidential," and "unknown" frequently appear. It is recognized that in many instances much information on a material safety data sheet would be unavailable or unknown, particularly when the test materials are newly synthesized compounds. However, some basic information should be available such as chemical class or family, solvents, and boiling point and this should be forwarded to the testing laboratory. For fear of divulging trade secrets, little usable information is passed onto the toxicology laboratory. These problems also exist for bioassay studies but, in general, are not as severe. A majority of clients now supply the testing laboratory with some chemical, health, and safety information. Many send material safety data sheets which identify the chemical and give adequate handling and precautionary information on which to make an assessment of risk for respirator selection. The best information tends to come from the larger chemical companies and institutions. However, there continue to be instances when little or no information is sent by the client. This precludes an accurate risk assessment. This is especially problematic in bioassay studies where the exposure potential for workers is greater than in *in vitro* studies. In these instances, respirator selection becomes complicated. Also, industrial hygiene air monitoring becomes difficult, if not impossible, to perform, and therefore precludes an accurate assessment of the degree of exposure. In order to safeguard the worker from these variables, respiratory protection should be based on maximum hazard from known chemicals that have been used before in similar situations. This approach should provide an extra margin of safety.

Proper assessment of respiratory hazards is essential to determine proper protective measures. For known chemicals which may present an inhalation hazard, respirator selection is based on a risk assessment that considers many factors. The "Joint NIOSH/OSHA Standards Completion Program, Respiratory Decision Logic" [27] provides a systematic approach to respirator selection. The purpose of the decision logic is to ensure technical accuracy and consistency in the selection of respirators and to provide necessary criteria to support this selection. It is basically a step-by-step elimination of inappropriate respirators until only those which are acceptable remain. Criteria include: permissible exposure limits for the chemical (OSHA PELs, ACGIH TLVs, and NIOSH recommendations), warning properties for gases or vapors, eye and skin irritation potential, LFL (lower flammable limit), IDLH (immediately dangerous to life and health) concentration, and physical and chemical properties [28] of the substance. Other considerations are sorbent limitations of cartridges and canisters and toxicological, health, safety, and research information on the chemical. Conditions under which the respirator would be used greatly influence the selection process. Such conditions include routine use, entry into and exit from unknown concentrations, firefighting, and escape. Also considered are industrial hygiene air-sampling data (when available) and work conditions. Although use of this information will greatly assist in choosing the appropriate respirator for the situation, there are many instances, particularly with newly synthesized chemicals, in which much of this data will not be available. In these situations, professional judgment, based on the best available information and hazard assessment techniques, must be relied upon.

MEDICAL ASSESSMENT

After the hazard has been assessed and the appropriate respirator selected, it is necessary to assess the health status of the wearer. A physical examination including a pulmonary function test is performed by the medical department on each prospective respirator user. The results of these tests, together with the medical history, are reviewed by a physician in order to ensure that the employee is capable of wearing respiratory protective equipment. The respirator user's medical status is then reviewed periodically. Adequate medical supervision of respirator users is indispensable in determining the extent of individual stress tolerance and in preventing adverse physiological consequences[2, 6].

It has been determined that persons with certain medical disorders and conditions may be at risk when wearing a respiratory protective device. Because of the added stress placed on the cardiopulmonary system, some pathological conditions (especially those associated with hypoxemia) should preclude the use of respirators. Limitations on the use of these devices would be the presence of other cardiovascular or systemic diseases which might be exacerbated [6].

Of prime importance to the industrial physician is the need to evaluate subjects with pulmonary and cardiovascular disorders which may prove detrimental to their health and safety or that of other workers if they are required to wear a respirator [29]. The following clinical conditions are among those most likely to be investigated by the examining physician in determining an individual's fitness for respirator use [6]:

- chronic obstructive and restrictive lung disease: chronic bronchitis, emphysema, pneumoconiosis, fibrothorax, asthma, etc.
- ischemic heart disease: coronary insufficiency and myocardial infarction
- benign and accelerated hypertension
- hemorrhagic disorders: vascular hemophilia, hypersplenism, thrombocytopenia, purpura, etc.
- thyroid disorders or cystic fibrosis
- epilepsy: grand mal, focal, etc.
- diabetes mellitus
- cerebrovascular accidents
- facial abnormalities
- kidney diseases
- conductive and sensorineural hearing loss
- serious defects in visual acuity
- ruptured eardrum

In addition, other factors should be investigated such as claustrophobia or anxiety during the wearing of a respirator [6]. It is not unusual that claustrophobic reactions might not be detected when a device is first worn or during the fit-testing procedure. For the industrial toxicology laboratory, most respirator users would not be likely to have many of the above-mentioned medical problems. This might be attributed to their young age and nonexposure to typical industrial settings. The importance of claustrophobia, anxiety, and other psychological factors should not be overlooked in a medical assessment. As yet, the physician is unable to discern the psychological traits best suited to the use of a respirator, especially in critical situations. Without such screening, persons psychologically unsuited to wearing respirators may be in situations in which they become a danger to themselves and others [29]. These psychological problems, particularly claustrophobia, may be relatively more frequent for laboratory workers than the physiological problems. Therefore, prospective respirator users must show evidence that the wearing of respiratory protective devices will not produce undue physical or psychological stress or risk.

By reason of the design features necessary to provide protection, the respirator imparts a significant physiological load on the user's pulmonary system [30]. In a recent review it was concluded that the primary means by which respirator wear manifests itself is the production of an altered pulmonary response to work [29]. This altered response is a result of the increased resistance to inspired and expired flow produced by the respirator. How well an individual responds to an altered pulmonary response indicates whether he or she can wear a respirator [31].

Medical surveillance, including bioassay surveillance when applicable, of respirator wearers should be carried out periodically to determine if respirator wearers are receiving adequate respiratory protection. A physician should determine the requirements of the surveillance program. Also, a physician should determine what physical and psychological conditions are pertinent for the wearing of the different types of respirators. The respirator program administrator or his or her designee, using guidelines established by a physician, should determine whether or not a person can be assigned a task requiring the use of respirators [7].

Fit-Test Procedures

Each employee who is medically able to wear a respirator must be fit-tested with the respirator to ensure proper fit. Simply stated, respirator fit is the ability of the device to interface with the wearer in such a way as to prevent the workplace atmosphere from entering the facepiece [5]. If contaminated air enters the facepiece via an inadequate face-to-facepiece seal, exposure occurs. However, in the real world, respirators have limitations on providing and maintaining a tight face-to-facepiece seal.

Many characteristics of the face can adversely affect the seal of a respirator facepiece [6]. Some of these include facial hair [32], the shape and size of the nose, small chin, missing dentures, hollow temples or cheeks, scars, or excessive wrinkles that may provide a channel for contaminated air to enter the breathing zone [6]. The large variety of human facial characteristics makes face mask design a difficult problem. Thus, a properly fitting face mask depends upon proper design and sizing [33]. The designer must endeavor to produce equipment which will fit the contours of as large a number as possible of an infinite variety of human faces [34]. It should be noted that while the facial and head dimensions of the civilian Caucasian male population are now reasonably well known, the female and non-Caucasian industrial population is not. Furthermore, an increasing segment of these groups is required to wear respirators, but anthropometric surveys to provide the necessary design criteria are unavailable or include a different population than the one at risk [33]. The design of a respirator has a great deal of influence on the relative degree of comfort experienced by the wearer. An uncomfortable mask will be adjusted less tightly than a comfortable one. The results of one study showed a positive correlation between comfort and respirator performance [35]. Another showed that the performance of half-face respirators was directly related to the tension of the head band straps [36]. Los Alamos researchers have demonstrated that many activities associated with normal work can also adversely affect a respirator's performance. These include smiling, talking, moving one's head, and deep breathing associated with heavy work [32]. Thus, it can be seen that there are many problems involved with attaining and maintaining a tight face-to-facepiece seal.

All respirators, regardless of type, allow a small amount of outside air to leak into the facepiece. This will vary with class of respirator (positive- or negative-pressure) and type. Therefore, to effectively use respirators as a means of hazard control, assessment must be made of the exposure resulting from a less than perfect fit. Such a fit can be considered satisfactory upon successful completion of the fit-test procedures. There are three major methods used to assess respirator fit: positive and negative pressure checks, qualitative fit-tests, and quantitative fit-tests. Each method has its uses and limitations, advantages and disadvantages. Initial steps in the fit-testing are the pressure checks. The positive pressure check involves having the user close off the exhalation valve with his or her hand and gently exhale into the mask. The fit is considered satisfactory if a slight positive pressure can be built up inside the facepiece without any evidence of outward leakage of air at the face-to-facepiece seal. The negative pressure test involves closing off the inlet openings of the respirator and then inhaling to create a negative pressure inside the facepiece. If the facepiece remains in its slightly collapsed condition and no inward leakage of air is detected, the fit of the respirator is considered satisfactory. These tests are particularly useful to indicate which respirator might fit the individual best. Because of the differences in facial structures, no single brand of respirator is likely to fit all individuals adequately. Therefore, at least two or three different brands should be checked for best fit and comfort. Also, respirators of different sizes should be stocked. Because the pressure tests are capable of detecting only major leaks, they are considered to be the least precise fit-test procedure. The best use of the pressure tests is as a screen to determine which respirators should be checked by the qualitative or quantitative method.

respirator for the individual. These include qualitative and quantitative methods. The qualitative method is the more frequently used method in industry because it is fast, economical, and provides a good indication of proper fit. After the wearer has put on the best-fitting respirator as determined by the pressure tests, the next step in the fit-test procedure involves challenging the face-to-facepiece seal with tracer chemicals. Typically the qualitative test consists of the organic vapor and particulate smoke tests. In the organic vapor tests a swab moistened with isoamyl acetate (banana oil) is moved at a distance of a few inches from the face in a circular motion around the face-to-facepiece seal. If no odor is noticed by the wearer, the seal is considered satisfactory. The next step is the particulate smoke test. A particulate smoke is generated by means of a ventilation smoke tube which is moved similarly about the seal. If the wearer notices no odor and experiences no nose or throat irritation or coughing, then he or she has successfully been fit-tested for that type and brand of respirator. Other qualitative fit-tests can be used, but these are the easiest and fastest.

Quantitative fit-tests are performed infrequently in industry today [5] because they are costly and time-consuming and require specially trained people to perform the tests [37]. The quantitative fit-test is designed to measure the amount of leakage of a tracer substance into the facepiece. Though there are commercially available devices and equipment for this purpose, no uniform methods or instrumentation requirements exist [5]. A typical method involves putting the wearer in a test atmosphere containing a known concentration of the tracer. The test subject wears a specially modified respirator that has a sampling probe attached to the facepiece. The percentage penetration of the tracer is determined by measuring the concentration of tracer outside the facepiece and comparing that to the concentration inside the facepiece. Dioctylphthalate (DOP) is commonly used as a tracer. Sodium chloride aerosols, ethylene gas, and refrigerant 12 have also been used. Quantitative methods do give a precise assessment of facepiece leakage.

At the present time much controversy centers on which testing method is best for respirator fit assessment. There are many who advocate the quantitative methods. However, for the industrial toxicology laboratory, qualitative fit-test methods are more practical and cost-effective and should be adequate. In an industrial setting, however, airborne levels tend to be higher, thereby warranting more precise determination of actual respirator leakage such as that which can be measured through quantitative test procedures.

ISSUANCE AND TRAINING

As part of the respiratory protection program, all employees who are issued respirators must receive initial and periodic training. This training must cover the need for and selection of respirators based on instructions regarding the nature of the hazard; statement on medical limitations restricting the use of respirators; instructions on proper use, care, and maintenance of the respirator; and instructions on coping with emergency situations. The initial and periodic training should be done by a health and safety professional such as an industrial hygienist, safety professional, or health physicist, or by a specially trained person. However, on a day-to-day basis, the supervisor must make certain that respirators are used, cleaned, and maintained properly by the people in his or her charge.

A formal program of instruction, conducted by competent persons, for all respirator users includes the opportunity to handle the respirator, have it fitted properly, and test its face-to-facepiece seal. Proper inspection, maintenance, and repair of respiratory protective equipment is mandatory to ensure success of any respiratory protection program [7]. Instruction in the disassembly and assembly of the respirator, inspection for worn or deteriorated parts and replacement of those parts, and proper cleaning techniques must be emphasized in the training. The goal is to maintain the equipment in a condition providing the same effectiveness it had when it was received from the manufacturer [3]. Trained employees have a greater degree of confidence in their respirators and in their ability to use them properly. Proper training, supplemented by pamphlets, eliminates misinformation and improper practices [38]. Supervisors, as well as workers, must be instructed in all aspects of respiratory protective equipment in order that these devices be used in the safest, most effective manner.

PROGRAM ADMINISTRATION

The development and implementation of a respiratory protection program presents a challenge to the management of an industrial toxicology laboratory. Successful programs are generally administered by one responsible individual (ideally a health and safety professional) who has overall responsibility and authority for the program [3]. However, the major requisite for a functioning and effective program is the wholehearted support of management from the chief executive to the first-line supervisor.

Many needed and well-intentioned respiratory protection programs have been implemented and failed for various reasons. A respiratory protection program, if it is to be effective, requires careful planning and diligent execution. The program must be practical and flexible enough so that people working in a hazardous atmosphere will use the equipment properly and follow the rules readily [39].

The formula for implementation is practical and will work for any personal safety equipment program in any size organization. The basic ingredients are [39]:

1.   thorough evaluation of the hazard and need for protection
2.   strong management support
3.   local union support (when applicable, e.g., for support staff such as engineers and maintenance personnel)
4.   mandatory supervision
5.   complete and honest personal communication with all personnel involved
6.   comprehensive training and educational program in the use, care, and maintenance of the safety equipment
7.   an effective system of evaluating the program

As with any aspect of work, the first-line supervisor is the key individual upon whom the success of the program hinges. It is he or she (along with line and staff management) who must sell and encourage the use of respirators in defined areas or for certain operations. Verbal encouragement is not enough; employees must see management follow the same rules—that is, wear the equipment when it is required [39]. Perhaps the greatest objection to the use of respirators is the degree of supervision required to obtain compliance [40]. A major reason for this is that many workers are more concerned with immediate dangers than with chronic problems that might develop from a lack of respiratory protection. If a person is going to wear personal protective equipment, he or she must be convinced that it is necessary. In the industrial toxicology laboratory, support for health and safety programs, in particular a respiratory protection program, must also come from the scientific staff. Chemists, toxicologists, veterinarians, molecular geneticists, and engineers are held in high regard by technical and nontechnical support staffs. What these professionals consider important tends to be passed on to others. Their active support and participation, especially by assisting health, safety, and medical personnel in problem solving, can be a tremendous asset.

Feedback on how well the program is functioning is necessary if management is to attain effective respiratory protection. Program improvements and elimination of deficiencies cannot be effective unless the program is monitored and evaluated on a continuing basis. Aucoin [39] lists the following techniques to be used in evaluating the effectiveness of the respirator programs:

1. Wearer acceptance: The effectiveness of a respiratory protection program can be largely determined by the degree of worker acceptance. Numerous factors affect the worker's acceptance of respirators. These include comfort, ability to breathe without objectional effort, adequate visibility under all conditions, provisions for wearing prescription glasses if necessary, ability to communicate, ability to perform all tasks without undue interference, and the facepiece fit. How well these problems are resolved can be determined by observing wearers during normal activities and by soliciting their comments. This is the responsibility of the operating supervisor, health and safety professional, and program administrator.

2. Evaluation of respirators in use: Respiratory protection is no better than the respirator in use, even though it is worn conscientiously. Frequent random inspections are conducted by responsible individuals to assure that respirators are properly used, cleaned, and maintained.

3. Evaluation of protection afforded: Biological testing and the periodic physical examinations provide a basis for medical evaluation of the effectiveness of the respirators. Positive evidence of exposure is followed up by the industrial hygienist to determine any relationship to inadequate respiratory protection.

In conclusion, with management support, careful planning, and diligent execution, there is no reason why the objective of a fully functioning and effective respiratory protection program cannot be met. However, we must not forget to actively enlist the understanding and support of the worker. Without this a truly effective program designed to protect the health of workers cannot be achieved.

SUMMARY

The toxicology laboratory has recently emerged as a significant industry. As a result, increasing numbers of people are employed in an occupation which health and safety professionals consider a unique working environment. That is, no other industry offers to the worker an environment in which there is risk of exposure to such a wide variety of chemical substances. Airborne contaminants produced by many common work operations constitute perhaps the single greatest job-related health hazard to laboratory workers. Therefore, major efforts must be made to recognize, evaluate, and control this hazard. Although engineering controls and prudent work practices are the primary approaches to minimizing worker exposure, there are conditions where respirators must be used to supplement other controls in reducing risk. OSHA regulations obligate the employer to provide employees with respirators when needed. This chapter's purpose was to provide information and guidance to the reader who may need to develop, implement, and administer a respiratory protection program in an industrial toxicology laboratory. The establishment of a respiratory protection program that meets OSHA requirements presents a challenge to laboratory management. Many problems can arise for which there are no quick easy answers. Successful programs are generally administered by one person who has overall responsibility and authority for the program. However, the major requisite for a functioning and effective program are the support of management from chief executive to the first-line supervisor and that of the respirator user.

DISCLAIMER

The material presented in this chapter is intended for persons concerned with establishing and maintaining a respiratory protection program. It presents certain information for guidance purposes. However, it is not intended to be all-inclusive in content or scope. In all cases, the current federal regulations, as published in the *Federal Register* and later collected in the *Code of Federal Regulations*, should be carefully studied and those regulations followed explicitly. Only these regulations define the specific requirements that are in force. In addition, the scientific literature must be consulted for up-to-date evaluation of various types of respiratory protective equipment.

ACKNOWLEDGMENT

I would like to express my appreciation to the management and staff of Litton Bionetics, Inc., for their support and preparation of the manuscript.

REFERENCES

1. Sansone, E.B., A.M. Losikoff, and R.A. Pendleton. "Sources and Dissemination of Contamination in Materials Handling Operations," *Am. Ind. Hyg. Assoc. J.* 38(9):433–442, 1977.
2. Reist, P.C. and F. Rex. "Odor Detection and Respirator Cartridge Replacement," *Am. Ind. Hyg. Assoc. J.* 38(10):563–566, 1977.
3. "Establishing and Maintaining an Effective Respiratory Protection Program," National Safety News Reprint, 111. 17–63, April 1971.

4. Olishifski, J.B. "Methods of Control," in *Fundamentals of Industrial Hygiene*, J.B. Olishifski, Ed. (Chicago: National Safety Council, 1979), p. 628.

5. Wilmes, D.P. "Respirator Usage: A Rational Program," *Haz. Mat. Manag. J.* 2(2):18–26, 1981.

6. U.S. Nuclear Regulatory Commission. "Manual of Respiratory Protection Against Airborne Radioactive Materials," NUREG-0041 (Springfield, VA: National Technical Information Service, 1976).

7. Lundin, A.M.,, "Respiratory Protective Equipment," in *Fundamentals of Industrial Hygiene*, J.B. Olishifski, Ed. (Chicago: National Safety Council, 1979), pp. 709–756.

8. Meiners, A.F. "Preparation of Carcinogen Monographs," in *Safe Handling of Chemical Carcinogens, Mutagens, Teratogens and Highly Toxic Substances*, Vol. 1, D.B. Walters, Ed. (Ann Arbor, MI: Ann Arbor Science, 1980), p. 295.

9. American Industrial Hygiene Association and the American Conference of Governmental Industrial Hygienists Joint Committee on Respirators. "Table of Sorbents for Contaminants Listed in ACGIH 1970 Threshold Limit Values," *Am. Ind. Hyg. Assoc. J.* 32(6):404–409, 1971.

10. Hitchcock, R.T., P.C. Reist, and S.R. Coover. "A Respirator Cartridge for Use in Removing Methanol Vapors," *Am. Ind. Hyg. Assoc. J.* 42(4):268–272, 1981.

11. Henry, N.W. and R.S. Wilhelme. "An Evaluation of Respirator Canisters to Acrylonitrile Vapors," *Am. Ind. Hyg. Assoc. J.* 40(12):1017–1022, 1979.

12. Nelson, G.O. and C.A. Harder. "Respirator Cartridge Efficiency Studies: IV. Effects of Steady-State and Pulsating Flow," *Am. Ind. Hyg. Assoc. J.* 37(12):797–805, 1972.

13. Nelson, G.O. and C.A. Harder. "Respirator Cartridge Efficiency Studies: V. Effects of Solvent Vapor," *Am. Ind. Hyg. Assoc. J.* 35(7):391–410, 1974.

14. Nelson, G.O. and C.A. Harder. "Respirator Cartridge Efficiency Studies: VI. Effects of Concentration," *Am. Ind. Hyg. Assoc. J.* 37(4):205–216, 1976

15. Nelson, G.O., A.N. Correia, and C.A. Harder. "Respirator Cartridge Efficiency Studies: VII. Effects of Relative Humidity and Temperature," *Am. Ind. Hyg. Assoc. J.* 37(5):280–288, 1976.

16. Nelson, G.O. and A.N. Correia. "Respirator Cartridge Efficiency Studies: VIII. Summary and Conclusions," *Am. Ind. Hyg. Assoc. J.* 37(9):514–525, 1976.

17. Freedman, R.W., B.I. Ferver, and A.M. Harstein. "Service Lives of Respirator Cartridges Versus Several Classes of Organic Vapors," *Am. Ind. Hyg. Assoc. J.* 34(2):55–60, 1973.

18. Henry, W.W "Respirator Cartridge and Canister Efficiency Studies with Formaldehyde," *Am. Ind. Hyg. Assoc. J.* 42(12):853–857, 1981.

19. "Respiratory Protection," U.S. Code of Federal Regulations, Title 29, Chapter XVII, Part 1910.134, 1974.

20. National Institute for Occupational Safety and Health. "NIOSH Certified Equipment List as of July 1, 1978," Publication No. 79-107 (Washington, D.C.: U.S. Government Printing Office, 1978).

21. National Institute for Occupational Safety and Health. "A Supplement to the NIOSH Certified Equipment List," Publication No. 82–106 (Washington, D.C.: U.S. Government Printing Office, 1982).

22. Beaumont, G.P. and C.H. Garrido. "Respirator Cartridge Test System and Test Results for Benzene and Acrylonitrile," *Am. Ind. Hyg. Assoc. J.* 40(10):883–887, 1979.

23. Miller, G.C. and P.C. Reist. "Respirator Cartridge Service Lives for Exposure to Vinyl Chloride," *Am. Ind. Hyg. Assoc. J.* 38(10):498–502, 1977.

24. "Compressed Air for Human Respiration," Pamphlet G-7, Compressed Gas Association, Inc., New York.
25. Pritchard, J.A. "A Guide to Industrial Respiratory Protection," Los Alamos Scientific Laboratory, Los Alamos, N.M., Contract No. W-7405-Eng. 36, 1977.
26. Hack, A.L., O.D. Bradley, and A. Trujillo. "Respirator Protection Factors: Part II-Protection Factors of Supplied-Air Respirators," *Am. Ind. Hyg. Assoc. J.* 41(5):376–381, 1980.
27. Leidel, N.A. and SCP Respirator Committee. "Joint NIOSH/OSHA Standards Completion Program, Respirator Decision Logic," National Institute of Occupational Safety and Health, Cincinnati, OH, August, 1976.
28. *American National Standard Practices for Respiratory Protection*, ANSI Z88.2-1969, American National Standards Institute, 1430 Broadway, New York, NY 10018.
29. Raven, P.B., A.T. Dodson, and T.O. Davis. "The Physiological Consequences of Wearing Industrial Respirators: A Review," *Am. Ind. Hyg. Assoc. J.* 40(6):517–534, 1979.
30. Johnson, A.T. "The Energetics of Maskwear," *Am. Ind. Hyg. Assoc. J.* 37(8):479–488, 1976.
31. Raven, P.B., A.W. Jackson, K. Page, R.F. Moss, O. Bradley, and B. Skaggs. "The Physiological Responses of Mild Pulmonary Impaired Subjects While Using a 'Demand' Respirator During Rest and Work," *Am. Ind. Hyg. Assoc. J.* 42(4):247–257, 1981.
32. Hyatt, E.C., J.A. Pritchard, C.P. Richards, and L.A. Geoffrion. "Effects of Facial Hair on Respirator Performance," *Am. Ind. Hyg. Assoc. J.* 34(4):135–142, 1973.
33. Stein, R.L. "Selected Head and Facial Dimensions of Mine Rescue Team Personnel," *Am. Ind. Hyg. Assoc. J.* 39(7):576–578, 1978.
34. Hughes, J.G. and O. Lomaev. "An Anthropometric Survey of Australian Male Facial Sizes," *Am. Ind. Hyg. Assoc. J.* 33(2):71–78, 1972.
35. Moore, D.E. and T.J. Smith. "Measurement of Protection Factors of Chemical Cartridge, Half-Mask Respirators Under Working Conditions in a Copper Smelter," *Am. Ind. Hyg. Assoc. J.* 37(8):453–458, 1976.
36. Hyatt, E.C., J.A. Pritchard, and C.P. Richards. "Respirator Efficiency Measurements Using Quantitative DOP-Man Test," *Am. Ind. Hyg. Assoc. J.* 33(10):635–643, 1972.
37. Revoir, W.H. and L.R. Birkner. "Current Problems in Respiratory Protection," *Haz. Mat. Manag. J.* 1(6):14–19, 1980.
38. Packard, L.H., H.L. Brady, and O.F. Schumm. "Quantitative Fit Testing of Personnel Utilizing a Mouthpiece Respirator," *Am. Ind. Hyg. Assoc. J.* 39(9):723–730, 1978.
39. Aucoin, T.A. "A Successful Respirator Program," *Am. Ind. Hyg. Assoc. J.* 36(10):752–754, 1975.
40. Alpaugh, E.L. "Particulates," in *Fundamentals of Industrial Hygiene*, J.B. Olishifski, Ed. (Chicago: National Safety Council, 1979), p. 194.

PART III

Safety Monitoring and Management

CHAPTER 12

Practical Aspects of Packaging and Shipping Test Chemicals For Research

Richard L. Trammell and
Lawrence H. Keith
Radian Corporation, 8501 Mo-Pac Boulevard,
P.O. Box 9948, Austin, Texas 78766

Douglas B. Walters and
Andrew T. Prokopetz
National Toxicology Program, P.O. Box 12233,
Research Triangle Park, North Carolina 27709

INTRODUCTION

As government and independent testing of potentially hazardous chemicals increases, it becomes increasingly important to develop safe, practical methods for packaging and shipping chemicals for research. Each year thousands of pure chemicals are shipped for mutagenic and carcinogenic testing and for other research-oriented purposes. Likewise, thousands of analytical standards of diluted chemicals are shipped to government and independent analytical laboratories to be used as reference standards for a variety of purposes.

What makes these materials important for toxicology testing also places them in shipping categories that are intensely regulated. For this reason, the packaging and labeling of research chemicals must be in accordance with established government regulations.

To develop a program to guarantee safe transport of research chemicals, there are three important aspects which should receive major consideration. The most important of these is packaging to ensure safe handling. Second, this program must involve safe transportation of the materials to their destinations. Finally, certain documentation must be developed to give personnel immediate access to all needed information. This is especially important when shipping coded samples that must not be readily identified.

The following sections describe methods and considerations which have been developed at Radian Corporation for contracts with the National Toxicology Program (NTP) and the Environmental Protection Agency (EPA). These procedures, while not the only methods used for packaging chemicals, are examples of proven methods which achieve the desired level of safety.

PACKAGING PROCEDURES

Packaging methods usually vary based on the physical state of the compounds involved. However, all packaging methods should be designed to assure the complete containment of the chemicals throughout shipment. This is extremely important since employees of the transportation industry generally are not familiar with handling hazardous materials and the appropriate precautions. In addition, the manner in which compounds are packaged determines how they can be shipped and what carrier may be used.

Chemical Packaging

We generally use two methods of packaging. Solids or liquids are placed in screw-cap glass bottles which have a Teflon®-lined cap. One-pound mercury bottles having extra thick glass walls are used as an extra safety precaution when packaging compounds from the NTP chemical repositories. Glass hypovials with Teflon®-faced septa have also been used and found effective when shipping small quantities of relatively nonvolatile materials, but these are unsuitable for shipment and storage of volatile materials because the lack of an air-tight seal cannot be readily determined.

After transferring a sample to the primary shipping container, the outside of the bottle and cap is completely decontaminated by washing with one or more appropriate solvents before securing the cap with tape. The container is labeled with all pertinent information and wrapped in absorbent paper. It is then heat-sealed into two polyethylene bags, cushioned in bubble-wrap plastic packing, and placed in a metal can and sealed [1]. We have conducted durability tests with tracer dyes to determine the survivability of the primary shipping containers packaged according to these procedures. A "worst case" destruction was carried out by running over each container oriented end-on or edge-on with a three-quarter ton pickup truck. In all cases, the primary glass container survived intact, as did the two polyethylene bags in which the primary container was sealed [1, 2].

The second method of packaging research chemicals involves placing standard solutions of diluted chemicals into small glass ampuls which are flame-sealed. These ampuls are enclosed in styrofoam blocks, as shown in Figure 12-1, heat-sealed into two polyethylene bags and placed in bubble-plastic mailing envelopes. The styrofoam blocks are specifically designed for the size and type of ampul used so that the ampul fits snugly in the blocks. This prevents unnecessary movement during shipment which might damage the ampuls.

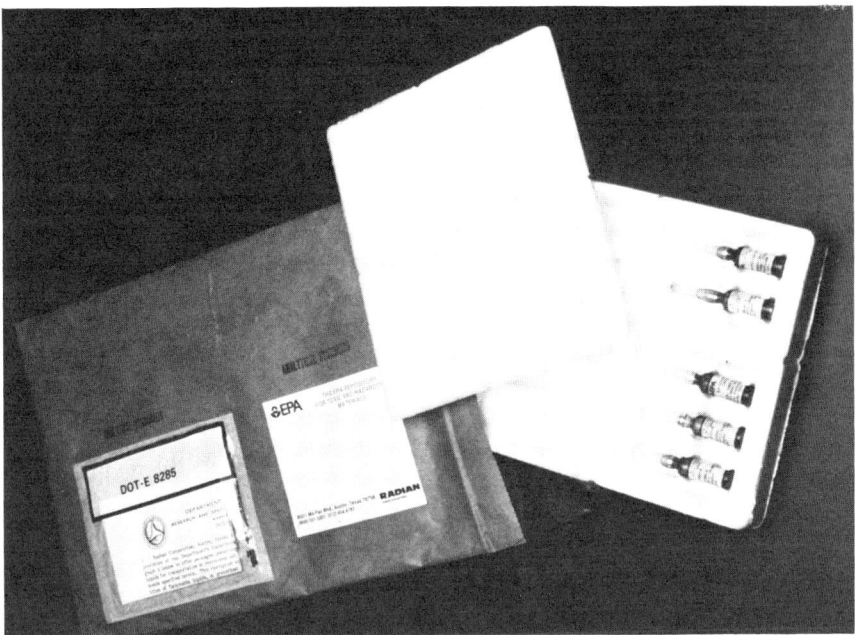

Figure 12-1.   Packaging of glass ampuls for shipment.

After the primary containers have been wrapped and sealed, they are placed in an appropriate Department of Transportation (DOT) shipping container which is large enough to leave room for additional packing material. A copy of all appropriate documentation always accompanies the samples in the shipping container. All individual containers are separated and surrounded with packing material such as styrofoam "peanuts" or vermiculite. The documentation, including a cover letter or detailed packing list, is placed on top of the packing so that it can be readily found by receiving personnel. The shipping container, free of all extraneous or erroneous markings, is then securely sealed and a shipping label affixed. All required DOT labels and markings, which give transportation personnel necessary handling information, are then placed on the shipping container in a clean, legible manner.

Proper Shipping Class Determination

The required DOT labels and markings are determined by first looking up the proper shipping name of the material in the hazardous materials table in the DOT regulations on hazardous materials [3]. If the specific compound is not listed in this table, then the compound must be placed in a specific hazard class pertaining to its hazardous properties. The hazard classes are generally listed as "not otherwise specified" (NOS) groups for the specific hazard. If no specific hazard can be determined, the compound may be shipped as nonregulated material.

Often a compound will have certain hazards that are not clearly definable as DOT hazard classes. This is seen in the selection of an NOS hazard class for a compound which has been shown to produce irritating effects. The DOT definition of an irritating material is a liquid or solid which, upon contact with fire or when exposed to air, gives off dangerous or intensely irritating fumes. A less regulated hazard class involving an irritating type of compound is "Other Regulated Material (ORM)-A." This category includes any material which has an anesthetic, irritating, noxious, toxic, or other similar property and which can cause extreme annoyance or discomfort to passengers and crew in the event of leakage [3]. Caution must be used in deciding which of these hazard classes is more appropriate. Other hazard classes such as poisons and corrosives have equally nonspecific definitions.

When shipping restricted hazardous materials, proper shipping names of the compounds must appear on the exterior of the shipping containers. Since this will reveal the identity of the compounds to receiving personnel, it is necessary to designate a receiver at the destination who is not associated with the investigator when shipping aliquots that are coded for testing as blind samples. This receiver unpackages the samples from the outside container before transferring them to the investigator. This prevents the investigator from determining the identities of the compounds and also offers an opportunity for someone to verify the contents of the shipment at the time of receipt.

TRANSPORTATION

The second important aspect of a program to ship research chemicals is their safe transport. When transporting chemicals, there are three things that must be considered. First, it is desirable to use the most timely and cost-effective mode of transportation. Second, DOT regulations are primarily designed for the safe transport of large quantities of materials. The labeling requirements which are part of these regulations readily inform the transportation personnel of the precautions they must take and the regulations they must follow. Finally, chemical shipments for research generally consist of relatively small quantities which may be restricted to expensive and time-consuming transportation. However, there are certain explicit exemptions in the regulations in regard to limited quantities that can be used when applicable. These exemptions primarily refer to packaging and labeling requirements.

Types of Shippers

Transportation methods for small quantities of toxic and hazardous chemicals packaged to conform to all appropriate DOT regulations have been evaluated at Radian Corporation. A study was conducted to determine shippers, shipping costs, and time en route. The four most frequently used shippers are:

1. United States Postal Service (USPS)
2. United Parcel Service (UPS)

3.   Federal Express
4.   various common carriers

We found several problem areas associated with each of these shippers [1]. The United States Postal Service accepts no class A points, irritants, and materials with flash points below 20° F for shipment. Though all chemicals are restricted to shipment as registered mail, the use of this shipper is not desirable due to the inexperience of personnel in handling hazardous materials. The United Parcel Service accepts no poisons, corrosives, explosives, or radioactive materials for shipment. While UPS delivery times are slightly longer than normal mail service (7–10 days), this mode is the least expensive of the four modes discussed.

The third major shipper, Federal Express, is preferable to the other four shippers. Federal Express has two levels of service, priority 1 and priority 2. Priority 1 service, which guarantees overnight delivery, is more expensive than the other shippers; Priority 2 service, which guarantees two-day delivery, is approximately one-half the priority 1 cost. Additionally, Federal Express requires that all poisons be packaged according to DOT exemption E-8249 or equivalent, which requires a packaging method which is much more stringent than normal DOT requirements. This is designed to safely allow consumable items and packages containing poisons to be shipped on the same vehicle or aircraft. This exemption and other similar ones are granted to specific companies for their own exclusive use; however, DOT E-8249 also exists for general public use. The packaging materials for use under this exemption must be purchased through Lawrence Packaging Supply, Newark, NJ 07107. Since it is not desirable to ship packages which might end up sitting in a warehouse over the weekend (which may be hot in the summer or cold in the winter), no shipments should be made on Fridays unless totally necessary.

The final type of shipper is common carrier companies. These shippers can be especially useful in shipping large quantities of chemicals since costs for shipments over a wide range of weights are usually very similar. However, using these shippers for small quantities of research chemicals results in an economic disadvantage. Additionally, problems often result from labor disputes, flammables being held up until an all flammable load is made, and poisons being "bumped" from a truck containing consumables. In addition to these types of carriers, there are several air forwarding companies that transport chemicals on commercial airlines. While these are preferable to common carriers, problems can result. Even though a forwarder has accepted a package for shipment, it is the prerogative of the pilot on these airlines to "bump" a package which contains poisons, dry ice (due to possible carbon dioxide buildup), or any other material which he or she feels might endanger the passenger or crew. Because of this, these forwarders generally do not guarantee delivery time. It also can be difficult to trace the route of a package, especially if it is "bumped" from a regularly scheduled flight.

In addition to these domestic chemical shippers, there are several carriers which are part of the International Air Transport Association (IATA) that transport chemicals overseas. Transport of hazardous chemicals by members of IATA is controlled by IATA's Dangerous Goods Regulations, which are very similar to those by DOT [4]. Shipment of research chemicals overseas creates the potential for additional problems related to tracking and verifying the delivery of the chemicals. It is crucial that all documentation be prepared accurately and that the shipment be closely tracked to verify delivery within a reasonable amount of time. Additionally, carriers with well-established routes to the destination should be used to minimize freight transfers between carriers.

While there are many possible choices for a commercial carrier for a chemical shipment, no person may carry a hazardous material, as described in the DOT regulations in the cabin of a passenger-carrying aircraft according to Section 175.85(a) of the DOT regulations [3]. This is necessary to ensure the safe handling and transport of hazardous materials and to prevent exposure to unsuspecting passengers and crew members. Additionally, when hazardous materials are carried on any aircraft, the pilot must be notified in writing through proper documentation that these materials are being carried.

Special Precautions

Though these procedures are applicable to the majority of chemicals, there are certain times when special procedures must be used during transportation. Some chemicals used in research are unstable under normal shipping conditions. Special precautions must be taken to assure that no decomposition occurs during transport for these cases. Samples that require refrigeration must be shipped in insulated shipping containers with dry ice or ice packs to maintain the required temperature. Shipping wet ice is not practical because of problems caused by water in the containers. Refrigeration need only be used when evidence shows that a compound might decompose during the relatively short period of transport.

In addition to temperature sensitivity, compounds susceptible to air oxidation require storage under an inert atmosphere. For this purpose, both argon and nitrogen can be used but argon is preferable due to its heavier-than-air properties. A great number of compounds are also photosensitive and must be protected from light during transport and storage. These compounds can be shipped either in amber glass primary containers or wrapped securely to prevent exposure to light. While in most cases special procedures are not needed, airtight seals are always sought to maintain sample integrity and to prevent exposure to vapors.

Finally, it is sometimes necessary to either chemically or by other means stabilize a chemical before it can be accepted for shipment. According to section 173.21(b) of the DOT regulations, no material capable of decomposing at a temperature of 54.4°C or less with the evolution of heat or gas can be offered for shipment without being stabilized or inhibited [3]. Chemical stabilization is preferable, though refrigeration can be used as a stabilizer when approved by the associate director for operations and enforcement, Material Transportation Bureau of DOT. An example of a compound requiring stabilization is N-Ethyl-N-nitrosourea (ENU) which decomposes to diazoethane (a compound which is expressly prohibited from shipment by any method) in alkaline solutions and near ambient conditions [5, 6]. A dilute acetic acid solution is typically used as a stabilizer, though refrigeration could be approved if questions concerning the safe transport of ENU within a few days could be answered. These include the melting point and initial decomposition temperature of the compound, the force an explosion would generate, and the exact conditions under which the decomposition becomes violent. This information is not available for ENU. As this example shows, extreme caution must be taken before shipping compounds requiring stabilization, especially compounds that are prepared in-house without necessarily being inhibited.

DOCUMENTATION

As part of any program to package and safely ship research chemicals, documentation must be developed to provide immediate access to information about potentially dangerous compounds. This is especially important when shipping chemicals that must be tested as coded samples. When a shipment from Radian involves coded samples, the documentation includes a safety and handling document for each chemical. This documentation does not identify the compound yet supplies all the information needed to safely handle it under normal circumstances. An emergency procedures document is also included. This is a sealed document which identifies the compound and supplies first aid and cleanup recommendations. If the compounds are shipped uncoded, a chemical data sheet giving all pertinent information about the chemical is included.

Items included in Radian's safety and handling documents are recommendations for personnel protection; the acute hazards associated with the material; recommendations for spills and leakage cleanup; storage precautions; and chemical and physical properties such as solubility, physical state, and color. Color is especially important because if a light yellow liquid is shipped and a brown liquid is received, the material is immediately assumed to have decomposed and is replaced. Occasionally false alarms occur when compounds with melting points close to room temperature are shipped; the solid that leaves Radian may convert to a liquid at the receiving laboratory and vice versa. This is why it is necessary to supply accurate information concerning chemical and physical properties in the safety and handling document.

A sealed emergency procedures document that contains all pertinent information required in an emergency always accompanies the safety and handling document. This includes the compound identification, the acute hazards of the compound, symptoms of exposure, first aid recommendations, and recommendations for cleanup of spills and leakage. Both the safety and handling document and the emergency procedures document should always accompany a coded sample, so that the information is readily accessible in an emergency. Uncoded shipments do not require separate handling instructions and emergency procedures; therefore, all the required information may be contained on a chemical safety data sheet.

Another recommended support document that should be provided to better track a shipment is a receipt acknowledgment card to confirm that a package reached its destination and describe the condition in which it was received. Instructions to the receiver, in the case of coded samples, should also be included so that the receiver can inspect and transfer the samples to the principal investigator within the shortest period of time. Finally, instructions to the principal investigator, in the form of a cover letter or shipment inventory list, should be included so that the investigator will know for what purpose the samples are being sent. This information often is supplemented by a letter five to seven days in advance of the shipment, notifying the investigator of the planned shipment.

CONCLUSIONS

When developing a program to package and safely ship chemicals for research, special precautions must be taken to assure that those who handle the materials will be protected. The procedures that are used must guarantee the complete containment of the material. Once this has been accomplished, proper packaging and labeling of these containers help assure that no personal exposure will occur during transport by providing transportation personnel with the appropriate handling instructions. This is important since these personnel are not usually trained in handling hazardous materials.

Additionally, all laboratory personnel at both the originating and receiving locations should be trained in handling highly toxic and carcinogenic materials and the laboratories should be designed to meet OSHA regulations governing toxic materials. It is these personnel who will have the highest risk of exposure. The primary objective when shipping research chemicals is to assure their safe, timely transport with minimal risk to the environment and involved personnel.

REFERENCES

1. Ward, J.T., C.H. Williams, Jr., C.D. Wolbach, L.H. Keith, and D.B. Walters. "Transportation of Materials from Radian Corporation's Hazardous Materials Laboratory," in *Safe Handling of Chemical Carcinogens, Mutagens, Teratogens and Highly Toxic Substances, Vol. 1,* D.B. Walters, Ed. (Ann Arbor, MI: Ann Arbor Science, 1980).
2. Walters, D.B., L.H. Keith, and J.M. Harless. "Chemical Selection and Handling Aspects of the National Toxicology Program," in *Environmental Health Chemistry: The Chemistry of Environmental Agents as Potential Human Hazards,* J.D. McKinney, Ed. (Ann Arbor, MI: Ann Arbor Science, 1980).
3. "Hazardous Materials Table and Hazardous Materials Communications Regulations," U.S. Code of Federal Regulations, Title 49, Parts 100–177, 1981.
4. *Dangerous Goods Regulations,* 24th ed. (Montreal: International Air Transport Association, 1982).
5. Druckrey, H., R. Preussman, S. Ivankovic, and D. Schmahl. "Organotrope carcinogene Wirkungen bei 65 verschiedenen N-Nitroso—Verbindungen an BN-Ratten," *Z. Krebsforsch.* 69: 103–201, 1967.
6. *IARC Monographs on the Evaluation of the Carcinogenic Risk of Chemicals to Humans, 17* (Lyon: International Agency for Research on Cancer, 1978), pp. 191–215.

CHAPTER 13

Bulk Chemical Management For Chronic Toxicity Studies

Steven W. Graves, E.J. Woodhouse, and K.M. Stelting
Midwest Research Institute,
Kansas City, Missouri 64110

C.W. Jameson
National Toxicology Program, P.O. Box 12233,
Research Triangle Park, North Carolina 27709

INTRODUCTION

Midwest Research Institute (MRI) currently serves as the analytical chemistry resource to the toxicity testing efforts of the National Toxicology Program (NTP). The project at MRI supports several types of *in vivo* animal studies whose main thrust is "to identify those chemicals considered toxic to humans and that must be controlled to prevent disease"[1].

Bulk chemical management, chemical analyses, and chemical/vehicle studies make up the major activities of the analytical chemistry resource. The bulk chemical management operation was created to handle the administrative and support aspects of the program. This separation of "nonchemical" functions allows chemists to concentrate on their technical responsibilities, thereby providing a more efficient operation.

The primary goals of bulk chemical management are:

1. To provide chemicals of appropriate purity, physical state, and amount for the various toxicity studies supported.
2. To ensure that chemical handling is done safely using the correct facilities, protective clothing, equipment, and techniques.
3. To document project activities in compliance with quality assurance requirements of the NTP.

PROCUREMENT	DOCUMENTATION	CHEMICAL HANDLING	SHIPMENT
• Experimental Design	• Procurement and Distribution	• Receipt/Interim Storage	• Classification
• Source Identification	• Safety and Toxicity	• Physical Manipulation	• Packaging
• Purchase	• Literature	- Protocol Design	
	• Analytical	- Staff Briefing	
		- Particle Size Reduction	
		- Homogenization	
		- Sampling	
		- Repackaging	

Figure 13-1.   Major tasks of bulk chemical management.

PROCUREMENT

Procurement of test chemicals is the first element of bulk chemical management. The three phases of procurement are experimental design, source identification, and purchase.

Experimental Design

The experimental design of a toxicity study specifies information pertinent to several factors relating to procurement. First, it specifies the selection criteria for a test compound. Some of the more common selection criteria are a potential for widespread exposure, structural similarity to known carcinogens, and possible cocarcinogenic (synergistic) effects. The chemical purity required to satisfactorily test the hypothesis may vary according to the primary selection criteria for the test chemical. For example, if a proposed cocarcinogenic mechanism is to be studied, a high purity material is required. Using a high purity material lessens the possibility of effects due to impurities rather than to the major component being studied. In contrast, the product of commerce may be needed when a compound is chosen because there is widespread exposure to it. In this case, concern is focused on the effect of exposure to the commercial product rather than to a single substance.

The experimental design also specifies the scope of a toxicity study. It details the number and species of animals required, the duration of the study, the dose level, and the route of administration. These factors are essential in determining the physical state and amount of chemical to be procured.

The case of p-nitroaniline, a recent procurement, illustrates the use of experimental design information. This compound, a solid dyestuff intermediate, was selected because a significant potential for worker exposure exists. This exposure potential called for the product of commerce to be procured for toxicity testing. The experimental design for the study specified a standard, lifetime toxicology testing with acute, prechronic, and chronic components. Two hundred rats and mice were to be tested. A daily maximum tolerable dose (MTD) was established to be 300 mg/kg body weight from previously published results. From this information it was calculated that $\sim$ 26 kg of p-nitroaniline were required as follows:

Amount (kg) = 2 [MTD (mg/kg-day = animal) $\times$ number of animals $\times$ average
body weight (kg) $\times$ number of days] 10^{-6} kg/mg
= 2 $[300 \times 200 \times 0.3 \times 730] \times 10^{-6}$
$\simeq$ 26 kg

The doubling factor assures sufficient chemical for bulk chemical and chemical/ vehicle studies by the analytical resource and acute and prechronic toxicity studies by the bioassayer. It also compensates for uncertainty in the MTD value.

For this study, gavage was specified as the route of administration because structurally similar chemicals had been unstable on feed, the preferred vehicle. The test material needed to be finely divided to facilitate the preparation of dose mixtures in water or corn oil, the protocol gavage vehicles. Based on these considerations, 25 kg of a powdered, technical grade material was procured.

Source Identification

After the initial procurement criteria are established, potential suppliers of the test chemical are identified. Standard publications, such as the *OPD Chemical Buyer's Guide, Directory of Chemical Producers, Chem Sources,* and the *Colour Index,* are consulted. A list is compiled and the suppliers are ranked so that those most likely to have the desired quantity and purity grade are contacted first. The volumes normally handled by potential suppliers, as indicated by which publication listed them, are a primary consideration in the initial ranking. The *OPD Chemical Buyer's Guide* lists primarily large-volume distributors and importers; the *Directory of Chemical Producers, U.S.A.* lists only large-volume U.S manufacturers, and *Chem Sources* lists mainly small-volume distributors and manufacturers. After the ranking a number of companies are contacted for representative market information including the price, purity, availability, packaging, and potential health hazards.

If a suitable supplier has not been identified at this point, the search is expanded to include government agencies, trade organizations, and manufacturers' associations. This step has proved valuable when a pure material is required but only the product of commerce, which is formulated, is available.

Custom synthesis is considered as the final alternative. Businesses known to have expertise in synthesizing the class of compound desired are selected from a list maintained for this purpose. Availability, synthesis schedule, and interest are determined. Bids are solicited from qualified sources.

If a source for a test chemical cannot be located through this process, the NTP is informed and chemical procurement activities cease pending further instructions.

Purchase

A supplier is generally selected from the various sources according to the following criteria:

- Large-volume products of commerce are purchased from a manufacturer whose process is used to produce most of the chemical.
- High-purity chemicals are selected on the basis of price, availability, and unit quantity.
- Custom-synthesized materials are ordered from the lowest bidder who can supply them in the desired purity within the specified time frame.

Once the supplier is identified, the purchase is completed using a standard purchase order. Purchase orders for NTP test chemicals are specially coded, however, to alert receiving personnel that these materials require handling according to a specified protocol.

Purchase is not always straightforward. Just because an item is available commercially does not mean it can be readily purchased by anyone who is interested in buying it. For example, complications can arise when (1) the quantity desired is not compatible with the supplier's normal package size (e.g., 20 kg of a compound desired that is sold only in tank car quantities); (2) the item is sold under contract to brokers who supply to specific end users; (3) the cost to set up an account is more than the profit to be gained by the supplier; or (4) the manufacturer is reluctant to have the product tested. In these cases, extensive interaction, sometimes involving intervention by the NTP, is required to successfully complete the procurement.

DOCUMENTATION

Documentation, the second element of bulk chemical management, has two objectives. The primary objective is to meet NTP quality assurance requirements for toxicity testing. It impacts bulk chemical management by requiring an extensive tracking effort to provide traceability for individual batches of chemicals and maintenance of records to establish the scientific validity of data in each analytical report. The secondary objective is to provide a literature base for the preparation of safe handling protocols.

Two files are maintained to accomplish the primary objective. One file focuses on procurement and distribution activities. This file, which is established at the time of the initial purchase of each chemical, contains the following information:

- procurement memo, which authorizes the purchase, specifies the purity grade and quantity, and lists acceptable suppliers

- copy of the purchase order
- receipt form completed on arrival of the chemical
- bill of lading, if available
- chemical handling data consisting of a sample removal form, which lists bulk chemical handling operations to be performed, and a mixing and sampling procedure form, which documents the chemical handling procedures used
- sample log, which shows the distribution history of the test chemical (number, identity, and amount of all samples removed and location of the remaining material)
- shipping authorization memo, which provides instructions for shipment to a bioassay laboratory
- copies of all shipping papers required
- receipt verification from the consignee

The second file details the results of each task completed by the analytical chemistry resource. This analytical file contains:

- task authorization memo defining the proposed work for that task
- all information pertinent to chemical handling, receipt, and storage of the specific batch of material tested
- notebook entries, charts, graphs, and other raw data from the laboratory work required to complete the task
- a copy of the final analytical report
- a copy of the transmittal letter accompanying the analytical report

These files are audited randomly by an independent MRI quality assurance unit to confirm that all quality assurance requirements of the NTP are satisfied.

The secondary objective is attained by a thorough compilation and evaluation of literature on the toxicity, pharmacology, reactivity, and stability of each test compound. An abstract of this information, the prior to opening container (PTOC) form, shown in Figure 13-2, is prepared by the project safety officer prior to the arrival of the initial batch of chemical. This document serves as reference for the preparation of chemical handling procedures, determination of appropriate protective clothing for the requested tasks, emergency procedures, and storage requirements.

CHEMICAL HANDLING

Chemical handling, the third element of bulk chemical management, is a unique operation. This operation has such a diversity of type and quantity of chemical handled that no counterpart is known to exist in industry or research. MRI's initial involvement, nearly nine years ago, was limited to homogenization of small samples prior to analysis. It has grown to include a variety of manipulative tasks (e.g., sizing, homogenization, sampling, repackaging, and purification) performed on approximately 100 batches of chemicals per year ranging in size from milligram to multikilogram amounts.

PTOC DATA SHEET

```
┌─────────────────────────────────────────────┐
│ Compound Name                                 │
│ MRI No.              L A B E L                │
│ NCI No.                                       │
└─────────────────────────────────────────────┘
```

HEALTH HAZARD RATING:
```
        ┌──────────────────────┐
        │                      │
        │      L A B E L       │
        │                      │
        │                      │
        └──────────────────────┘
```
OSHA STANDARDS FOR EXPOSURE:

TOXICITY:

            Animal   Human

    1. LD Data: 1. LD Data:

                                         2. Symptoms of Acute Exposure:

    2. TD Data

                                       3. Symptoms of Chronic Exposure:

    3. IRDS Data:

CARCINOGENICITY:

Figure 13-2. Prior to opening container (PTOC) form.

PHYSICAL PROPERTIES:

    1. m.p.:   2. b.p.:   3. Flash Point:

    4. Density: 5. Volatility:

    6. Solubility:

    7. Stability:

BULK CHEMICAL HANDLING PRECAUTIONS:

SPILLS:

    1. Protective Clothing:

    2. Containment and Cleanup:

    3. Decontamination:

    4. Disposal:

STORAGE:

Figure 13–2. *(continued)*

EMERGENCY FIRST AID PROCEDURES:

In case of exposure, immediately summon qualified medical assistance. Use the following procedures until help arrives.

    1. Inhalation:

    2. Skin:

    3. Eyes:

ANALYTICAL HANDLING PRECAUTIONS:

DOT HAZARD CLASSIFICATION:

Prepared by: _____   Approved: _____
               Project Safety Officer   Principal Investigator

      Date: _____   Date: _____

STAFF BRIEFING:

           Chemical Characterization   Chemical/Vehicle

Figure 13–2. *(continued)*

REFERENCES:

Figure 13–2.   *(continued)*

Facility

The safety of bulk chemical handling operations has always been of primary concern. This concern has led to the construction and recent renovation of a facility designed solely for bulk chemical handling. The current facility, whose floor plan is given in Figure 13–3, occupies an area ~ 50 x 20 feet. It includes:

1. Storage areas for packaging materials, shipping supplies, chemical handling equipment, and chemicals.
2. Transition area from "clean" areas to potentially contaminated areas.
3. Bulk chemical and sample handling areas suitable for a wide range of sample types and sizes.

Access and egress are controlled to minimize the possibility of personnel exposure and contamination of clean areas. Unlimited access and egress by authorized personnel are allowed between storage areas and the adjoining hallway. Access and egress between the bulk chemical handling area is decontaminated. Access and egress for the sample handling and equipment storage areas are permitted only when the chemical handling area are allowed only through the bulk chemical handling area, which must in turn be entered via the transition area. Other exits from the chemical handling areas are used for emergency purposes only.
icity testing, the current design of the chemical handling areas emphasizes ease of decontamination. Noteworthy features of the bulk chemical handling area include:

*   A totally washable, waterproof design. Light switches and electrical outlets designed for outdoor locations are used. Ceilings, walls, floors, and hood surfaces are painted with an epoxy-based paint, which prevents permeation of the surface. Light fixtures are watertight. Doors are flanged at the,bottom to prevent escape of liquid into adjoining areas during decontamination.

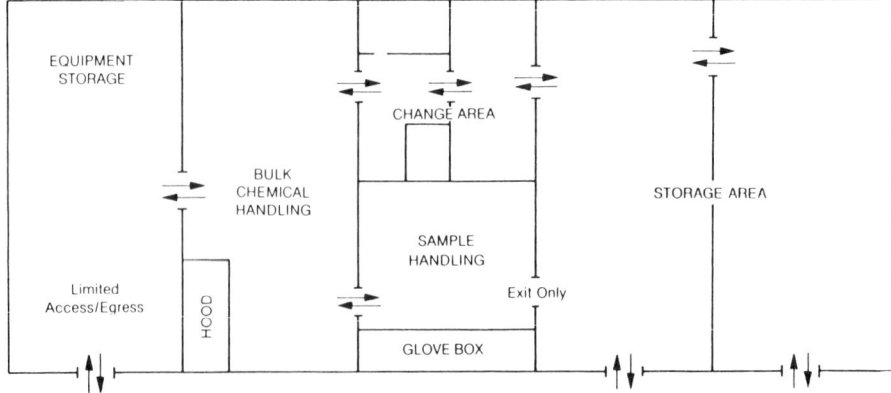

Figure 13–3.   Chemical handling facility.

- An air filtration system capable of removing airborne particulates. All exhaust air is passed through two particulate filters in series. The outer filter, which is easily replaced, removes the majority of particulates. An inner, high efficiency particulate air filter (HEPA) removes most solids which pass through the outer prefilter. The outer filter is replaced when it becomes visibly contaminated. The HEPA filter is replaced semiannually, unless an appreciable decrease in exhaust airflow is noted.
- Maintenance of work areas at a negative air pressure relative to storage areas, which are in turn at a negative air pressure relative to the adjoining hallways.
- A 350-gallon stainless steel sump to contain potentially contaminated wash liquids. This system allows liquids to be analyzed or decontaminated prior to release. Alternatively, waste liquids can be pumped into other containers for disposal by landfill or incineration.
- Location of all breathing air equipment except hoses and an air supply selection valve (normal or emergency) in an adjoining location, as shown in Figure 13-4. This eliminates tedious decontamination of the equipment between tasks.
- An emergency bell, which summons help from other locations.
- A small access door connecting the bulk chemical handling area to the glove box in the adjacent sample handling area.
- A hood modified to accommodate 55-gallon drums for the convenient repackaging of bulk liquids.

The sample handling area is used for handling smaller batches of test chemicals and analytical samples. All work in this area is performed in a glove box. Exit air from the glove box is vented through a HEPA filter when the worker is handling solids, or a charcoal filter when the worker is handling volatile liquids. Both filters are replaced semiannually. Interior surfaces of the glove box are coated with a strippable epoxy-based paint for easy decontamination in the event of a large spill. Waste liquids from the cleanup of equipment, containers, and surfaces in the glove box are trapped in plastic carboys for disposal.

Protective Clothing

Two types of protective clothing are considered acceptable for large scale operations in the bulk chemical handling room. A full-body, air-supplied chemical handling suit, as shown in Figure 13-5, is worn for all operations outside the hood except those involving nontoxic materials (e.g., sugar and gum tara). The suit is constructed of vinyl-coated nylon, which is impervious to most chemicals. Although cumbersome, hot, and difficult to work in, it offers maximum worker protection. The air supply maintains the suit at positive pressure relative to the working environment, preventing any particulates from entering, even in the event of a puncture. All seams are sealed with folds of suit material to minimize entry of liquids into the suit via a wick-

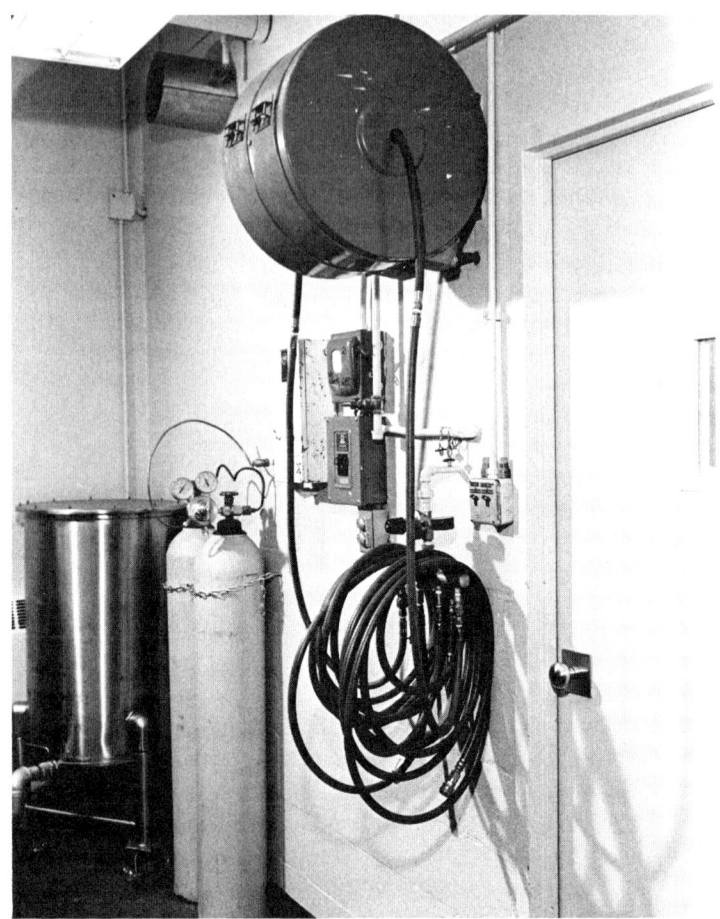

Figure 13–4. Air supply equipment.

ing mechanism. Since experience has shown that these suits are dependable but not foolproof, additional protective clothing is worn under the suit as a safeguard.

Disposable coveralls with attached hood and boots, rubber gloves, and a full-face, air-supplied respirator make up the second alternative, shown in Figure 13–6. This type of protection is used for all tasks performed in the hood and for handling nontoxic compounds outside the hood.

As shown in Figure 13–7, protective clothing for small-scale work in the hood or glove box consists of disposable coveralls with attached booties (shoe covers are worn if coveralls without booties are used), safety glasses, and latex gloves. This protective clothing is considered the minimum acceptable for any bulk chemical handling operation.

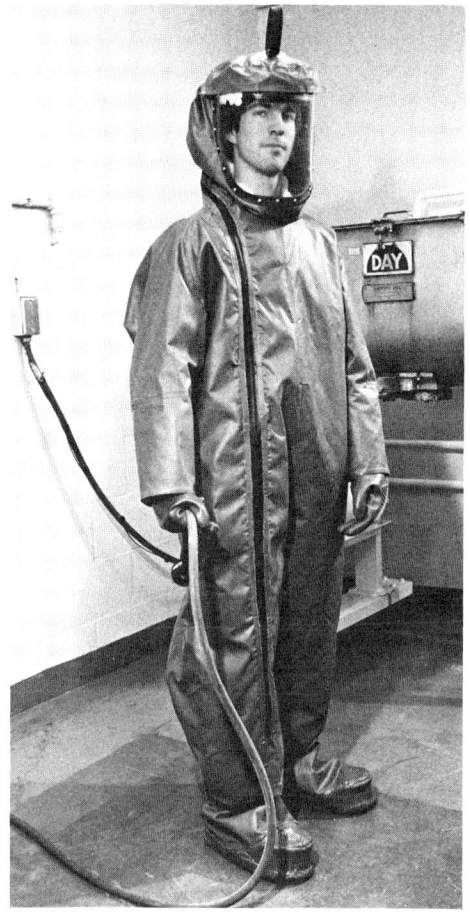

Figure 13–5.   Chemical handling suit.

Operations

Chemical handling operations begin with the arrival of a batch of test chemical. Project personnel are immediately notified by receiving personnel. The container is inspected, transported to the storage area, and stored as directed in the PTOC form for that chemical. If leaks or contamination of the container is found at this time, the chemical handling supervisor is summoned. The supervisor directs all required clean-up activities using instructions provided in the PTOC form as guidelines. When the chemical reaches interim storage, a receipt form documenting the arrival is prepared.

For every chemical handling operation, instructions are prepared, reviewed by the project safety officer, and prior to chemical handling, discussed in detail with the

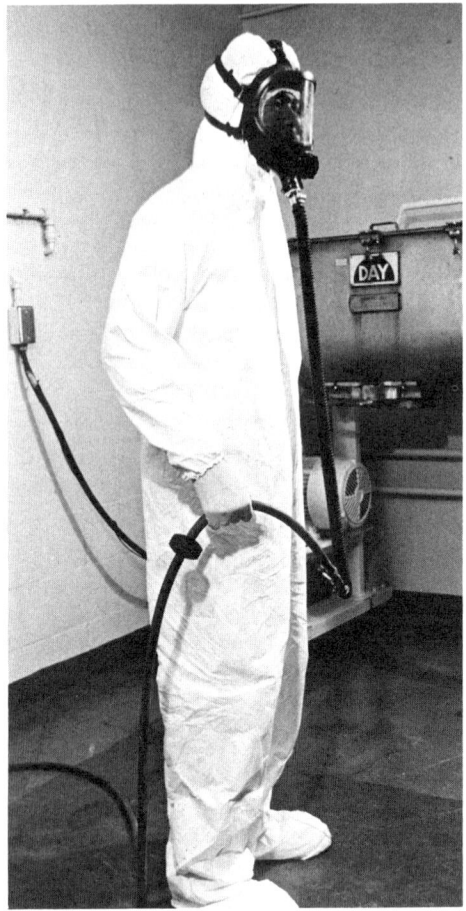

Figure 13-6. Protective clothing for low hazard operations.

assigned chemical handling technicians. These instructions cover the four major areas of chemical handling: particle size reduction, homogenization, sampling, and repackaging. In addition, they specify cleanup, decontamination, and waste disposal procedures. The potential hazard involved in each operation is carefully assessed, and protective clothing, equipment, and handling procedures are specified to provide maximum personnel protection, while allowing as much freedom of movement as possible. Most of the information used to prepare these protocols is abstracted from the PTOC form for the test chemical.

Bulk chemical handling operations routinely include particle size reduction, homogenization, sampling, and repackaging. Particle size reduction is required in three situations. The first is when the particle size of the chemical as received is too

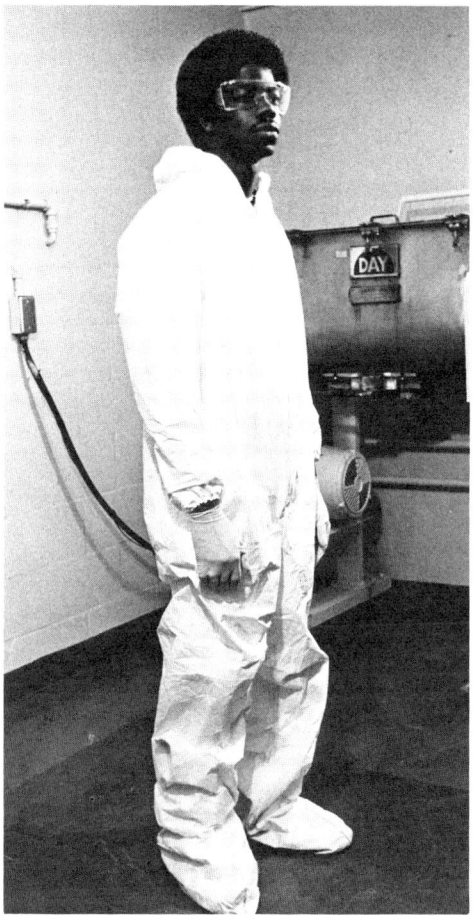

Figure 13-7. Minimum acceptable protective clothing for bulk chemical handling.

large to prepare a homogeneous feed blend. Table 13-1 shows the particle size needed to produce acceptable blends at several concentrations. The second situation is when the particle size of the compound is not small enough for successful homogenization of the batch. This precludes removal of representative samples for chemical analysis. Finally, particle size reduction is required for gavage studies in which the test compound must be suspended but the particle size received cannot be suspended at the desired concentration.

The particle size of large volume samples is reduced by using a Fitzmill, shown in Figure 13-8. The final particle size can be determined by a removable screen located near the exit chute. With this equipment, effective particle size reduction down to 120 mesh is possible for most solids. In some cases a maximum particle size

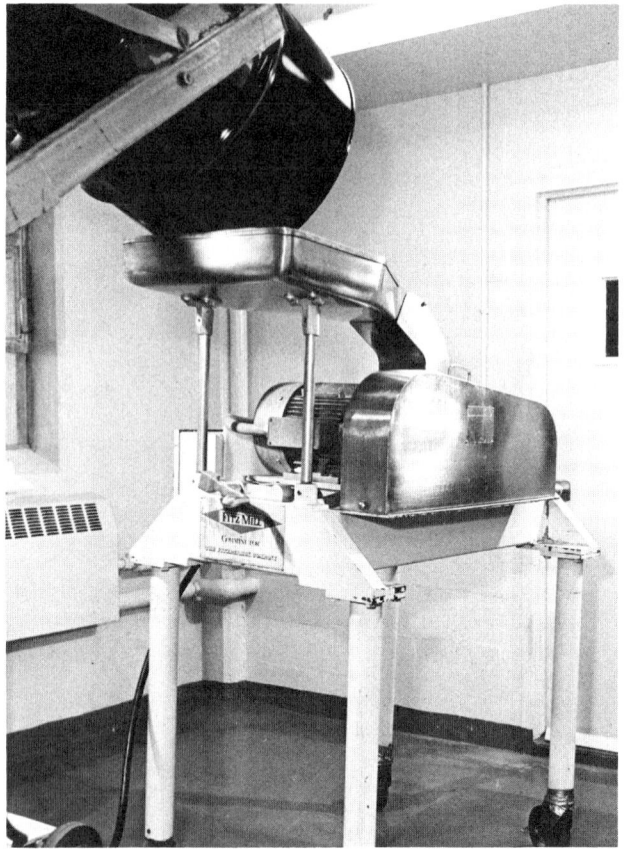

Figure 13-8. Fitzmill.

of 200 mesh can be obtained. The particle size of intermediate size samples is usually reduced with a carborundum ball mill and grinding medium. In this case, the final size distribution is dependent on the initial properties of the solid being ground. Small samples are ground with a mortar and pestle or a laboratory-size blender.

All samples except gases are homogenized prior to sampling. Solids weighing more than 30 kg are mixed using a Day ribbon blender as shown in Figure 13-9. Smaller batches of solids are homogenized by tumbling and rolling of the outer container on a ball mill roller or by a barrel tumbler. Liquids are blended by mechanical

Table 13-1.   Particle Size Requirements

Particle Size (Mesh)	Dosed-Feed Concentration (% w/w)
40–10	1–5
80–40	0.1–1
> 80	< 0.1

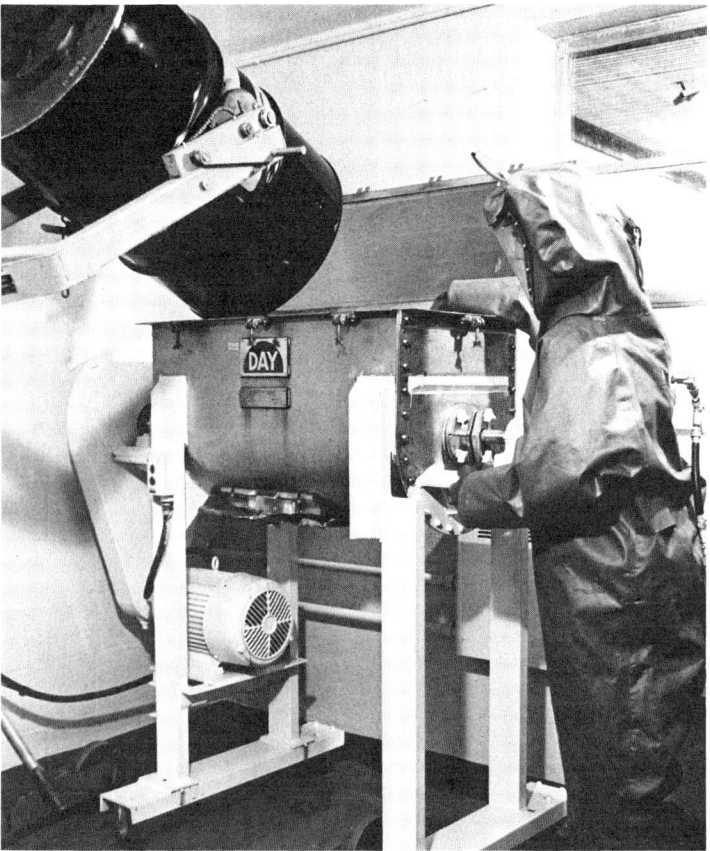

Figure 13-9.   Day ribbon blender.

stirring or tumbling and rolling of the outer container. Whenever possible, volatile liquids are homogenized in a closed system.

Random sampling is used to remove samples from the homogenized material. Samples are generally transferred to glass containers because of their inert nature; amber glass containers are used for light-sensitive compounds. Plastic containers are used occasionally, as required, to eliminate specific problems (e.g., brominated hydrocarbons which solidify at subambient storage temperatures, causing glass containers to shatter on melting).

Repackaging prepares the compound for shipment to the bioassay laboratory. Consideration is given to the stability of the chemical, U.S. Department of Transportation (DOT) shipping requirements, and the needs of the bioassayer in the operation. Potentially unstable chemicals are generally divided into small packages having a minimum of headspace, with inert gas placed in the headspace as required (e.g., for oxidizable materials). The DOT regulations are determined prior to repackaging to assure that the material can be shipped in the new container. Test chemicals which could present unnecessary hazards for a bioassay laboratory are repackaged into units more easily handled and stored (e.g., quantity sufficient to prepare a single dose blend). Each repackaged compound is transferred to a facility where it is stored in a manner suitable to maintain its integrity prior to shipment to the toxicology testing laboratory.

Cleanup is accomplished systematically after completion of bulk chemical handling for each test chemical. Any large spill is contained so it can be disposed of through regular waste disposal channels. Minor contamination of equipment, facilities, and protective clothing is removed by initially scrubbing with soap and water and rinsing with water. Residual test chemical is then removed using an appropriate solvent. An abrasive is used only if the test chemical is insoluble in common solvents. All solvents used for decontamination are contained in a large sump until an appropriate disposal or chemical treatment procedure is selected. Wastes from chemical handling operations are disposed of in accordance with current local, state, and federal regulations.

SHIPMENT

Shipment is the final element of bulk chemical management. Each test chemical is rechecked to assure that the packaging is consistent with its DOT hazard class. All possible precautions are taken to prevent leakage during shipment. Glass containers are wrapped in sorbent paper. All containers are sealed in plastic bags. Inert solid absorbent is placed in all liquid shipments. Sealed containers are often nested for shipment of hazardous materials.

Selection of a carrier is based on the required delivery timetable. Test chemicals requiring rapid delivery (e.g., must be shipped cool or are needed immediately) are shipped via a carrier that provides one-day service to most locations, handles most hazard categories, and has well-trained personnel. Where the delivery timetable is less restrictive, over-the-road common carriers are used. In these cases, cost, which generally parallels the size, is the determining factor. The U.S. mail service is not to be used because post office personnel are not trained to handle potentially hazardous materials. More importantly, incoming mail is normally handled differently than freight arrivals, which could result in exposure of untrained and unsuspecting personnel in the event of a spill.

SUMMARY

The analytical resource program supporting NTP toxicity studies requires a strong bulk chemical management capability. Bulk chemical management tasks occur during all phases of this project. The goals of these activities are to enhance the scientific validity, safety, and efficiency of operations at the analytical resource laboratory and to assist the NTP in meeting its quality assurance requirements. To meet these objectives, the following tasks are required: (1) procurement of test chemicals compatible with the requirements of each study, (2) documentation of laboratory results obtained by the analytical resource laboratory, (3) documentation to authenticate and track each batch of test compound, (4) safe chemical handling to provide a homogeneous batch of chemical suitable for its future use, and (5) storage and shipment of samples to assure their integrity and on-time, safe arrival at the bioassay laboratory.

REFERENCE

1.   *National Toxicology Program Fiscal Year 1981 Annual Plan* (Research Triangle Park,NC: National Toxicology Program, 1981), p. 10.

CHAPTER 14

Safety Problems in a Chemical Testing Program

Harry Mahar and
Richard E. Shaff
Division of Safety, National Institutes of Health,
Public Health Service, U.S.
Department of Health and Human
Services, Bethesda, MD 20205

INTRODUCTION

In the last few years, there has been increasing evidence to suggest that a number of procedures routinely used in testing or research laboratories may release chemical substances into the work environment. These chemicals, whether they are under investigation to determine their physical, chemical, or toxic characteristics or are employed as reagents, may pose significant health risks to laboratory or support personnel who may be inadvertently exposed. Although several studies have implicated chemicals as a causal factor in the etiology of specific diseases in laboratory workers [1–3], scientific opinion remains divided as to the legitimacy of that relationship [4]. However, evidence suggesting that microbiological laboratory personnel are at increased risk to infection with the etiologic agents with which they work supports the position that laboratory workers can be exposed to materials they handle, manipulate, or use [5].

The biological significance of inadvertent chemical exposures sustained in a toxicological testing laboratory is often difficult to ascertain because two crucial factors may not be defined: the potency of the material involved and the extent of exposure. Potency is an inherent property of a chemical; it determines the magnitude of the biological response in the test system of interest at a given dose. If the material in question is not well characterized from a toxicological perspective, then any quantitative estimate of the health risk to personnel resulting from exposure to the material is tenuous.

In toxicological testing laboratories, the risk of personnel exposure to a material under test is dependent upon a number of factors, including the test system employed (e.g., *in vivo, in vitro*), the route of exposure to the animal, the size and duration of the study, the dosage employed, and the type of facility in which the study is conducted. Although it is difficult to quantify exposures that can be expected in all situations, it is possible to identify particular operations or activities in which the opportunity for exposure of laboratory personnel to test materials is greatest. Since the spectrum of toxicological testing studies share a number of common activities or phases, it is also possible to compare the relative magnitude of the exposure potential across these different experimental protocols.

The potential for personnel exposure to chemicals within a toxicological testing facility can be mitigated by the engineering controls, administrative controls, operational practices, and personal protective equipment employed. In order to reduce to a minimum the potential for personnel exposure to a chemical, the implementation of the most appropriate combination of these controls should be based not only on an identification of those areas or activities offering the greatest opportunity for personnel exposure but also on the effectiveness that the various options to control exposure provide.

POSSIBLE EXPOSURE ROUTES

The principal routes of exposure for laboratory or support personnel to chemicals are through inhalation or direct contact (e.g., dermal or ocular absorption), although inadvertent inoculation or ingestion may also occur. It is important to recognize that these exposures can result during the handling or manipulation of the test material or may occur because of contamination within the facility. Although exposures arising from general contamination probably result in relatively low incremental exposure doses, cumulatively they may constitute significant exposures to the personnel. In many cases, these repetitive, low-level exposures are not recognized by the investigator; therefore, no steps to control them are taken. For this reason, it is important to consider the exposure potential through all phases of an experiment, extending from the time of acquisition of the material to be tested through study termination and facility decontamination.

Table 14–1 describes a number of activities or phases typically encountered in a toxicological testing program. Since any of the several phases may offer the possibility of personnel exposure to the test agent (or other particularly toxic reagents involved in the study), each should be evaluated for this potential. Classical laboratory animal testing studies are typified in Table 14–1, although it is readily recognized that most of the phases are common to other types of toxicological testing efforts (e.g., *in vitro* or specialized systemic toxicity studies). Obviously, the areas of greatest concern in an animal study may be different from those in an *in vitro* protocol, but the generic approach to evaluating the problem is similar.

Table 14-1.   Typical Phases of an In Vivo Toxicological Testing Experiment

Activity	Examples
Test article acquisition	shipping/receiving; chemical synthesis or labeling
Chemical storage/dispensing	storage of bulk material; dispensing/aliquoting for analyses or mixing
Dosage preparation	preparation or mixing of test article into appropriate vehicle (e.g., feed, water, oil)
Dosage administration	actual administration of test article (e.g., dosage feed, gavage, injection)
Post-treatment animal holding	animal maintenance during dosing (if life-time study) or subsequent to dosing
	may include frequent handling, testing animal subsequent to dosing (e.g., neurobehavioral studies)
Examination/pathology	sacrifice, necropsy, tissue and slide preparations
Analytical chemistry support	analytical activities to determine purity and stability of test articles, or accuracy/homogeneity of dosage mixture
Data acquisition and storage	data records of experimental procedure, observations, or tests; includes both hard copy and magnetic tape
Study termination	decontamination/decommissioning the equipment, supplies, and facilities involved in the study
Facility and equipment maintenance	housekeeping, routine or emergency equipment servicing, and preventive maintenance program

DETERMINANTS OF EXPOSURE

A number of independent studies have demonstrated the ease with which a material under test can contaminate areas within a laboratory [6-10]. Exposure of personnel to the test material or a simulant may occur, even when strict work practices are employed in a modern, well-designed facility. The studies emphasize that many laboratory operations, and in particular those involving laboratory animals, can easily result in the distribution of test materials throughout a facility (albeit in small amounts). Several activities, including material handling operations, dosage preparation and administration steps, post-treatment holding of animals, and waste disposal have been shown to be problem areas, although other miscellaneous activities can also contribute to the exposure of laboratory personnel.

Material Handling

Activities involving the manipulation of pure or neat material typically provide a significant opportunity for its release into the work environment. Several studies conducted within bioassay testing facilities have shown that where procedural steps involved the manipulation of the concentrated solid material (e.g., chemical storage/dispensing, analytical chemistry laboratory) contamination of equipment, containers, and personnel (e.g., gloved hand) by the chemical was detected [6–8]. The fact that the test chemical was consistently found in these locations is all the more significant because in each case, personnel used good laboratory practices and conducted the work in well-designed, well-ventilated areas. Several other studies, using suitable tracer material to simulate chemicals under test, corroborate these findings [9, 10]. In each of the studies cited, contamination was typically found on the outer surfaces of the stock container, on floor and bench tops where it was handled, on the analytical balance used during quantitative transfers, on clothing or protective garments, and in adjacent areas or rooms. The last apparently resulted from the movement of contaminated persons or equipment through adjoining areas. Collectively, the studies demonstrate the ease with which solid test material can be released into the work environment and how widely it can be dispersed. Concentrated liquids appear less prone to form aerosols, although even careful transfer operations may still produce local contamination [11]. An often overlooked problem is the tendency for solid or liquid materials with even moderate vapor pressures (e.g., approximately 0.5 mm Hg) to volatilize in the laboratory or animal care areas. This event can result in exposure of unprotected lab personnel or test animals to possibly significant vapor concentrations of the test material [12].

Dosage Preparation and Administration

The procedures involved in the preparation of the dosage mixture and its subsequent administration to animals also provide the opportunity for personnel exposure to the test material. Dosage preparation procedures have the same potential for generation of aerosols as previously mentioned for material handling operations, where pure or concentrated test chemicals are quantitatively added to the appropriate vehicle (e.g., feed, water, corn oil) and vigorously mixed to ensure homogeneity of the blend. When large numbers of animals are under test for long periods of time, the dimensions of the contamination problem tend to be greater, since more test material is released into the dosage preparation area with each repetitive mixing operation. For these reasons, it is not unexpected that the dosage preparation areas within a testing facility typically have the worst contamination control problems of any area or activity involved in the study. Several studies have shown that animal holding areas become contaminated with the test material as the animals are being administered the agent [6–8]. In dosed-feed studies, filling or refilling the feed hoppers with the dosage mixture may create large amounts of aerosols. These aerosols, unless controlled with local exhaust ventilation, can result in contamination of the work area.

This is especially true when a meal "chow" is used. Gel diets offer a more attractive substitute, since the generation of aerosols when the material is dispensed or consumed by the animal is somewhat less than with solid feed.

Administration of the test agent to animals by other methods also can lead to contamination. Studies have shown that the administration of test compounds in drinking water can result in widespread contamination of the animal room and surrounding areas [7]. Handling and changing of individual cage water bottles can be a significant cause of contamination since spillage can easily occur. Administration of the material by gavage is generally regarded as a more controlled delivery method, and, if properly done, creates a minimum of aerosols. However, if volatile materials are administered by gavage, contamination of the workplace may occur by volatilization of the dosage mixture or by exhalation of the test material by the dosed animal. Studies have shown that detectable levels of a volatile test material (i.e., vapor pressure of 14 mm Hg at 20° C administered in a corn oil vehicle) occurred in the air in the animal dosing/holding room during gavaging activities, and that the levels peaked about one-half hour after termination of treatment [7]. Off-gassing from the animals or from the capped stock solutions was suspected as the causal factor, since the intubation and gavaging was performed under local exhaust ventilation. In contrast to large-scale animal studies, *in vitro* studies using cell or tissue cultures typically employ small amounts of test agent, so that less contamination occurs during dosage formulation. Contamination does occur, but can be controlled within primary containment equipment [13]. However, incubation of cultures treated with volatile materials may result in release of the contaminant vapor into the laboratory, unless the incubator is properly vented [14].

Post-treatment Animal Holding

A variety of studies have demonstrated the degree to which a chemical may be dispersed throughout an animal holding room. Based on the information to date, dosed-feed studies appear to have the greatest potential for causing contamination of the facility, followed by dosed water, gavage, and skin-painting studies. Parenteral administration tends to produce the least amount of contamination. Inhalation studies are a special case, since the animal is held in an environment in which the test agent is intentionally introduced. The pharmacokinetics of a chemical in the test animal species is an important consideration because of the possibility that the parent compound or biologically active metabolites may be eliminated in the urine or feces. In single-dose studies, this aspect is particularly important, since the animals need to be maintained under controlled conditions from the time of dosing to when the material has either been completely metabolized to innocuous by-products, or the active by-products have been eliminated from the body. Because of these considerations, the manipulation or testing of a treated animal outside the treatment or holding room (e.g., neurobehavioral tests), needs to be accomplished with due consideration for the potential for spread of contamination to other areas or equipment.

Waste Handling and Disposal

Waste handling and disposal activities associated with animal studies can produce significant amounts of contamination within the facility, while the various gaseous, liquid, and solid waste streams emanating from the site may likewise contain the test agent. Cleaning operations to remove bedding from cages, prior to washing, generate large amounts of contaminated aerosols. The majority of the particles in these aerosols are not of respirable size, but they do result in the contamination of surfaces near the waste handling site [7, 8]. Results of experiments using dyes to simulate chemicals under test indicate that typical automatic cage washers may not completely remove test materials from the cage surface, and, in fact, may redistribute the contaminant onto the surface of other items in the washer [10]. Procedures used in the cleaning of dosage preparation areas may produce solid and liquid wastes containing the test chemical in amounts of an order of magnitude greater than that associated with cage cleaning operations [15]. Based on analyses of wastewater from laboratories conducting long-term toxicological studies in animals, it has been estimated that up to 5% of the total amount of a test chemical administered may become a component of the facility's wastewater [15].

Given the degree to which the test chemical can be distributed throughout the facility, effective routine housekeeping procedures during the study and final decontamination of those areas, or of items dedicated to the study (e.g., animal rooms), are essential.

Miscellaneous Tasks

In addition to those already mentioned, several other activities associated with toxicological testing programs can provide an opportunity for exposure of personnel to the material under test. Servicing and maintenance of equipment directly involved in the study provides an opportunity for personnel exposure, if the equipment is not thoroughly decontaminated prior to servicing or if maintenance personnel do not wear appropriate protective equipment and clothing.

Servicing of such equipment, however, is usually recognized as potentially hazardous, so the necessary precautions are generally taken. Problems typically arise when the equipment or item is not directly involved in the conduct of the study or is in a remote location away from the animal colony, and therefore assumed to be uncontaminated.

Several monitoring studies of facilities in which chemicals were under test provide examples of contamination being present on items which had been removed from the animal holding area, or articles which had come in contact with such items. These articles were either ineffectively decontaminated prior to removal, or were not recognized as being contaminated and therefore removed without adequate cleaning; examples include logbooks and data sheets, personal respirators, necropsy tissue containers, and transport carts [7, 8]. Logbooks and data sheets pose an interesting dilemma: good laboratory practice requires that all pertinent data be recorded and retained for quality assurance purposes, yet many areas where such data records are generated are typically contaminated with the test article (e.g., dosage preparation). Original log sheets and animal data records have been found to be contaminated with the test article [7, 8].

CONTROL MEASURES

Toxicological testing programs, by their nature, involve the manipulation of potentially toxic chemicals. As described earlier, the opportunity for contamination and the spread of that contamination is significant in these operations and facilities. Therefore, in order that personnel involved in these operations are not exposed to the material, it is necessary that the opportunity for such exposure be eliminated or at least adequately controlled by the application of administrative controls and good work practices, sound engineering controls, and the judicious use of personal protective equipment. Any one of these controls alone will probably not provide adequate protection; however, when used in combination, a safe work environment can be attained.

Administrative Controls and Operational Practices

The first line of defense against personnel exposure in toxicological testing operations, or in any laboratory program, is the implementation of sound administrative controls and safe operational practices. Chemical testing programs are by their nature "dirty," yet if good laboratory practices are followed, contamination of personnel, equipment, and the facility will be significantly reduced.

The first step in establishing administrative controls in a program is to identify the hazards associated with the materials being used or the work being performed. The chemical, physical, and if possible toxic properties of the material to be tested must be assessed in order to determine the degree of risk involved at each stage of a testing program. Flammable, reactive, or corrosive materials may require special handling or storage procedures. Physical (e.g., volatility, electrostatic properties) and chemical characteristics may help to define appropriate handling, containment, and decontamination procedures to be used during the study.

Once this initial evaluation is completed, planning for routine operations and emergency situations (e.g., spills, fire) should be accomplished prior to the initiation of work, and all personnel involved in the study properly instructed. Such planning should include procedures for assisting or advising local fire departments, rescue squads, and hospitals whose support may be necessary during emergencies.

Work areas (i.e., where the compound is used or stored) must be identified and appropriate signage posted at each entrance to these areas. The warning signs should be concise, unambiguous and prominently displayed. These "controlled" areas should be entered only by those persons authorized access by the investigator responsible for the program. Service, maintenance, or housekeeping personnel who must enter the controlled areas must be fully apprised of the attendant risks, instructed in the proper procedures to follow, and provided suitable equipment. Any equipment or material removed from the controlled areas should be thoroughly decontaminated or properly disposed of.

Clerical and administrative personnel should not be permitted inside the controlled area. Instead notes, telephone messages, and other such items should only be directed into the controlled area to reduce the possible spread of contamination to the outside. If data books, notes, protocols, and other program-related documents are removed to clean areas for calculations, data analysis, and report or manuscript preparation, they must be thoroughly decontaminated. A computerized data entry system with the terminal inside the barrier and the computer outside is one solution to this problem, albeit somewhat expensive.

Standard practices or procedures should be developed and implemented which not only ensure the consistency of the experimental study, but also provide optimal protection of the staff. Work surfaces on which toxic materials are used or stored should be covered with stainless steel or plastic trays, dry absorbent plastic-backed paper, or other impervious materials. These protective surfaces and materials should be decontaminated or properly disposed of after completion of any procedure involving the test material.

Stock quantities of test materials should be stored in access-controlled, appropriately labeled storage areas or cabinets. The individual responsible for the area should maintain an inventory of the compounds stored, listing the quantities and dates of acquisition. In addition to the identity of the contents, individual storage vessels should also be appropriately labeled as to the hazard. Individual containers should be kept in impervious pans or trays large enough to contain the entire volume of the stored material, should breakage occur. Transportation of test materials inside the facility should be accomplished by using a durable secondary container. Contaminated materials should be bagged or otherwise suitably contained and labeled before transportation through the facility.

Procedures which suppress the generation of aerosols should be instituted. Wet mopping and the use of vacuum cleaners equipped with high-efficiency particulate air (HEPA) filters are recommended. Dry sweeping and dry mopping should be prohibited. Experimental areas should be cleaned frequently and, if necessary, special cleanup and decontamination procedures should be developed for each individual compound under study.

Vacuum lines and water aspirators must be protected to prevent the entry of toxic chemicals into the central vacuum or drain system. Absorbent or liquid traps and in-line HEPA filters should be installed on all vacuum service cocks. Unprotected utility systems may need to be thoroughly decontaminated prior to any servicing by maintenance personnel.

Eating, drinking, smoking, chewing of gum or tobacco, application of cosmetics, and storage of food, utensils, or food containers must be prohibited in areas where toxic chemicals are stored or used. Furthermore, good personal hygiene habits should be followed by all personnel in the program. Hands should be washed immediately on completion of any procedure involving the test material and whenever leaving the work area. Fingers should be kept away from the mouth, nose, and eyes. Thorough showering may be required before leaving the controlled facility. Immediate washing or showering is required after any overt exposure to the test material. Lastly, mechanical pipetting devices must always be used for any pipetting procedures. Mouth pipetting must be absolutely prohibited in any toxicological testing procedure.

The adequacy of any set of administrative controls or standard operating procedures is dependent upon their eventual implementation. When these procedures are ignored or circumvented, the effectiveness of the overall control program is compromised. Experience with microbiological laboratory safety programs has shown that failure to adhere to good laboratory practices may account for a significant number of laboratory-acquired infections [16].

Engineering Controls

Since activities or operations that generate contamination cannot be eliminated from a toxicological testing protocol, control of that contamination, preferably at the source, is essential. Engineering controls, which include certain design or operational parameters, and primary containment and local exhaust ventilation devices can be used to augment the protection against personnel exposure afforded by the implementation of good operational practices and administrative controls.

Design/Operational Parameters

Areas of the testing facility in which potentially toxic materials are stored or used should be selected so that the net movement of air within the facility is from areas of lowest potential contamination to areas of highest. In this way, any contaminated aerosols or vapors will tend to migrate to or be retained in those areas of strict access control. Air within the facility should not be recirculated unless it is demonstrated to be contaminant free. Energy conservation measures should be carefully evaluated to ensure that occupant health and safety are not compromised. In the design of an animal testing facility, or in the renovation of an existing one, it may be appropriate to consider various architectural design concepts (e.g., single- versus dual-corridor facilities, designs to simplify maintenance) [17, 18]. In addition, consideration should be given to the treatment (via filtration, reaction, absorption, adsorption, electrostatic precipitation, or incineration) of exhaust airstreams prior to discharge from the facility if there is the likelihood that the airstream will become contaminated with the test material.

Primary Containment Devices

Three principal primary containment devices are routinely used in chemical testing facilities: chemical fume hoods, biological safety cabinets, and glove boxes. The purpose of these devices is to contain the contaminant inside the unit and discharge the air, after treatment if necessary, to the outside. Evaluation of the hazard potential is necessary to determine which type of device should be used for any particular procedure in the program. The exhaust air from these units must be discharged in a manner that permits no re-entrainment into the supply air intake of the building or an adjacent facility.

Any procedures in which aerosols may be generated should be performed in a containment device. Opening of vessels and ampules, weighing, transferring, mixing, and diluting procedures should be done in a fume hood or other device providing local exhaust ventilation. If highly toxic materials are used, a glove box is recommended. Investigators should be aware of the contamination resulting from the transfer of solid and liquid materials in chemical fume hoods, and the need to decontaminate the internal surfaces of the hood and any equipment used in the transfer [11]. The administration of the dose to the test animal may need to be performed inside a fume hood or a biological safety cabinet. It is sometimes necessary to airwash the treated animal before returning it to the post-treatment holding area.

Toxicological test procedures involving cell cultures and microorganisms are more easily controlled, since virtually all work is conducted inside a biological safety cabinet, which provides both product and operator protection. Class II biological safety cabinets used in such studies are equipped with HEPA filters which supply sterile air to the work areas of the cabinet and remove particulate material from the exhaust air. Since these filters do not remove vapors or gases and a portion of the air is recirculated within the cabinet, they are not generally recommended for work involving volatile compounds. Class II Type A biological safety cabinets may recirculate HEPA-filtered air back into the laboratory. This mode of operation should never be used in such testing operations. Suitable provisions can be made for discharging the cabinet exhaust air to the outside (via the general ventilation system). Class II Type B biological safety cabinets also recirculate a fraction of the air within the cabinet (although substantially less than that recirculated within the Type A), so their use with volatile compounds should likewise be discouraged. The total exhaust biological safety cabinet, as the name implies, exhausts all the air after a single pass through the workspace within the cabinet, so no restrictions regarding the use of volatile materials are necessary. Both the Class II Type B and the total exhaust laminar flow biological safety cabinets require installation to allow for discharge of exhaust air to the outdoors.

Glove boxes provide the highest levels of containment and should be used whenever possible for handling highly toxic chemicals. Exhaust air from glove boxes should always be treated before discharge to the outdoors and should never be manifolded with other hoods.

Primary containment devices provide excellent protection for workers handling highly toxic compounds; however, they can be compromised if good work practices are not observed. Chemical fume hoods and biological safety cabinets must be properly located in the room so that their performance is not adversely affected by room air currents or pedestrian traffic. Airflow into the device should not be obstructed by items stored within the unit. Work should be conducted six to eight inches back from the face to ensure capture and containment of contaminants in the entering air stream. Contamination of the work surfaces should be avoided. Hoods and safety cabinets should be certified initially at installation, at least yearly thereafter and always after maintenance work is performed. Adequate face velocities must be maintained[19].

One specialized type of primary containment equipment used in toxicological testing is the inhalation chamber used to expose animals to a constant, controlled level of test material via the inhalation route. These chambers must be certified and routinely tested for leaks and must be exhausted to the outdoors. Treatment of the exhaust air is typically required. Specialized purging and monitoring devices are needed to ensure that the test material has been removed prior to opening the chamber. Other specialized containment devices have been designed for work involving animals and animal wastes. Individually ventilated cages, ventilated cage racks, and cages fitted with filter bonnets can reduce contamination in animal holding areas. The use of a ventilated cage dumping station in the cage wash area reduces the contamination potential in handling animal bedding.

Local Exhaust Ventilation

Local exhaust ventilation should be provided over any equipment or operation that cannot be accommodated in a primary containment device and which has the potential for aerosol production or other release of toxic contaminants. Local ventilation may be used to capture vapors or aerosols over analytical instruments, in dosage preparation areas, in cage dumping and cage washing areas, and in necropsy areas where test materials as well as other toxic vapors (e.g., formaldehyde) may be present. Equipment requiring local exhaust ventilation is sometimes also encountered in *in vitro* testing procedures. The incubation of cultures treated with volatile test chemicals is one example. Control measures in this case may require special local exhaust ventilation into either a chemical fume hood or the building exhaust.

Personal Protective Equipment

The use of personal protective equipment may be required to provide protection against exposure to toxic chemicals when engineering and operational controls are insufficient to adequately protect the laboratory worker. However, such equipment should not be relied upon as the sole basis of protection. For example, even properly fitted respirators are recognized as providing only a finite degree of protection that varies with the individual user and the type of respirator (e.g., air purifying or air supplied).

A risk assessment must be conducted in each area of the testing facility to determine what personal protective equipment may be needed. For example, in the analytical laboratory or with procedures conducted in a glove box, the need for personal protective equipment is minimal. However, in the posttreatment animal holding area, if ventilated cages or cage racks or local exhaust ventilation are not used, then maximum personal protective equipment is needed. This can only be determined by careful evaluation of the toxic properties of the test material, the experimental procedures, and the administrative and engineering controls available.

Protective clothing can consist of fully buttoned or wraparound lab coats, jump suits, scrub suits, or positive-pressure "space suits." Head and shoe covers may also be required. Protective clothing should not be worn outside the work area. Disposable clothing should be used whenever possible to reduce the spread of contamination to other areas and personnel. Overtly contaminated clothing should be removed immediately, and properly disposed of or decontaminated prior to laundering. When methods of decontamination are not known or are not applicable, disposable clothing should always be worn.

Gloves which are appropriate for both the task and the chemical being handled should be worn whenever the toxic material is handled. Disposable gloves should be discarded after each use and after any overt contamination. Selection of the proper glove material should take into account its resistance to penetration by the particular chemical or solvent in use [20–22].

Eye protection devices, appropriate to the hazards involved, should be available and used in the work areas. Chemical splash goggles, full-face shields, or full-face respirators may be required, depending on the test agent and the operation being conducted.

Finally, respiratory protection may be required in certain areas of the chemical testing facility if engineering controls are not adequate in reducing the potential hazards. This is especially likely in dosage preparation, dose administration, and posttreatment animal holding areas of the facility, although it may also be necessary in other areas. Respiratory protection can consist of half-face or full-face air purifying respirators or air supplied respirators (self-contained or air-line). If respiratory protection equipment is used, a respirator-use program must be instituted for all personnel (including maintenance and emergency personnel) who may enter the contaminated areas. The program must comply with the appropriate Occupational Safety and Health Administration (OSHA) standards [23].

SUMMARY

A number of studies have demonstrated the ease with which contamination can be generated during the conduct of toxicological testing studies. The presence of this contamination, both inside and outside the controlled testing environment, suggests the potential for employee exposure to the test agent and the possibility of cross-contamination between animals under study (e.g., different treatment levels, controls, other studies). Although the levels of exposure to which workers may be subjected appear quite low, cumulative effects of repeated exposures become significant, especially if the chemical in question is very potent.

There are a variety of options available to reduce or eliminate the potential for personnel exposure to test chemicals. These typically involve the use of appropriate design or engineering controls, operational practices and administrative controls, and personal protective equipment. It is through the judicious combination of these three options, tailored to the specific facility and procedure, that the potential for personnel exposure can be reduced. It is possible to compensate for deficiencies in one area (e.g., facility design) by providing tighter controls in the others.

Whichever methods are chosen, it is advisable to conduct periodic evaluations of the effectiveness of the control program, including monitoring for contaminants (or suitable surrogates) at various locations within the facility. In long-term bioassay studies, where the test chemical is administered to animals for the majority of their lifespan, this periodic evaluation is particularly instructive in order that weak links in the control program can be identified and corrected. These weak links may be caused by the gradual accumulation of a test agent released at low levels, or may result from a breakdown in standard operating procedures.

The various control measures described have been used in a broad variety of circumstances and have proved effective. This is not to say that these are the only methods to assure safe operations in toxicological testing facilities. What is important is to be aware of the many possibilities for personnel and facility contamination, and to consider which control measures will be most effective in protecting the facility, the program, and most importantly the personnel involved in the study.

REFERENCES

1. Li, I., J. Fraumeni, N. Mantel, and R. Miller. "Cancer Mortality Among Chemists," *J. Natl. Cancer Inst.* 43:1159–1164, 1969.
2. Olin, R. "The Hazards of a Chemical Laboratory Environment: A Study of the Mortality on Two Cohorts of Swedish Chemists," *Am. Ind. Hyg. Assoc. J.* 39:557–562, 1978.
3. Searle, C., J. Waterhouse, B. Henman, D. Bartlett, and S. McCombie. "Epidemiological Study of the Mortality of British Chemists," *Br. J. Cancer* 38:192–193, 1978.
4. National Research Council, Committee on Hazardous Substances in the Laboratory. *Prudent Practices for Handling Hazardous Chemicals in Laboratories* (Washington, D.C.: National Academy Press, 1981), pp. 247–256.
5. Richardson, J.H. and W.E. Barkley, Eds. *Biosafety in Microbiological and Biomedical Laboratories* (draft), Centers for Disease Control and National Institutes of Health, Public Health Service, U.S. Department of Health and Human Services (Washington, D.C.: U.S. Government Printing Office, 1983).
6. Health and Safety Committee Minutes, Carcinogenesis Bioassay Program, National Cancer Institute/National Toxicology Program, National Institutes of Health, Public Health Service, U.S. Department of Health and Human Services, Bethesda, January 5, 1981.
7. Unpublished data on chemical contaminant monitoring of bioassay operations, Carcinogenesis Bioassay Program, National Cancer Institute/National Toxicology Program, National Institutes of Health, Public Health Service, U.S. Department of Health and Human Services, Bethesda, May 2, 1980.
8. Unpublished data on chemical contaminant monitoring of bioassay operations, Carcinogenesis Bioassay Program, National Cancer Institute/National Toxicology Program, National Institutes of Health, Public Health Service, U.S. Department of Health and Human Services, Bethesda, August 31, 1979.

9. Sansone, E.B., A.M. Losikoff, and R.A. Pendleton. "Sources and Dissemination of Contamination in Material Handling Operations," *Am. Ind. Hyg. Assoc. J.* 38: 433–442, 1977.

10. Sansone, E.B., A.M. Losikoff, and R.A. Pendleton. "Potential Hazards from Feeding Test Chemicals in Carcinogen Bioassay Research," *Tox. Appl. Pharm.* 39:435–450, 1977.

11. Sansone, E.B. and A.M. Losikoff. "A Note on the Chemical Contamination Resulting from the Transfer of Solid and Liquid Materials in Hoods," *Am. Ind. Hyg. Assoc. J.* 38:489–491, 1977.

12. Sansone, E.B. and A.M. Losikoff. "Contamination from Feeding Volatile Test Chemicals," *Tox. Appl. Pharm.* 46:1–6, 1978.

13. Sansone, E.G., A.M. Losikoff, W.B. Lebherz, and J.A.Poiley."Assessment of Environmental Contamination Associated With a Mammalian Cell Transformation Assay," *In Vitro* 17(9):811–815, 1981.

14. Sansone, E.B. "Incubator Contamination," *Nature* 260:527, 1976.

15. Light, W.G., K. J. McNulty, and R.L. Goldsmith. "Development of Decontamination Procedures for Aqueous Chemical Carcinogens (Final Report)," submitted to Tracor-Jitco Inc., Rockville, Md, August, 1978.

16. Pike, R.M. "Laboratory-Associated Infections: Summary and Analysis of 3921 Cases," *Hlth. Lab. Sci.* 13:105–114, 1976.

17. Fox, D.G., Ed. *Design of Biomedical Research Facilities,* U.S. DHHS/NIH Publication No. 81-2305, National Institutes of Health, Public Health Service, U.S. Department of Health and Human Services, Bethesda, Maryland, 1981.

18. Sansone, E.B., and A.M. Losikoff. "Potential Contamination from Feeding Test Chemicals in Carcinogen Bioassay Research: Evaluation of Single- and Double-Corridor Animal Housing Facilities," *Tox. Appl. Pharm.* 50:115–121, 1979.

19. Committee on Industrial Ventilation. *Industrial Ventilation,* 16th ed. (Lansing, MI: American Council of Governmental Industrial Hygienists, 1980), pp. 5–23.

20. Weeks, R.W. and B.J. Dean. "Permeation of Methanolic Aromatic Amine Solutions Through Commercially Available Glove Materials," *Am. Ind. Hygiene Assoc. J.* 38:721, 1977.

21. Sansone, E.B. and Y.B. Tewari. "The Permeability of Laboratory Gloves to Selected Solvents," *Am. Ind. Hyg. Assoc. J.* 31:169–173, 1978.

22. Walker, E., M. Castegnaro, L. Garren, and B. Pignatelli. "Limitations to the Protective Effect of Rubber Gloves for Handling Nitrosamines," *Environmental Aspects of N-Nitroso Compounds* in E. Walker, M. Castegnaro, L. Gricuite, and R.E. Lyle, Eds. (Lyon, France: International Agency for Research on Cancer Scientific Publication No. 19, 1978) pp. 535–543.

23. U.S. Department of Labor, Occupational Safety and Health Administration. "Occupational Safety and Health Standards (29 CFR 1910)," 1910.134, Respiratory Protection (Washington, D.C.: U.S. Government Printing Office, 1981).

CHAPTER 15

Laboratory Hood Performance in Toxicity Testing Laboratories

E. Robinson Hoyle and R. Scott Stricoff
Arthur D. Little, Inc., Acorn Park,
Cambridge, Massachusetts 02140

Douglas B. Walters
National Toxicology Program, National Institute of
Environmental Health Sciences, P.O. Box 12233,
Research Triangle Park, North Carolina 27709

INTRODUCTION

Over the past several years an increasing amount of research has been conducted on ventilation systems in laboratories [1-3]. As a result of these efforts many guidelines and design criteria for laboratory ventilation systems have been produced [4-7, 8, 9, 10]. The standard laboratory fume hood is the primary exhaust system in any laboratory. In examining laboratory hoods, it is appropriate to discuss three areas: existing laboratory hood systems, their design, and performance criteria for these systems. The emphasis of this chapter is on hood performance criteria and on the development of a detailed hood evaluation and monitoring program. In conducting health and safety reviews of laboratories participating in the National Toxicology Program (NTP) bioassay program, two significant trends with regard to laboratory hoods are notable. First, many hood monitoring and maintenance programs are limited to the visible components of the system (i.e., the hood), ignoring the rest of the system (ductwork, fan, etc.). Second, many biologists and chemists work with improperly designed ventilation systems but are still held responsible for maintaining good hood performance to protect employees from exposure to hazardous chemicals. For these reasons this discussion concentrates not only on qualitative but also on general quantitative methods for monitoring the entire exhaust system from the hood to the fan and discharge stack. Quantitative monitoring techniques for specific equipment and ventilation systems are not described here, but are available from equipment manufacturers and the ventilation guidelines mentioned above.

LOCAL EXHAUST VENTILATION SYSTEMS

There are chemical fume hoods, biological safety cabinets, glove boxes, and a variety of miscellaneous exhaust enclosures found throughout the NTP bioassay program. First there is the common chemical fume hood—simply a sash with an opening and an exhaust slot. Chemical fume hoods most often come in 6-foot or 4-foot widths and can have supply air introduced inside or outside the sash.

Class II biological safety cabinets (BSC) are a bit more complicated than the normal chemical fume hood. In addition to a sash and an exhaust slot, there is also supply air or laminar flow. The BSC supply and exhaust air are HEPA (high efficiency particulate air) filtered, and in some cases the exhaust air is filtered and recirculated (class II type A) or the exhaust is partially or totally exhausted to the outside (class II type B). For the class II, type A BSC, 70% of the air is recirculated and 30% is exhausted out of the cabinet. The reverse, 70% exhausted and 30% recirculated, is true for class II, type B BSC. Due to the recirculation feature, volatile or highly toxic materials should not be used in the BSC. Both type A and B BSC exhaust the cabinet air back into the laboratory, unless special ducting is provided to the outside environment. The class II total exhaust cabinet (or 100% exhaust), although it is on the market, is still undergoing testing and has not been certified by the National Sanitation Foundation. Glove boxes, which are totally enclosed cases with glove ports, are used for handling materials that are extremely toxic.

Miscellaneous systems for bioassay facilities include small dosing hoods with plexiglass for easy vision (Figure 15-1), and even smaller recirculation desktop hoods with charcoal filters for use with solvents (Figure 15-2). Local exhaust ventilation systems include large walk-in hoods for P&K blenders (Figure 15-3), "elephant trunk" for gas chromatographs and spectrophotometers, and extraction hoods for extracting with large amounts of solvents.

As shown in Figure 15-4, there are five basic components to a local exhaust system: the laboratory hood; the duct work; an air cleaner, which can be a high-efficiency particulate air (HEPA) or charcoal filter; the fan; and the exhaust stack. In addition to the hood itself, it is important to understand the four other components which, although not as visible as the laboratory hood, are just as critical. The fan pulls the air through the hood; the duct work contains the air to protect the rest of the environment from the contaminant; the air cleaner removes the contaminant; and the fan exhausts the air through the stack up and above the roof level to avoid reentrainment of exhaust air into the general air supply system. If any one of these components malfunctions, the entire system fails. Consequently, if there is a hole in the duct work, the face velocity through the hood will be reduced. If the HEPA filter has too much particulate on it, there will be too great a pressure drop for the fan to provide the proper face velocity at the hood.

Design Criteria

Design criteria for laboratory local exhaust ventilation systems should include the following:

- Location of the hood in the laboratory to keep the hood away from traffic, and windows, and doors. General air supply and exhaust diffusers should not be placed where they will create drafts at the hood face.
- Introduction of auxiliary or supply air at the face of a chemical fume hood should be done so as to cause air to sweep down across the outside of the sash.
- The front edge or lip of the hood should be rounded to reduce turbulence. Rear exhaust slots and baffles should be fixed to avoid inadvertent closure.
- The duct connection to the hood should be designed to avoid sharp angles of introduction of other branches to within six duct diameters of the hood. This will reduce turbulent air patterns inside the hood.
- Air cleaning equipment should be appropriate for the type of contaminant. The equipment should be located for easy access to change or monitor filters. Differential pressure gauges should be located in the laboratory so that pressure drops, indicative of the need to replace filters, can easily be determined.

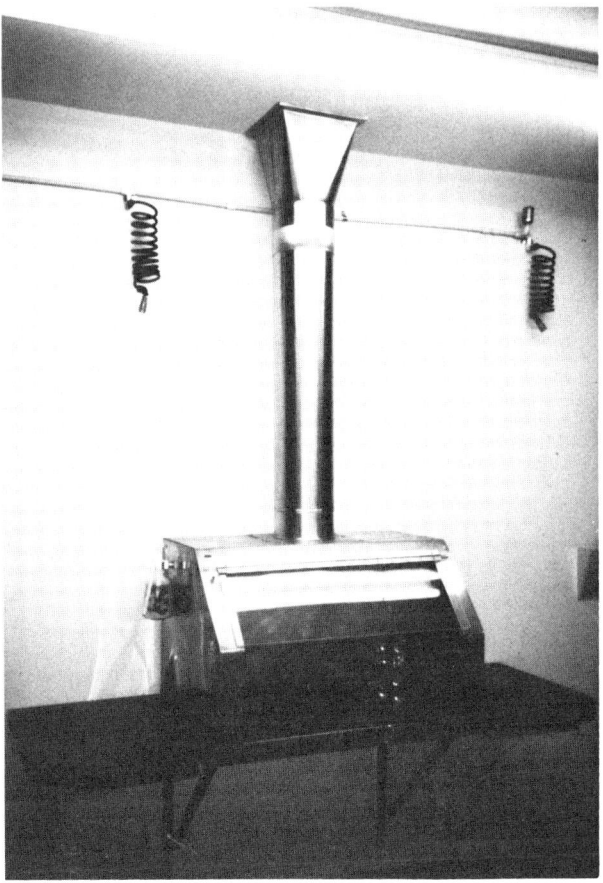

Figure 15-1.   Dose administration hood in bioassay *(in vivo)* testing laboratory.

- The fan should be located outside the building (on the roof) so a negative pressure can be maintained in the duct carrying contaminated air from the hood to the fan. Air cleaning equipment should be located ahead of the fan to reduce deterioration of fan parts due to the action of contaminants.
- Exhaust stacks should be placed above the roof line and away from air supply equipment.

Figure 15–5 is a poor example of an exhaust duct location at the rear of the exhaust slot of a hood. The duct should be introduced so that the exhausted air is evenly distributed inside the hood. (Figure 15–6). Ducts should not have sharp 90-degree elbows immediately before the connection to the hood. The hood on the left in Figure 15–7 was actually emptying its contaminated air into the hood on the right, due to the location of the duct and damper on the second hood. Improper location of the exhaust fan (on stand), in a manner making reentrainment of contaminant inevitable, is shown in Figure 15–8. Elevated exhaust stacks (Figure 15–9) above the roof line reduce the opportunity for reentrainment of contaminants, which can result in recycling contaminants back into the laboratory.

PERFORMANCE CRITERIA: HOOD MONITORING AND EVALUATION

Effective hood performance criteria should include: nondisruptive interior and exterior air patterns—from room makeup and exhaust air baffles and from the introduc-

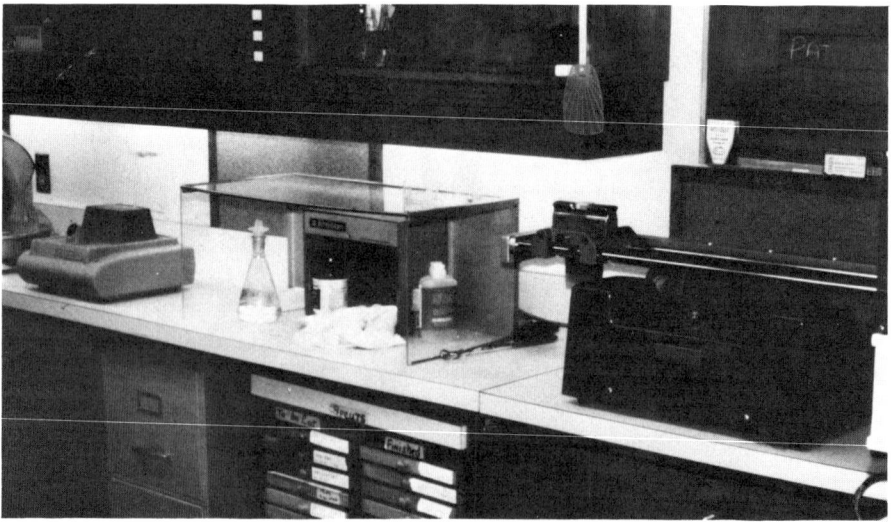

Figure 15–2. Desktop recirculation hood for solvent transfer.

tion of makeup air at the hood face; absence of capture or face velocity leakage from duct plenums, sashes on hoods, or from gloves on glove boxes; good working area downflow in a laminar flow system; use of pressure gauges for reading differential static pressure on either side of filters; and programmed routine maintenance of duct work, fans, and air cleaners. We will discuss these hood performance criteria in terms of a hood monitoring and evaluation program. The four basic elements of this program are: daily visual inspections, quarterly inspections, user training, and routine maintenance.

Daily Visual Inspection

Daily visual inspections should include observation and correction of any clutter in front of exhaust slots in fume hoods or biological cabinets. In Figure 15–10 too much

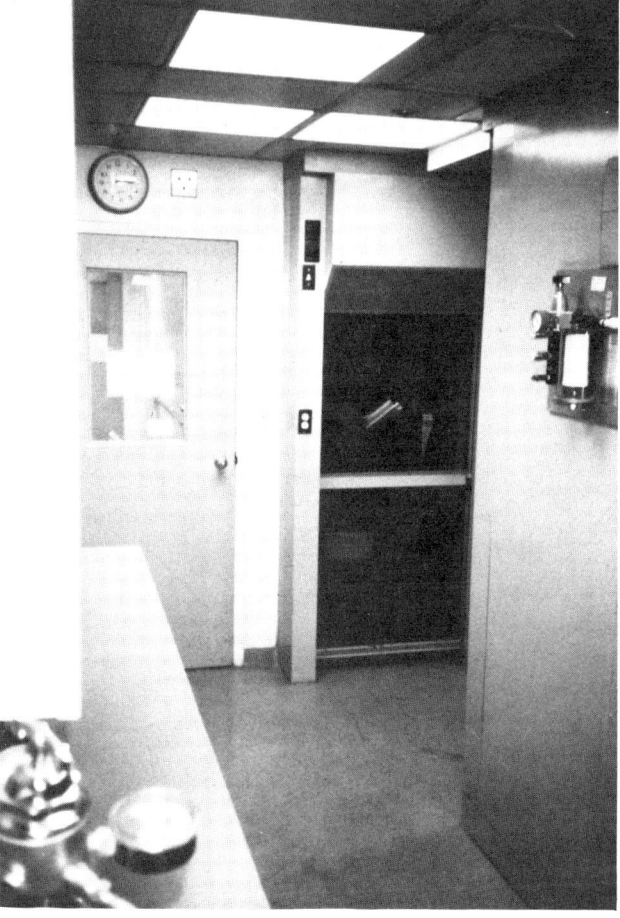

Figure 15–3.   Walk-in vented enclosure for large mixer.

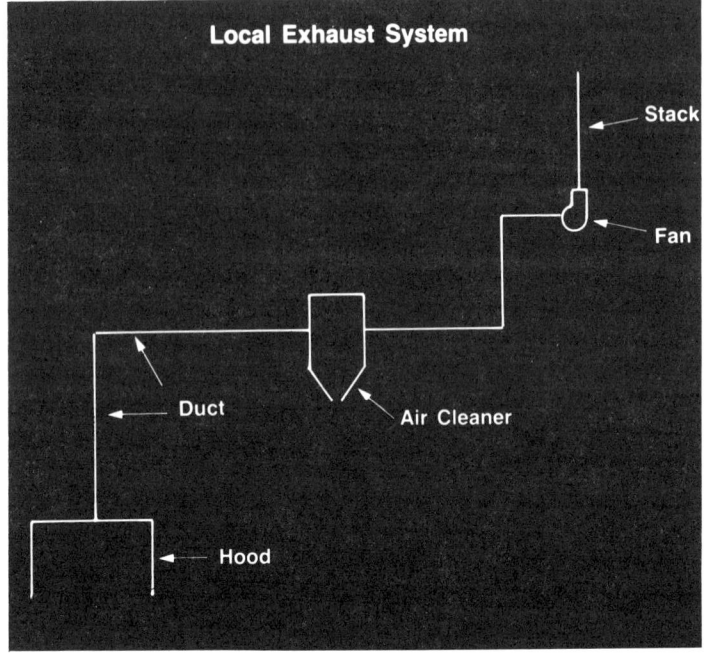

Figure 15–4. Local exhaust ventilation system.

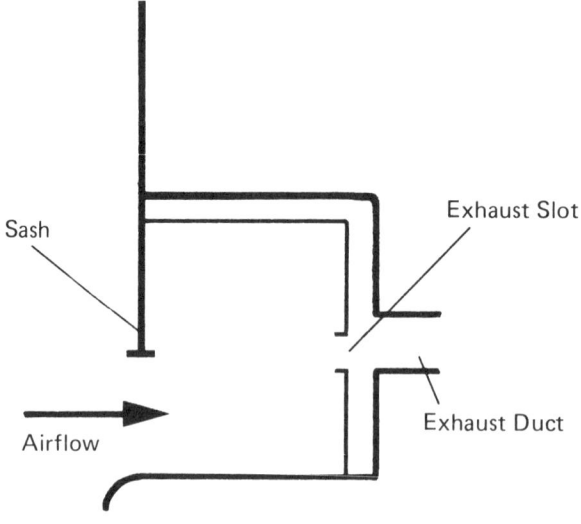

Poor Exhaust Duct Location

Figure 15–5. Laboratory hood: improper introduction of exhaust duct.

equipment is in front of the hood for operating personnel to effectively work at the hood face. Also, material blocking the exhaust slot should be taken away to avoid disrupting the capture velocity profile at the hood face. Figure 15–11, where solvent bottles are cluttered throughout the hood, is an example of this problem. Any pressure gauges that are at the hood where the user can see them should be checked to make sure that they are within a normal operating range. If static pressure is high, the filter or air cleaner may be overloaded. If it is low, the entire system may be shut down due to a mechanical failure.

A simple air check can be made for biological safety cabinets and laboratory hoods. Tissue paper can be placed at the face or near the slot, and if the tissue paper moves toward the rear of the hood, the exhaust is operating. In a glove box a similar test can be made with tissue paper inside the box held by the gloves up near the exhaust slot. The operator should be careful not to allow tissue paper to fly up the exhaust as it can block the filter and reduce airflow.

Quarterly Inspection

The second component of a hood monitoring program should include quarterly inspections conducted by qualified personnel. The first part of this quarterly inspection should include smoke tests with either smoke candles or smoke tubes. The proper method for using a smoke tube to analyze air patterns in front of the hood face is shown in Figure 15–12. A smoke tube, in some cases titanium tetrachloride, should

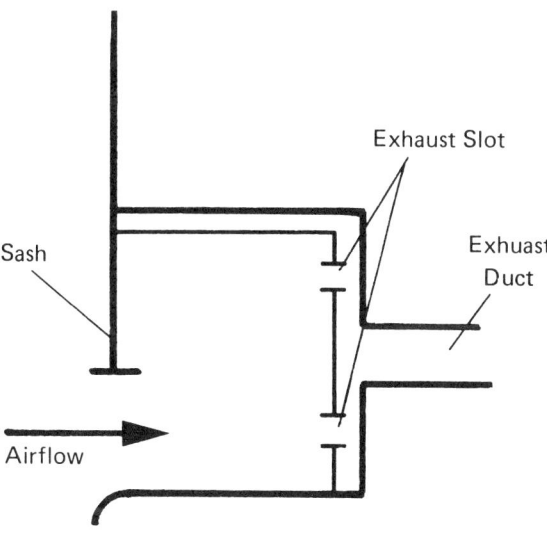

Good Exhaust Duct Location

Figure 15–6.   Side view of laboratory hood: proper location of exhaust duct.

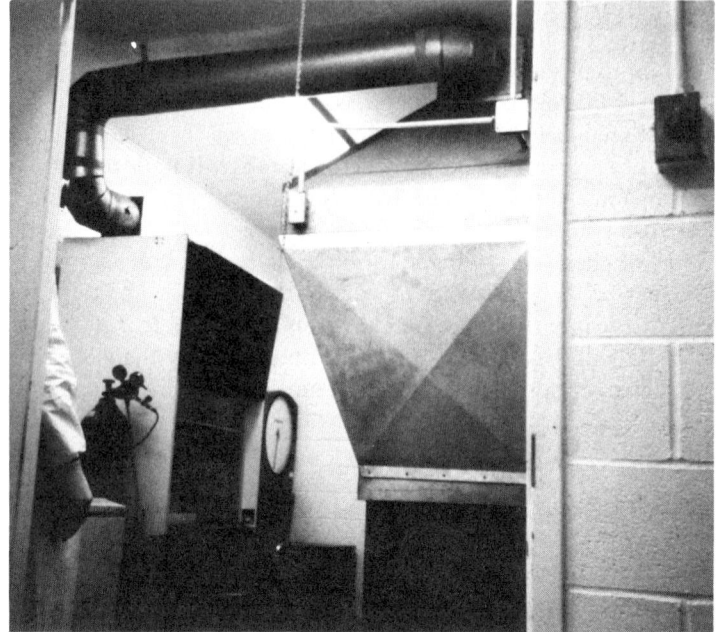

Figure 15-7. Incorrect connection of two laboratory hoods.

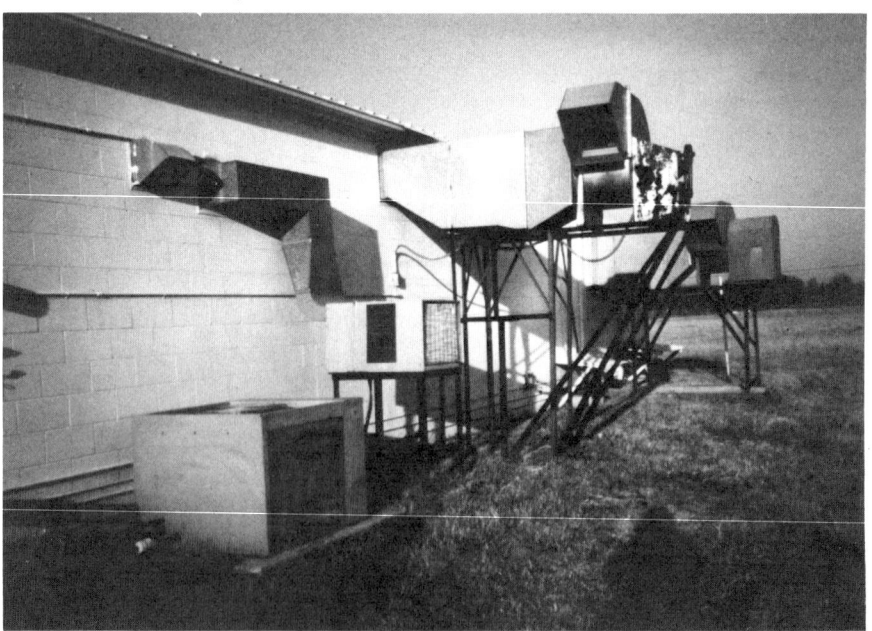

Figure 15-8. Example of reentrainment of contaminants from exhausted and supply air systems.

be placed 1 foot to 1.5 feet away from the face, moving slowly across the length of the sash. Gradually the tube should be moved closer while maintaining the horizontal movement to check for any turbulence or dead spots at the face. This can also be performed well inside the hood to check for any leakage or dead spots. This is an important test because in some situations equipment or special modifications to a laboratory hood may create air turbulence. As can be seen in Figure 15–13, a storage shelf was placed in the normal chemical fume hood with the solvents stored well above the exhaust slot. When smoke was introduced into the hood a large curl was found where the smoke curled up toward the solvent bottles and out toward the sash. It was found that if the sash was not pulled down to an 8-inch operating height the smoke actually curled outside the hood and was not recaptured.

Smoke candles and tubes are particularly useful in dose preparation hoods where neat chemical is weighed or mixed. In these hoods, analytical or top-loading balances and small blenders may block the exhaust slots and create undesirable air patterns which affect the capture efficiency of the hood. Similar smoke tests can be done with biological safety cabinets. Sashes and gaskets can be checked for leakage, and laminar downflow and inflow patterns can be observed by placing the smoke tube in the center of the working area and observing the smoke movement. BSC sashes which do indicate leakage may create a problem if any vapor or particulate is recirculated (class II type B) inside the hood.

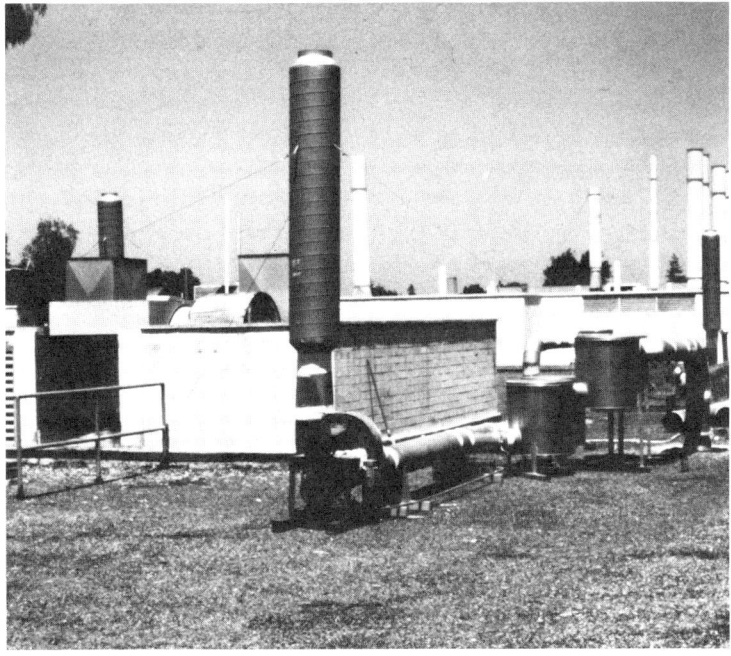

Figure 15–9. Exhaust stacks elevated above roof level.

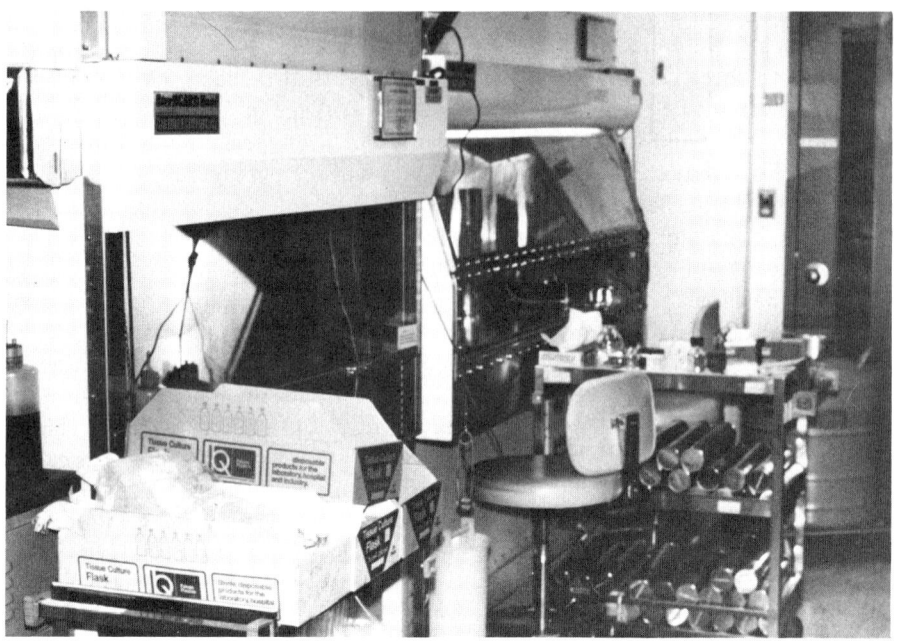

Figure 15–10.   Clutter in front of laboratory hoods.

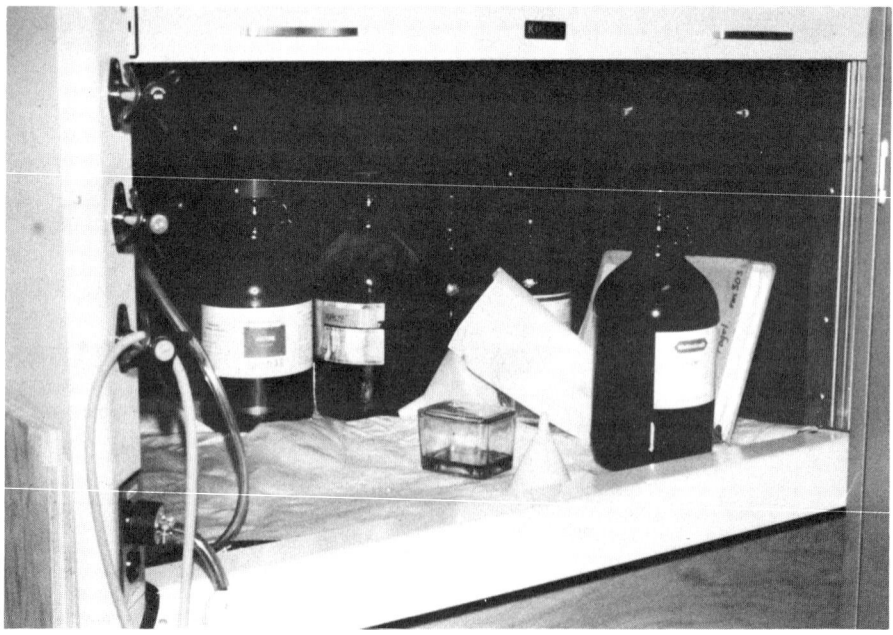

Figure 15–11.   Solvent containers blocking the laboratory rear slot exhaust.

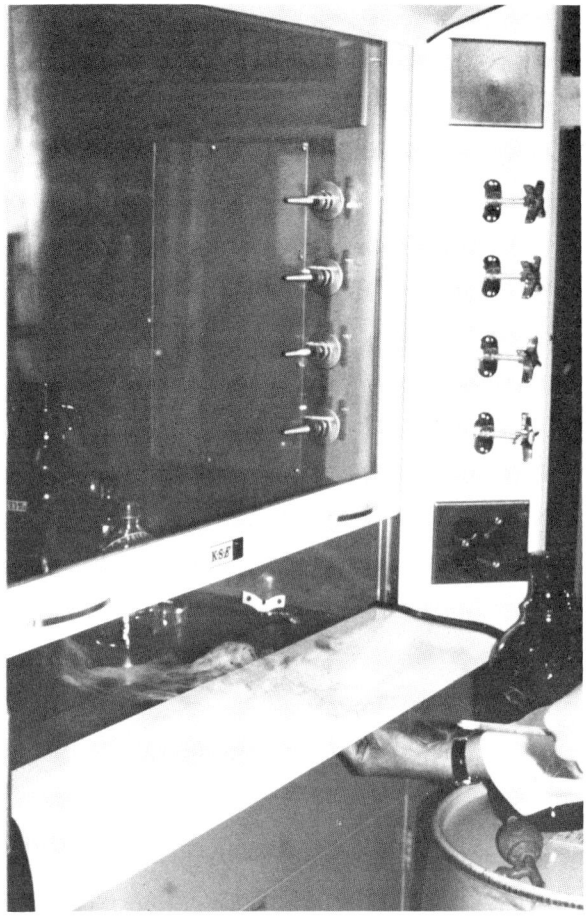

Figure 15–12.   Qualitative smoke evaluation of laboratory hood exhaust.

The second portion of the quarterly inspection is a quantitative measurement of the face or capture velocity. For fume hoods these measurements should be taken with mechanical vane velometer or thermal anemometer. Face velocity should be measured with the sash either in the fully open position or at the normal operating height. At the operating height three measurements should be made across the open area. When the sash is fully open, six readings should be performed (Figures 15–14 and 15–15). The average of these six (or three) readings will be the face velocity of the hood. It is important to follow the recommendations of the manufacturer of the hood for the requirements in measuring the face velocity. Usually manufacturers recommend that no auxiliary supply air should be present during measurements. In other words, any makeup air introduced at the hood should be turned off when measuring exhaust velocity. If several hoods are connected together, maximum

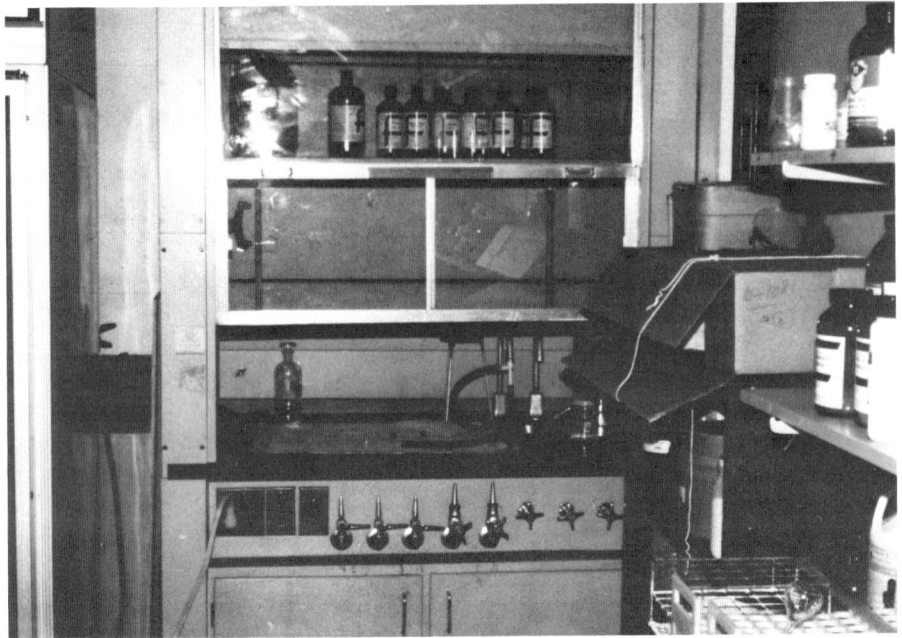

Figure 15-13.   Laboratory hood with poorly located storage shelf.

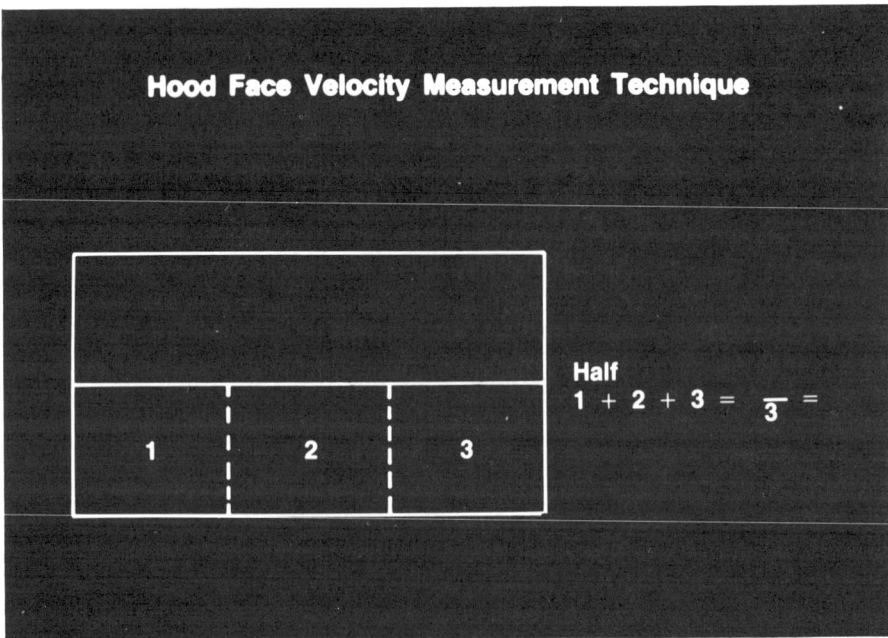

Figure 15-14.   Quantitative laboratory hood evaluation with sash half open or at operating height.

"worst" conditions should be simulated for measuring the face velocity. Consequently, if two hoods are in a series both sashes should be open to make sure that minimum exhaust volumes are present. If several hoods in several different rooms are all connected on the same system, the sashes should be open in all hoods during the measurements.

As mentioned earlier, introduction of the makeup air can have a dramatic effect on turbulence at the face. Figure 15–16 shows a laboratory chemical fume hood with the makeup air introduced at the top: air is sent directly down across the face into the hood. As shown in Figure 15–17, the sash when totally opened does not capture the smoke which was generated in the hood. This is because the makeup air is short-circuited at the top into the laboratory hood. Shown in Figure 15–18 is the same hood with the sash at a lower operating height where all the smoke that is generated in the hood is properly captured.

Currently in NTP laboratories a face velocity of 100 feet per minute (fpm), plus or minus 20%, is recommended. This level should be met at an operating height of 8–10 inches. As emphasized throughout this discussion, this 100 fpm should not be the only evaluation parameter. This level is acceptable in fume hoods if design criteria (no traffic, dust design, etc.), smoke tests, and other performance criteria are satisfied.

The face velocity requirements for biological safety cabinets are more dependent on manufacturers' recommendations. As mentioned above, there are a variety of different BSCs used in the NTP program. In addition to the class II type A and B hoods, there are the class II type B total exhaust (or no recirculation) cabinets. For

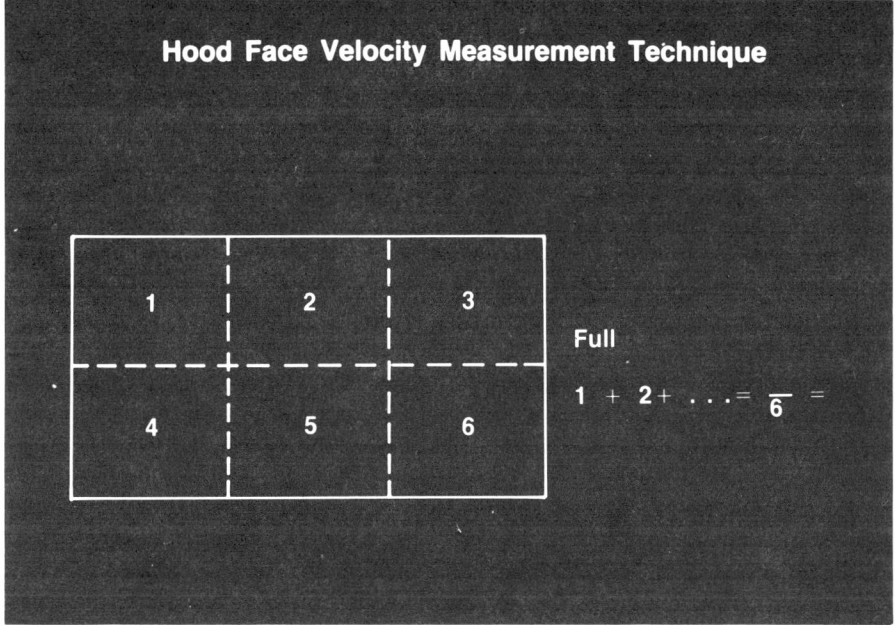

Figure 15–15.   Quantitative laboratory hood evaluation with sash fully open.

the class II type A and B cabinets, inflow measured without the laminar flow (downflow) should be at 100 fpm, plus or minus 20%. Downflow, depending on the manufacturer's recommendations, should be in the area of 50–80 fpm at the working surface. As can be seen in Figures 15–19 to 15–21 proper inflow-downflow balance in a biological safety cabinet is critical to performance. The hood in Figure 15–19 was certified by qualified personnel as operating properly when a velocity of 100 fpm was achieved at the face at the normal work operating height. However, as can be seen from Figures 15–19 and 15–20, the inflow (not the laminar flow) was not operating properly. Smoke escaped out into the room 5 or 6 feet, as well as through the sash and the top of the hood. Closer visual inspection revealed that the exhaust slot at the rear of the hood had vibrated shut and was closed. What the professionals and the user were measuring was the downflow from the air introduced at the top of the cabinet. Figure 15–21 indicates how the hood should work properly when the exhaust slot is open.

Finally, with biological safety cabinets, class II type B total exhaust hoods cannot be tested for inflow because in some cases the downflow (laminar flow) cannot be turned off. Consequently, a quarterly inspection must rely on a series of smoke measurements to observe air patterns, daily visual inspections, and also downflow measurements with a velometer in order to satisfy a semiquantitative evaluation of this type of hood.

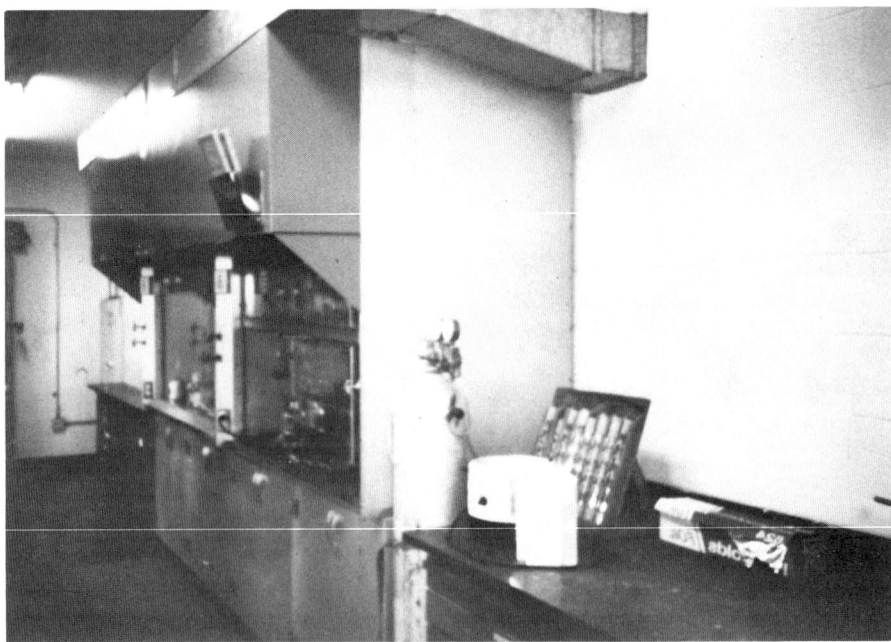

Figure 15–16. Chemical fume hood with auxiliary supply air introduced at top.

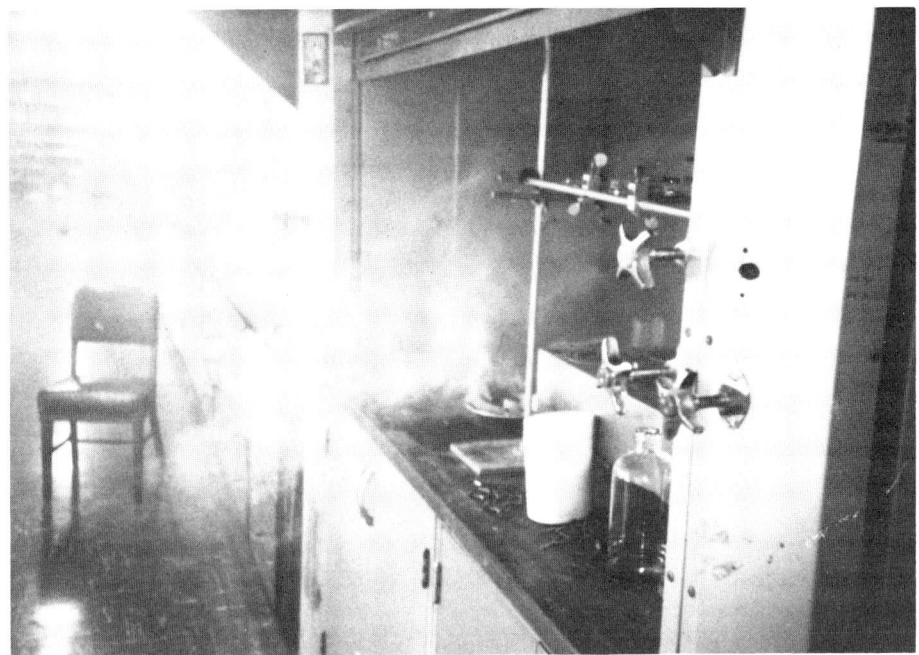

Figure 15–17. Smoke escaping from hood with sash fully open.

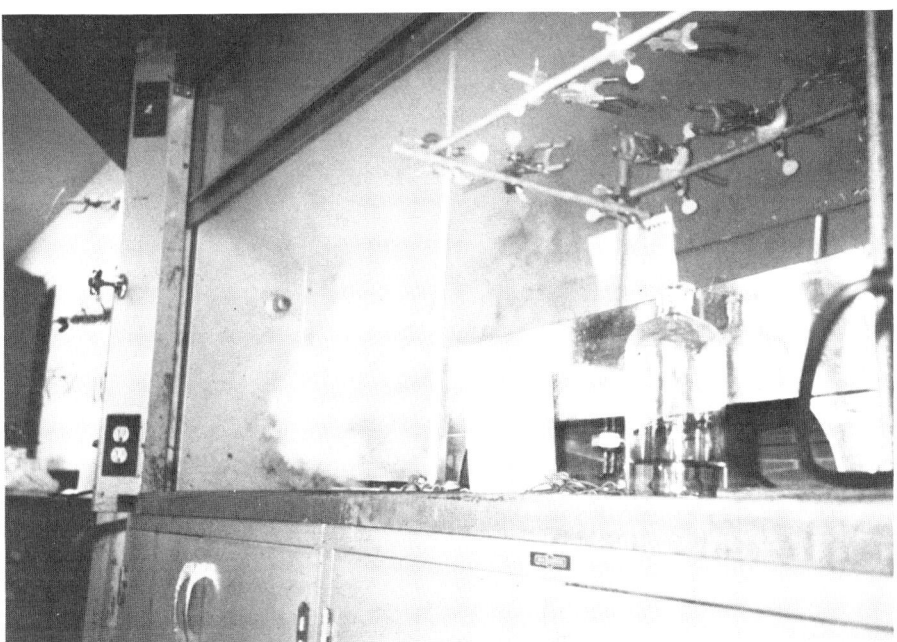

Figure 15–18. Smoke capture with sash at operating height.

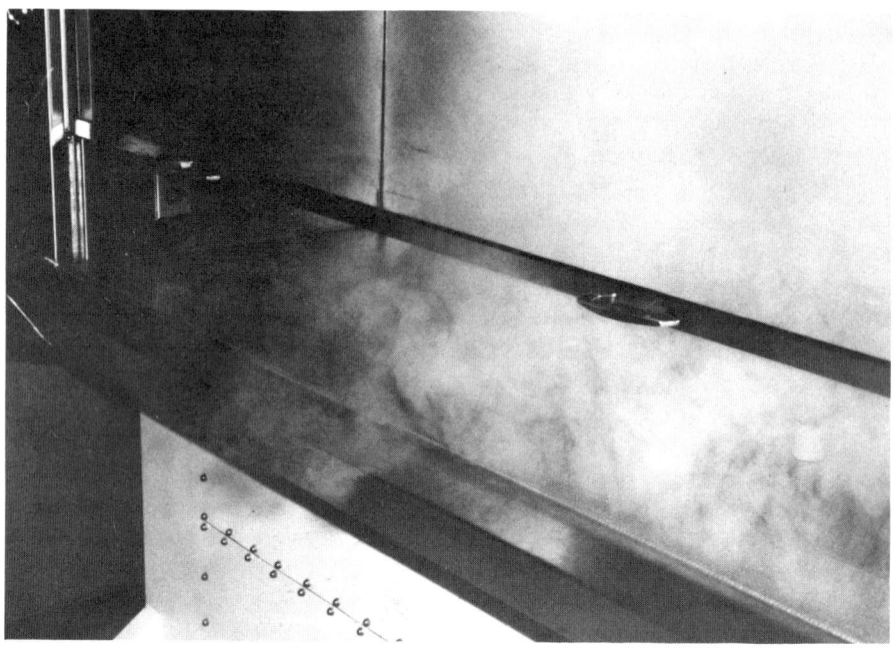

Figure 15–19.   Biological safety cabinet (Class II Type B) with poor capture efficiency.

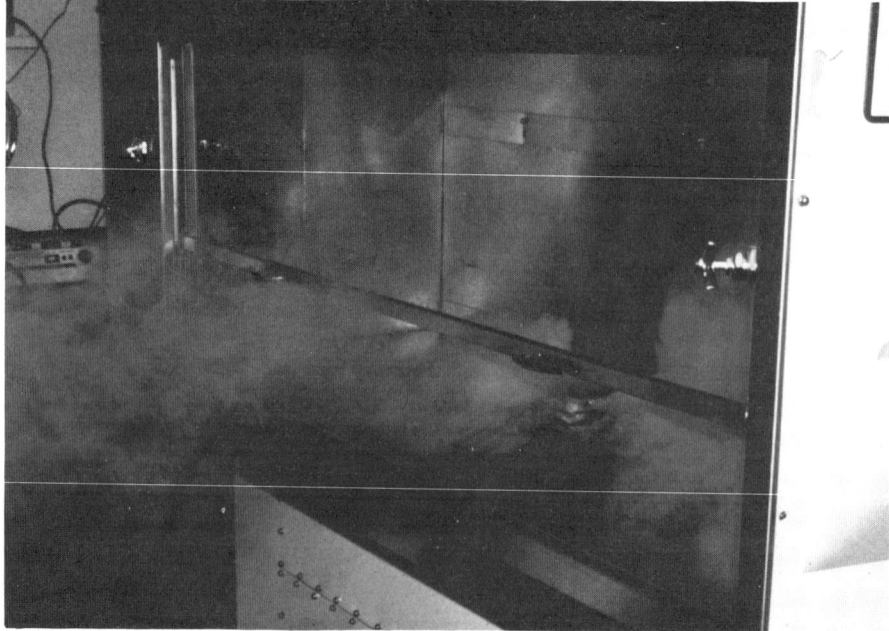

Figure 15–20.   Biological safety cabinet with poor capture efficiency.

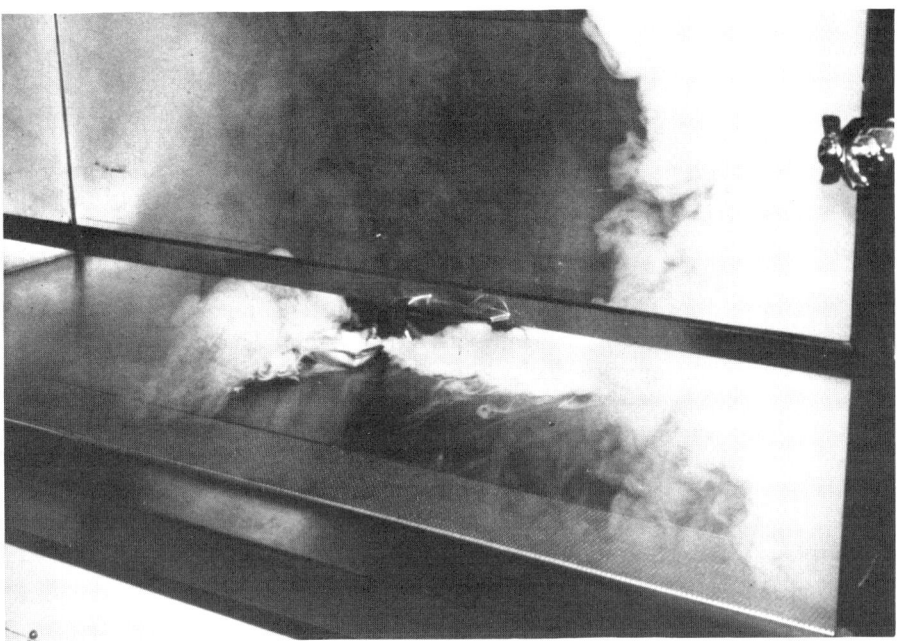

Figure 15–21.   Biological safety cabinet with good capture efficiency.

A glove box can be evaluated by a number of different methods on a quarterly basis. The airflow in the exhaust duct attached to the hood can be measured. Depending on manufacturers' specifications, this should range from 30 to 50 cubic feet per minute (cfm). In addition, the air velocity at the side door can be measured and the area of the door can be calculated. The face velocity multiplied by the area gives the volume of air (cfm) exhausted. In addition, smoke tests can be done inside the gloves and inside the glove box to make sure the gloves do not leak and the box is under negative pressure.

Training

The third component of the hood monitoring and evaluation program is user training. The user or technician must be trained on the proper use of the entire exhaust system. Any pressure gauges that are present, work practices, and maintenance programs should be reviewed with the technician. A good example of a work practice is to locate the work area at least 8 to 9 inches from the front hood edge to avoid any sort of turbulence at the face.

The hood user should understand monitoring programs—the most important, of course, is the daily visual inspection—but also should understand quarterly inspections, as well as any fan maintenance. The more informed the hood user is, the greater the likelihood that he or she can spot and correct any sort of problems which occur in the hood.

Finally, user training should include any sort of recordkeeping on the hood including face velocity measurements, and smoke pattern distribution so other personnel are easily informed.

Routine Maintenance

The last component of the hood evaluation program is routine maintenance performed by the maintenance department. This function should include such things as lubrication of fan moving parts, a check for belt slippage, blade deterioration, and some sort of periodic check on fan speed.

A routine maintenance program should include a visual check of all duct work for damage by corrosion from contaminants inside the duct work or by liquid or solid condensates. Damper or blastgate lubrication is also necessary. Unused hoods or duct work should be removed. In many cases systems in older laboratory buildings are retrofitted leaving old pieces of duct work on laboratory hoods, which may affect the connected hoods. In Figure 15-22 there is an improper seal where this duct meets the hood. In the same hood (Figure 15-23) an old duct was left cut off by a blast gate. This should have been taken out completely in order to assure proper performance of the hood.

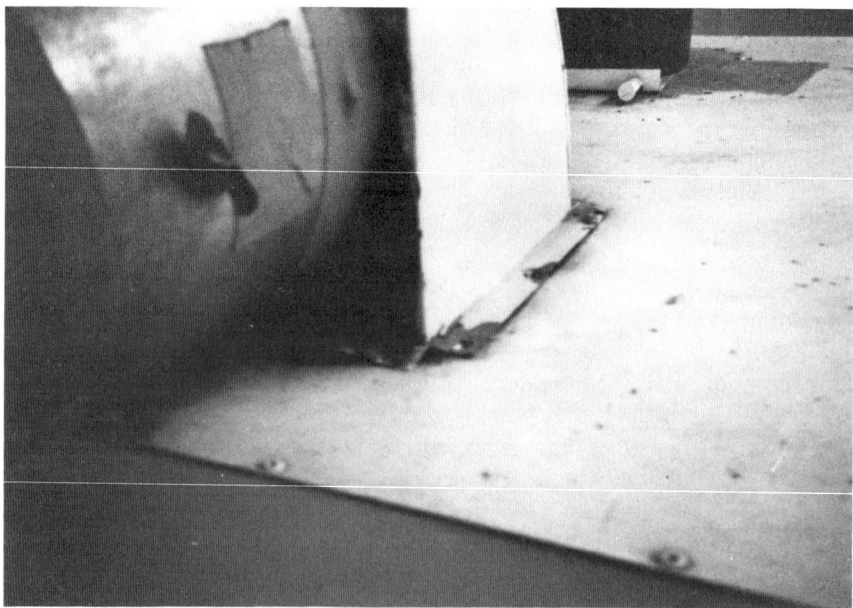

Figure 15-22. Poor seal for exhaust duct/hood connection.

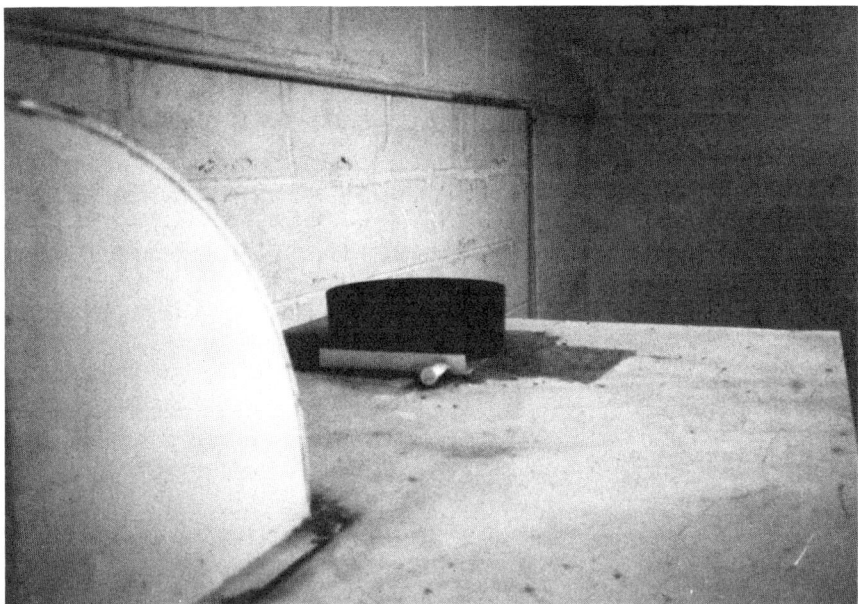

Figure 15-23.   Old duct remaining on top of a chemical fume hood.

Finally, routine maintenance should include a check of air cleaning equipment for contaminant buildup on filters, and any sort of leak checks. Leak checks for HEPA filters include dioctyl phthalate (DOP) testing; for charcoal filters, chloro-fluorocarbon testing gas.

The last portion of this routine maintenance program should include a quantitative assessment of the class II type B total exhaust hoods. This procedure would involve a pitot traverse of the supply duct to determine the exhaust volume, and then the supply volume can be determined by measurement of the laminar flow. The supply volume divided by the exhaust volume taken out by the area face is equal to the face velocity. This test for class II type B total exhaust hoods should be done on an annual basis by qualified personnel. Typically manufacturers recommend annual certification of all BSC's by qualified technicians. These annual checks include decontamination, cabinet leak checks and DOP testing of the HEPA filters.

CONCLUSION

In summary, a complete hood monitoring and evaluation program should include daily visual and quarterly inspections, as well as a good user training program and routine maintenance performed by qualified personnel. These four components should include the entire exhaust system from the hood to the exhaust stack. This multicomponent program should decrease hood malfunction and fully protect laboratory personnel from chemical exposure.

REFERENCES

1. Caplan, K.J., and G.W. Knutson. "The Effect of Room Air Challenge on the Efficiency of Laboratory Fume Hoods," *ASHRAE Trans.* 83 (Part I): 141–156, 1977.
2. Gaffney, L.F., et al. "Field Testing and Performance Certification of Laboratory Fume Hoods," U.S. Environmental Protection Agency, Washington, D.C., and CLV Industries, Inc., Cambridge, MA, paper presented at American Industrial Hygiene Conference, May 1980.
3. Fuller, F.H. and A.W. Etchells. "The Rating of Laboratory Hood Performance," *ASHRAE J.* 49–53, October 1979.
4. Industrial Ventilation: A Manual of Recommended Practice, Committee on Industrial Ventilation, American Conference of Governmental Industrial Hygienists," 17th ed., 1982.
5. "National Sanitation Foundation Standard No. 49 for Class II (Laminar Flow) Biohazard Cabinetry," The National Sanitation Foundation, Ann Arbor, MI, 1976.
6. "Recommended Industrial Ventilation Guidelines," U.S. Dept. of Health, Education and Welfare, HEW Pub. No. 76-162, The National Institute of Occupational Safety and Health Contract No. CDC-99-74-33, prepared by Arthur D. Little, Inc., Cambridge, MA, G.P.O., 1976-657/5543, January 1976.
7. U.S. Department of Labor, Occupational Safety and Health Administration. "Subpart 2: Toxic and Hazardous Substances 1910.1000-1910-1045," in *General Industry*, rev. (Washington, D.C.: U.S. Government Printing Office, 7 November, 1978).
8. Stuart, D.G., M.W. First, R.L. Jones, Jr., and J.M. Eagleson Jr. "Comparison of Chemical Vapor Handling by Three Types of Class II Biological Safety Cabinets," *Particulate and Microbial Control* 2(2):18–24 (1983).
9. "Scientific Apparatus Makers Association Standard LF10-1980, Laboratory Fume Hoods," Scientific Apparatus Makers Association, Washington, D.C., 1980.
10. Chamberlin, R.I. and J.E. Leahy. "A Study of Laboratory Fume Hoods," U.S.E.P.A. report from contract No. 68-01-4661, 1978.

CHAPTER 16

Industrial Hygiene Monitoring of Chemical Contaminants at Bioassay Laboratories

J.J. Beres
IBM, 9500 Godwin Drive,
Manassas, Virginia 22110

INTRODUCTION

Exposure of personnel to bioassay test chemicals is of continuing concern in toxicological testing laboratories. Personnel, in the course of performing the work required, are potentially exposed to a variety of chemical substances. The substances are encountered in many phases of the operation including receipt, storage, preparation, testing, and disposal. In order to determine the degree of hazard to personnel handling chemicals, a thorough industrial hygiene investigation is necessary to determine where the hazards exist and what chemicals are of primary concern. Although there are many facets of such a survey that are important, the following will deal primarily with exposure monitoring as a means for determining the degree of chemical exposure.

ROUTES OF EXPOSURE

In order to properly monitor a particular work situation, it is necessary to consider what the possible routes of exposure are. In work dealing with toxicological testing, exposure is possible through four different avenues: inhalation, skin contact, ingestion, or injection.

Inhalation of chemicals may occur where the breathing air has been contaminated with a test gas, volatilized liquid sublimed solid, or with an aerosolized liquid or finely divided solid. Skin contact occurs either directly during the handling or transfer of a chemical, or indirectly by touching surfaces (bench tops, walls, notebooks, etc.) that have been contaminated with a chemical. Ingestion of a chemical directly is not very likely. However, if food, drink, chewing gum, cosmetics or other similar items are allowed and used in the laboratory, these may become contaminated and a chemical may thus be ingested indirectly. Injection may occur in a variety of ways, including accidental injection with a syringe containing a chemical, through the bite of an animal that has the substance in its mouth, or through a laceration with a piece of broken glassware that has contained the chemical.

SELECTION OF AREAS

Although the size and specific facilities available at bioassay laboratories vary, certain kinds of facilities are common to most full-service laboratories. These are listed below:

office/administrative	corridors
receiving/shipping	cage dumping areas
chemical storage	equipment washing/sanitization
dosed vehicle storage	necropsy room
general supplies storage	histology/pathology
dosage preparation room(s)	showers/restrooms
analytical laboratory	lunchroom
maintenance/utility rooms	laundry
animal housing rooms	waste handling/storage/disposal

Areas of primary concern regarding personnel exposure are those where test or other chemicals are transferred from one container to another, utilized in an open vessel, or mixed with other substances. These areas include dosed vehicle preparation facilities, cage dumping, animal rooms, and necropsy, histology, and pathology facilities. If containment in such locations is poor, chemicals may spread or be carried to other areas, even office and administrative areas. Thus any area in a laboratory should be viewed as a potential exposure area. In addition, spills of chemicals may occur in shipping and receiving or in transportation from one part of a facility to another. Incidents of this type may cause serious problems unless plans for emergency response are made beforehand.

In dosage preparation operations, pure chemicals, some with potentially carcinogenic, mutagenic, or teratogenic properties, are mixed with predetermined quantities of feed, water, gavage vehicle, or skin penetrant solution. If the test chemical is a volatile liquid, there may be a buildup of harmful levels of vapors in the mixing room. If the test chemical is a solid, and especially a fine and powdery one to be mixed with feed, suspension of dust is highly likely. Contaminated air may then quickly move to other areas of the laboratory. The actual degree of hazard both inside and outside the room would depend on the limitations of the facility for performing this type of work adequately, the control equipment in use, and the operating procedures utilized, including work practices during chemical transfer and equipment cleanup operations.

Cage dumping is a high-dust generation area by nature of the task involved. Cages filled with dirty bedding and litter are emptied into a refuse container which may also be scraped to remove additional dirt. Test chemical present in the soiled litter, especially where dosed feed was involved, may be suspended into the air in the process of dumping the cages. The concentration may be significant in a very localized area near the worker performing this job. Controls for this operation are often of inadequate design due to the freedom of movement required by the operator. Even in those cases where controls are good, the final step of removing the bag from its holder and closing it is done in a haphazard manner causing dust from the bag to enter the technician's breathing zone.

Animal rooms are that part of the facility where the animals are both housed and dosed. The mode of dosing is important in the consideration of employee exposure and spread of chemical contamination. For example, skin painting and gavaging, if done under a hood, controls evaporation of test chemical during administration. However, in a feeding study, localized ventilation is usually not practical and whole room ventilation becomes necessary for controlling aerosolized test chemical. Since the room then in effect acts as a large hood, particulates may be deposited on surfaces, and test chemical may potentially be transferred to the technicians working in the rooms and further carried into other areas, thus contaminating them also.

In the necropsy room, dosed animals brought in after testing may contain some test chemical on their bodies either through contact with dosed feed or from excreted unmetabolized chemical. However, exposure to test chemical may be expected to be minimal, and the chemical of prime concern here will probably be formaldehyde, which is used as a tissue preservative. Formaldehyde is suspect as a potential carcinogen and has an Occupational Safety and Health Administration (OSHA) permissible exposure limit of 3 parts per million (ppm) by volume in air on a time-weighted average basis; the National Institute of Occupational Safety and Health (NIOSH) is recommending the limit be lowered to 1 ppm as a ceiling.

Formaldehyde, xylenes, and alcohols are required in processing tissues and in staining and producing microscope slides. All of these organic solvents readily evaporate and produce potentially toxic concentrations of airborne vapors. Here again, concentrations will vary depending on the efficacy of ventilation controls, on standard operating procedures, and on how well these procedures are followed.

SELECTING CHEMICALS TO MONITOR

When developing an exposure monitoring strategy, it is necessary to determine which chemicals are to be monitored. If time and resources were unlimited, the ideal situation would be to monitor all operations and all chemicals. However, this is usually not the case. Thus, it is necessary to select those chemicals which are suspect as being the most toxic, which are expected to be at relatively high concentrations due to the proerties of the chemicals (volatility, aerosol-forming potential, etc.), and/or which are present in operations that present potentially high exposure conditions.

Operations that are similar and are conducted under the same conditions, for example, dosed-feed mixing, may be monitored by sampling the chemical which is expected to produce the highest airborne concentrations. For example, a very fine, dusty solid would more likely be dispersed into the air during mixing operations than a coarse granular solid. Thus, by sampling for the chemical that is a fine solid, an upper concentration or exposure level may be established. If this upper concentration is acceptable for all similar compounds that are mixed in this manner, additional monitoring may be unnecessary.

As noted previously, test chemicals are not the only ones of concern. Certain substances such as formaldehyde or xylenes used in support operations also require investigation. As part of an overall industrial hygiene evaluation, it is necessary to perform a chemical inventory and determine where the chemicals are used, in what quantities, and under what conditions. This information simplifies the targeting of chemicals and specific jobs for exposure monitoring.

MONITORING TECHNIQUES

In determining potential for exposure and direct contact with chemical substances, it is necessary to take both air and wipe samples. Air samples are needed to determine airborne concentrations of gases, vapors, and aerosols; wipe samples, to determine the potential spread of a solid or of nonvolatile liquid chemicals by surface contamination and subsequent contact.

Air samples can be taken in a number of ways: with direct reading instruments calibrated for a particular substance, with passive dosimeters, or with a sampling train consisting of a calibrated pump which draws air through a collecting medium such as an adsorbent or absorbent solid, a filter, or a liquid solution. Samples may be taken in a specific fixed location (area samples), or the sample may be placed on a person and worn throughout a job to evaluate a time-weighted average exposure (personal sample). Usually a combination of area and personal samples provides the most useful information for an exposure evaluation.

Direct reading instruments are available for monitoring some of the more common substances; however, they may not be available for some of the more exotic chemicals being tested. Passive dosimeters, if appropriate to a particular substance, may not be adequate due to the long sampling times required to obtain detectable results if airborne concentrations are low. Overall, sampling trains provide the best means for determining exposure or potential exposure to airborne chemicals. This is because sampling media used in the trains are either readily available or may easily be prepared for a wide variety of substances, and because relatively large volumes of air may be sampled even over short periods of time by adjusting air collection rates and sampling train configurations.

Wipe samples can be taken with filters, cotton swabs, or other appropriate materials in evaluating surface contamination. Wetting the sampling medium with an absorbent solution aids in more efficiently collecting the chemical. Care is necessary in collecting wipe samples since cross-contamination may easily occur. A strategy should be developed prior to taking the samples to minimize contaminating a wipe, for example, with gloves containing chemicals from previous samples.

Factors that are important in deciding upon a monitoring strategy are the expected concentration of a chemical, the availability of monitoring techniques for a particular chemical, ease of analysis of the samples, interferences that may be expected from other chemicals, and the amount of time and the cost involved in the development of a method when necessary.

INTERPRETATION OF RESULTS

A large number of the most commonly used chemicals are regulated by OSHA for airborne exposure. In addition, NIOSH has recommended new standards for substances based on recent investigational data. A third group, the American Conference of Government Industrial Hygienists (ACGIH), publishes a revised list of threshold limit values (TLVs) for chemical substances in the workroom environment on a yearly basis. These standards may be used for comparisons to the exposure data generated through chemical monitoring.

Unfortunately, there are many substances undergoing bioassay testing which have no established exposure standards. In these cases internal standards must be established based on the best available toxicological data or based on comparisons with substances of similar chemical or metabolic activity.

There are no standards for surface area contamination. The primary purpose for wipe samples is to determine how well an area is being cleaned and whether or not supposedly clean areas such as sterile corridors or office areas are being inadvertently contaminated. Air samples may also be taken in these "clean" areas to determine if a particular chemical is contaminating them due to an inefficiency in engineering controls in the areas of generation or to poor work practices.

PART IV

Waste Management

CHAPTER 17

A Risk Assessment Program for Toxicology Laboratory Waste Disposal

**Robert G. Nemchin and
Joseph A. Coco**
Office of Occupational Safety and Health,
Litton Bionetics, Inc., 5516 Nicholson Lane,
Kensington, Maryland 20895

INTRODUCTION

The purpose of this chapter is to provide guidance to industrial toxicology laboratory managers on matters of hazardous waste disposal. Decisions on proper disposal of these types of wastes in the most cost-beneficial manner are not easy despite federal and state regulations. The problems of proper disposal are especially difficult for materials which may be contaminated with only "trace" quantities of hazardous chemicals. The regulations do not address these problems. In order to make sound decisions in these situations, management must have a scientifically based decision-making tool. This risk assessment approach should assist management in the decision-making process on matters of public health and environmental concern.

The toxicology laboratory has emerged as a major "industry" in response to federal toxic substances legislation which mandates the safety testing of chemical substances destined for industrial or consumer use [1]. Toxicology laboratories, singly and collectively, are viewed as having a significant potential impact on the environment because of the nature of their operations and of the kinds of waste that may be generated. Within the laboratory sector, the toxicology laboratory is considered by health and safety professionals as a rather unique working environment and as such has unique waste disposal problems. Few other industries must deal with such a wide array of chemical substances, ranging from seemingly innocuous food additives to pharmaceuticals, biocides, and explosives. Additionally, the quantities of chemicals handled during normal operations can vary from a few milligrams for genetic screening to hundreds of kilograms for chronic carcinogenicity studies. Because of the way these materials are utilized, the volume of potentially contaminated waste from these testing operations can be several orders of magnitude greater than the volume of the chemical as it was originally received. The kinds of waste (excluding wastes resulting from accidental spills) typically evolving from toxicology laboratory processes are as follows:

- cage bedding
- disposable caging
- filter tops
- animal diet
- containers
- process water
- dosing solutions
- paper, plasticware

Decisions on how to properly deal with these types and quantities of wastes in the most cost-beneficial manner are not always easy to make. Federal environmental legislation, such as the Resource Conservation and Recovery Act (RCRA), imposes constraints on how certain types of hazardous wastes may be disposed. If one examines these regulations to find specific answers to the toxicology laboratory waste disposal needs, there is an astonishing lack of information. Because of this, it is not surprising that there may be a tendency for some laboratories to utilize disposal methods that may not be environmentally sound, even though the discarded waste may be assumed to consist of nothing but "trace quantities" of chemicals. Paradoxically, the very studies being conducted by the laboratory may prove that the chemical under test eventually should be regulated as a hazardous material and that its wastes be regulated also.

There is another factor to be considered in addressing the toxicology laboratory's hazardous waste disposal problems. As expected, the increasing volume of this waste has created a substantial impact on laboratory operating costs. It has been estimated that the cost of disposing of hazardous wastes in a secure landfill ranges from $50 to $400 per metric ton while the cost of incineration ranges from $75 to $2,000 per metric ton [2]. Consequently, the cost of disposal may outweigh any consideration of potential environmental risk in the decision-making process. Additionally, many toxicology laboratories may not be equipped to properly handle their hazardous wastes. These factors may then tend to cause some laboratories to rely on unacceptable disposal methods. The onus of potential environmental contamination then becomes a liability which the toxicology laboratory management must be prepared to accept.

In order to avoid this consequence, it would be desirable to be able to apply a meaningful risk analysis prior to disposal. In the extreme, one can consider either incinerating all chemically contaminated laboratory waste or discarding it all to a conventional sanitary landfill. It becomes obvious that the cost for the former method would be prohibitive for most laboratories. Also this kind of expenditure does not necessarily ensure public safety (e.g., heavy metal compounds are not destroyed by incineration). However, with prudently applied risk analysis combined with waste segregation techniques, a significant portion of the waste that is being incinerated or transported to a secure landfill could be handled confidently by a conventional sanitary landfill.

RISK ASSESSMENT

The potential for damage to the public health and to the environment from mismanagement of hazardous waste justifies the need for the implementation of an effective hazardous waste management program [3]. In planning management programs for waste disposal alternatives, it is necessary to consider all the options which are applicable to a particular waste. Depending upon such factors as composition, volume, and economics, proper waste disposal for industry typically involves one or more of the following acceptable methods [4]:

- recycling or reuse of recoverable waste for safe and useful purposes
- removal of toxic or hazardous components by treatment or by waste segregation prior to disposal
- reduction of waste volume by segregation, evaporation, or treatment, or by process modification
- conversion of toxic wastes to nonhazardous forms by chemical, thermal, or biological treatment, stabilization and fixation, or some other method
- burial of highly toxic wastes and residuals in specially designed hazardous waste disposal sites (secure landfills)
- burial of innocuous, stabilized, or detoxified wastes in sanitary landfills, under special precautions

In practice, many of these waste disposal alternatives are not viable options for the industrial toxicology laboratory. In addition, many of the physical and chemical methods that are used for treatment of hazardous wastes [2] are not practicable for these types of wastes. Guidelines and recommended procedures for the disposal of waste laboratory chemicals have been published. These procedures emphasize chemical reaction or degradation as a means of producing a less dangerous or innocuous waste. Similar procedures have also been compiled for the degradation of chemical carcinogens [6]. However, because these procedures generally apply to small quantities of chemicals, their applicability to large quantities of chemically contaminated wastes of various types is very limited. Thus, the toxicology laboratory is left with three options: disposal (long-term storage) in a secure landfill, destruction by high-temperature incineration, and disposal in a sanitary landfill (for innocuous wastes). The question then is to decide which option to use. Regulations such as RCRA address typical industrial waste products and process streams. Wastes contaminated in the part-per-million range are not addressed. Is the waste still hazardous in this range? How do we know when a waste is hazardous? What risk does the waste pose? Is it "safe" to send it to a sanitary landfill instead of the more costly secure landfill?

Should it be disposed of in the most environmentally sound and most expensive way—incineration? These are extremely difficult questions to answer unless the problem is approached in a systematic, holistic manner.

In order to answer these questions, a foundation must be laid down upon which a framework for making hazardous waste disposal decisions can be devised. Consider the definition of "hazardous waste" as defined by RCRA:

> a "hazardous waste" is a solid waste, or combination of solid wastes which, because of its quantity, concentration, or physical, chemical, or infectious characteristics, may: (a) cause or significantly contribute to an increase in mortality or an increase in serious irreversible, or incapacitating, reversible illness; or (b) pose a substantial present or potential hazard to human health or the environment when improperly treated, stored, transported, or disposed of, or otherwise managed.[1]

We can consider this a guiding definition for determining whether a waste is hazardous in a qualitative sense: either it is or it is not according to this operational definition. Of course all hazards are not of equal magnitude; i.e., some wastes are more hazardous than others. In any case, the hazardous aspect of a waste refers to an inherent property of the waste to do harm or damage. *Risk comes into play when there is a potential exposure to a hazard.* Similarly, all risks are not of equal value. Informed decision making requires that the hazards and attendant risks of a waste be defined and measured.

In order to make the proper waste-disposal decisions, toxicology laboratory management must have the tools to systematically define and measure the hazards and risks associated with the various types of contaminated wastes emanating from their operations and select the appropriate cost-beneficial disposal options that will minimize the risk to workers and the public. Assessment cannot be done without these initial steps. In the absence of specific guidelines, the assessment of risk must be based on a combination of sound scientific information and informed professional judgment. Realistically, the assessment of risk is viewed as an activity used as a management tool. The ultimate determination of the "safety" of a waste is a value judgment based on the acceptability of the assessed risk [7]. Exercising this level of judgment is difficult unless management has available a clearly defined set of criteria and a methodology for delineating risk. The approach must be well thought out, practicable, and cost-effective and should have broad applicability. This risk assessment can then be utilized as part of the overall decision-making process.

Attempts to define hazards and measure risk are not new. Insurance companies and safety engineers have been doing this for years. For discrete events such as deaths due to coronary heart disease or motor vehicle accidents, expressions of risk have been embodied in various statistical methods such as probability. Unfortunately, traditional statistical methods are not easily applied to defining environmental risk, i.e., subtle environmental effects are not easily predicted. Various approaches have been used. The most frequently used approach has involved some type of waste classification scheme. Classifications of waste have been developed using one or more of several available techniques. The overall objective of this particular approach to risk assessment has been to predict the potential impact that a particular waste may have when placed in a landfill environment. Listed below are three examples of waste classification systems that have been used [8]:

1.   Listing of waste types. This approach is based on the concept of identifying or defining "hazardous waste" by generic name or by materials which may be contained within a particular waste mixture. This concept is applied solely by making a distinction between the two broad categories of hazardous and nonhazardous wastes.
2.   Listing of waste criteria. In this approach, quantitative data are obtained through waste sampling and testing according to specific criteria which are applied to all wastes. These criteria are used collectively as a "gauge" for predicting the degree of environmental impact that may be caused by the disposal of certain wastes.
3.   Waste rating/ranking. This is a mathematical ranking system approach incorporating the use of weighting factors. These factors are assigned to waste criteria based on their relative importance with respect to potential adverse impact on the environment. Through a mathematical combination of the weighted criteria, a single numerical rating is obtained. This rating can then be compared to a set range of values to determine if a particular waste is acceptable or unacceptable for disposal at a certain site.

Because of some of the disadvantages of the first two approaches, there have been attempts to use the waste rating/ranking method. One example of this is the "Hazardous Index" [8] used by the State of Texas. However, because it considers only solubility and toxicity of waste (based on LD_{50} values) its applicability is limited. Other more sophisticated approaches have been developed [9], but are difficult to use and interpret. Most of these risk assessment methods tend to be too narrow in scope or too limited in applicability to the types of wastes generated by toxicology laboratories.

In order to provide a practical decision-making tool for toxicology laboratory waste management, a semiquantitative, multiparametric risk assessment methodology has been developed. It is based upon the hazard rating/ranking method, but also incorporates some of the best features of other methods. In this method, a *hazard index* (HI), which is a composite measure of the waste material's capacity to do harm or damage, is determined for each chemically contaminated waste. The methodology attempts to integrate the relative importance of several intrinsic potential hazards of a chemical substance with the total quantity of the waste and concentration of the contaminant within that waste. This leads to a determination of the relative *cumulative risk* (R_c) which correlates the hazard index with the frequency of discharge to the environment. It is this R_c value that can be utilized as one factor in the decision-making process in arriving at an acceptable disposal option.

THE MULTIPARAMETRIC METHOD

The determination of hazard levels can be approached using the previously mentioned techniques. All these techniques, to be viable, must consider measurements that (1) define the conditions of exposure, (2) identify the adverse effects, (3) relate exposure with effect, and (4) arrive at an estimate of the overall risk [7]. Hence, any derived hazard index is *a priori* a complex expression which embodies terms for describing the probability of exposure as well as the severity of the consequences of such exposure [10,11]. The mathematical relationship between these terms has been expressed as follows [7]:

$$\text{frequency} - \text{severity index} = \text{severity of risk} \times \text{frequency of injury} \qquad (1)$$

This equation adequately depicts discrete, acute accidents or injuries, but for chronic, more subtle hazards, expressing the risk is not so easily derived. However, we can utilize this fundamental concept to derive model equations for developing a risk assessment method.

In an analogous manner we can restate equation (1) as follows:

$$\text{risk} = \text{level of hazard} \times \text{exposure potential} \qquad (2)$$

In this case, the level of hazard can be equated with the intrinsic hazard characteristics of the chemical or combination of chemicals in the waste, i.e., its hazard value (described below). The exposure potential is determined by the concentration of the hazardous substance(s) in, and the total quantity of, the waste.

Hazard Value (Single Component Systems)

The first step in this method requires the determination of a *hazard value* (H_v) for each of several different hazard parameters. The hazard parameters selected are as follows:

- flammability
- reactivity
- corrosivity
    to skin
    to materials
- mammalian toxicity
- sensitivity (immunologic)
- irritant
- anesthetic
- carcinogen (incl. genotoxicity)
- aquatic toxicity
- phytotoxicity

These particular parameters were selected because of a need to consider as many hazard characteristics as possible. Additionally, these terms are commonly used in the literature and as key words, serve to facilitate computer literature searches.

Each H_v is the product of a specific *hazard rating*, H_r, and a *weighting factor*, W, for each parameter. Individual H_r's for each parameter are obtained by comparing an assigned level of hazard for the chemical against a published rating scale or other applicable standard. The weighting factor takes into account the relative importance (potential severity) that each hazard parameter has with respect to the others, and to normalize the several different rating scales. The next step is to determine the total hazard value, identified as ΣH_v, for the specific chemical in the waste. Thus ΣH_v is the sum of the individual weighted terms and represents an intrinsic composite value for the level of hazard of the specific chemical, one that is unique and independent of its concentration or quantity in the waste. Referring back to the basic risk assessment equation (equation 2), ΣH_v is equivalent to the level of hazard.

Bioconcentration is not included in the determination of ΣH_v and for various reasons is considered later in the discussion.

Table 17-1.   Hazard Value Determination $H_v = WH_r$

Hazard Category	Rating Scale	Weighting Factors (W)	Hazard Rating (H_r)	Hazard Value (H_v)
Flammability[a]	0–4	35		
Reactivity[a]	0–4	30		
Corrosivity[b]				
To skin	0 or 1	140		
To materials	0 or 1	120		
Mammalian toxicity[c]	0–5	32		
Sensitizer	0 or 1	100		
Irritant[b]	0 or 1	100		
Anesthetic	0 or 1	100		
Carcinogen[d]	0–5	40		
(incl. genotoxicity)				
Aquatic toxicity[e]	0–4	40		
Phytotoxicity	0 or 1	40		
			$\Sigma H_v =$	

[a]NFPA No. 704, "Recommended System for the Identification of the Fire Hazards of Materials," National Fire Codes, Vol. 11, pp. 5–22, 1980.

[b]"Corrosive Materials: Definition and Preparation," U.S. Code of Federal Regulations, Title 49, Part 173.240, 1976.

[c]Spector, S.W., Ed. *Handbook of Toxicology* (Philadelphia, PA: W.B. Saunders, 1956), Vol. I.

[d]An Adaptation of the carcinogen ranking scheme of Squire. Squire, R.A., "Ranking Animal Carcinogens: A Proposed Regulatory Approach," *Science* 214:877–880, 1981.

[e]Verschueren, K.: *Handbook of Environmental Data on Organic Chemicals* (New York: Van Nostrand Reinhold Co., 1977), p. 47.

Table 17-1 illustrates a typical worksheet used for ΣH_v determinations. The left-hand column lists the hazard categories. The second column lists the reference hazard rating scales, with the higher numbers representing the greater hazard. These hazard rating scales are obtained from the literature. The appropriate references are cited at the bottom of the table. For those hazard parameters where no published rating scales could be found, zero or one has been assigned. The third column shows the weighting factors applied as a multiplier to the hazard level rating assigned to the chemical (fourth column). These assigned hazard level values are derived from the literature (e.g., safety data sheets). In practice, it is necessary to consult several different information sources to obtain data on a specific chemical for each hazard parameter. The fifth column is the product of columns three and four and represents the weighted hazard value for that parameter. The sum of these values is ΣH_v.

Hazard Index

A hazard index (HI) can be quantified by modeling an expression analogous to equation 2 relating the chemical's total hazard potential (ΣH_v) to its concentration (or dilution) in the waste and the total quantity of the waste. Additional factors which modify the value of HI are the bioconcentration factor, a measure of the tendency for some chemicals to selectively accumulate in biota, and the chemicals' odor characteristics. This relationship is represented by equation 3 as follows:

$$HI = \Sigma H_v(k) + P_r \qquad (3)$$

where ΣH_v = severity (or hazard potential)
   k = exposure potential
   P_r = public relations or nuisance factor

The value k is defined as:

$$1 + \log D_f + \log Q + \log BCF \qquad (4)$$

where D_f = dilution factor (10^{-x}) of the chemical contaminant in the waste (10^0 = undiluted)
   Q = quantity (10_y) of contaminated waste (in grams).
   BCF = bioconcentration factor (10_z)

The value P_r is defined as:

$$\frac{(\log Q)^2 (\log O_v)^2}{2 + (-\log D_f)} \qquad (5)$$

Where O_v = odor index of the chemical (10_n).

HI is thus a dimensionless value when expressed in this form.

It is felt that the inclusion of the bioaccumulative capacity of the biota for certain organic chemicals was essential in order to properly assess the risk of selecting the ordinary landfill as a disposal option. A semiempirical correlation has been shown to exist between the BCF and the octanol/water partition coefficient, i.e., the selective partitioning (ratio) of an organic chemical between octanol and water phases at equilibrium [12].

The assumption is that most organic chemicals are transported and selectively accumulated by biota into their lipid constituents. Apparently this correlation is linear [13,14], resulting in a regression line described by the following equation:

$$\log BCF = 0.76 \log K_{ow} - 0.23 \qquad (6)$$

where K_{ow} = octanol/water partition coefficient. This relationship was used for calculating BCF from published K_{ow} values.

Where literature values for K_{ow} were not available for particular organic compounds, K_{ow} may be obtained from the linear relationship that exists between K_{ow} and the organic compound's water solubility [15,16].

$$\log K_{ow} = -0.862 \log S + 0.710 \qquad (7)$$

where S = water solubility of the organic compound. These equations seem to hold for a large number of organic compounds (including pesticides), and their applicability is more than adequate for the risk assessment method discussed here. It is of interest that a correlation between K_{ow} and toxicity has also been shown [17].

The public relations factor P_r is likewise felt to be an essential consideration in discarding a chemically contaminated waste to an ordinary landfill. In our multiparametric method, P_r embodies the importance of odor on the ultimate acceptability of conventional disposal. This odor factor, is dependent upon the quantity of the waste as well as the dilution of the chemical within it. In the eyes of the public, hazard and risk are often associated with materials that have strong or peculiar odors. Unfortunately, public perception is that the worse something smells, the more dangerous it is. Obviously, this correlation is not necessarily true. For example, benzene, a known leukemogenic agent, has a rather pleasant odor. However, in viewing an overall risk assessment and disposal strategy, it is prudent for laboratory management to heavily weigh the potential nuisance value of its waste along with its more obvious hazard characteristics, for the former may be the deciding factor against landfill disposal even though the waste's hazard characteristics indicate otherwise.

The odor index O_v is the ratio of a chemical's vapor pressure (or volatization potential) to its odor recognition concentration detected by 100% of a group of individuals comprising a test panel [18]. The apparently subjective organoleptic odor-intensity assessment method is remarkably consistent and a means by which odor can be quantified. The odor indices for about 300 organic chemicals have been published [19]. Additionally, O_v values are dependent upon such characteristics as chemical class, molecular weight, molecular configuration, and functional groups. Thus, if the chemical of interest is not specifically listed but its chemical structure is known, O_v can be predicted to within two or three orders of magnitude. Since the recorded O_v

values vary over a 10^{11} range, two or three logs difference is not a very large error. For extremely malodorous chemicals, the contribution of the P_r term to HI (equation 3) is large when the odor index, quantity of waste, and concentration of chemical contaminant in the waste is large. Conversely, if the chemical has low odor characteristics and the quantities are small or diluted, the effect on HI is negligible.

The hazard index equation is so formulated that plotting HI as a function of k results in a straight line of slope ΣH_v and intercept P_r. When P_r is small, the slope passes close to or through the origin. This relationship is graphically illustrated in Figure 17-1, where a family of slopes have been generated for several hazardous chemicals selected to demonstrate divergent hazard characteristics. From this plot,

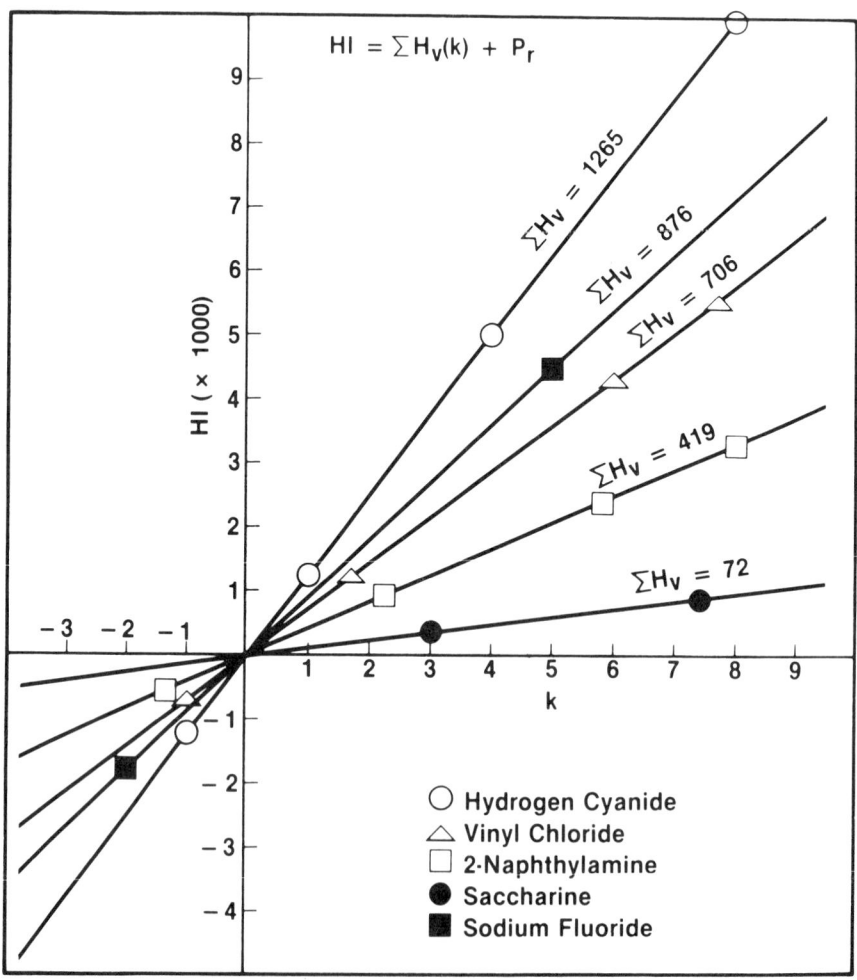

Figure 17-1. HI versus k for selected chemical substances. P_r values are negligible so that all plots pass through the origin.

an HI value may be obtained for any combination of chemical concentration and quantity of waste (as embodied in k) as a point along the ΣH_v slope for the chemical of interest. Vinyl chloride, 2-naphthylamine, and saccharin are known carcinogens. These three substances represent a wide range of carcinogenic potency. Sodium fluoride is a toxic substance but at extremely low concentrations (approximately 1 mg/ml) is used to fluoridate public water supplies.

RELATIVE CUMULATIVE RISK

The hazard index is an expression of the relative potential hazard associated with a chemically contaminated waste. The concept of risk is encountered when waste discharge occurs. Accordingly, the model must be expanded in order to account for the risk as a function of the frequency of disposal.

The relative cumulative risk (R_c) to the public is directly related to the relative hazard, HI, and the exposure potential, identified by the disposal rate, D_r. The equation for R_c follows the same general form as most risk assessment equations:

$$R_c = HI(D_r) \tag{8}$$

D_r is expressed as the number of times the waste is discarded annually. Taking the logarithm of both sides of equation 8, the data can be plotted as shown in Figure 17-2. This plot is analogous to the environmental indexes described independently by Ott [20]. For a single annual discharge, $D_r = 1$, $R_c = HI$. For a single daily discharge for 365 days, $\log D_r = 2.56$. Ostensibly, in the limit ($D_r \rightarrow \infty$), the disposal rate becomes equivalent to a continuous waste stream. The values of R_c are also dimensionless.

In order to utilize the R_c plot, HI is interpolated (or calculated) from Figure 17-1 for any given set of D_r and Q along the ΣH_v slope. That is, for any given value of k, there is an equivalent value for HI. Thus, plotting the specific HI versus its disposal rate gives a point on the R_c plane. This value is compared to an arbitrarily selected reference index in order to determine whether the risk of sanitary landfill disposal would be acceptable.

The reference index selected here is that of determining the relative cumulative risk of disposing of saccharin, a weak carcinogen, which is consumed by the general public. For saccharin, $R_c = 5 \times 10^3$. This could be expressed as the risk associated with discharging approximately 100 pounds of animal diet dosed with 280 ppm of saccharin at a rate of once per week or 52 times per year ($\log D_r = 1.7$). This saccharin content is equivalent to approximately 12 gallons of diet soda, disposed of at the same rate. The assumption here is that any combination of HI and D_r yields the same R_c. For example, since $\log R_c = \log HI + \log D_r$, $\log R_c = 3.5$ when $\log HI = 3.5$ and $\log D_r = 0$; when $\log HI = 0$ then $\log D_r = 3.5$. Chemical wastes having $R_c \leqslant 10^{3.5}$ could be considered eligible for landfill disposal. For chemical wastes where $\log HI = 3$ and $\log D_r = 3$; $R_c = 10^6$. This risk value indicates that it would be preferable to handle this waste using a more rigorous disposal mode. Consequently, any point fal-

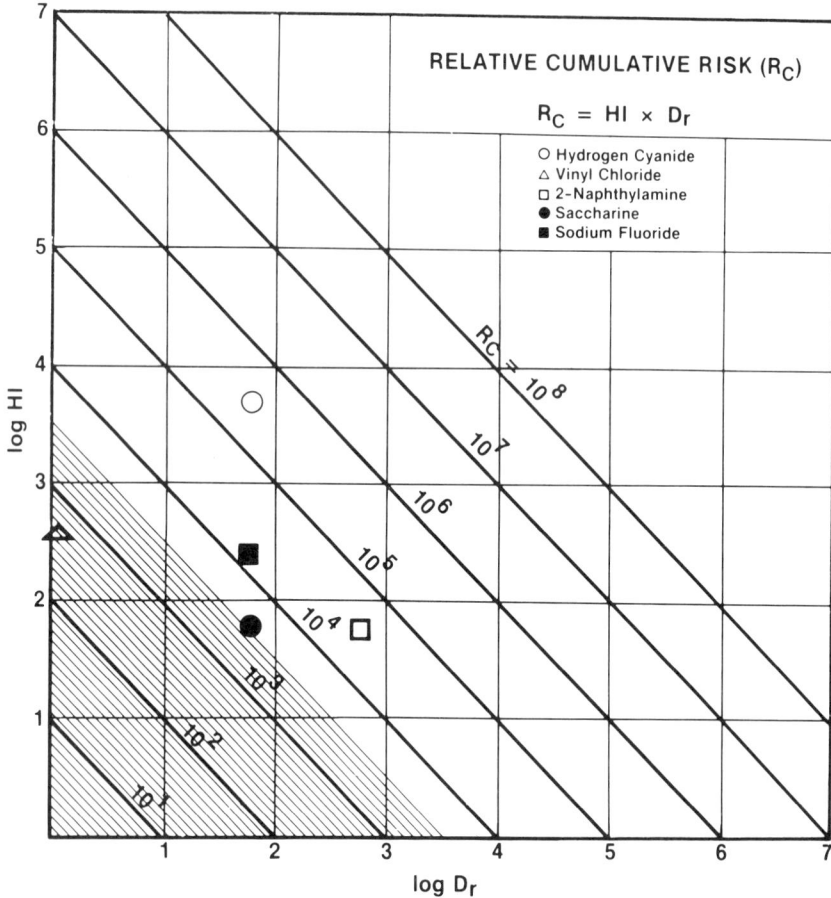

Figure 17-2. R_c plot of chemical substances for selected HI values and discharge rates. The area subtended by the cross-hatching is considered as the acceptable risk zone.

ling outside the zone of reference (i.e., $R_c > 10^{3.5}$) would be expected to present an adverse cumulative risk to the public. Other reference indexes could be selected besides saccharin.

This model is purposely limited and does not take into consideration the degradation of the chemical, once discharged, by sorption, chemical, photolytic, or microbial action, or in the case of volatile substances, evaporation. Similarly, we have dealt only with a single hazardous component system. The model can be extended to consider the relative risk of wastes containing two or more hazardous components. This fundamental risk assessment model also may be extended to show a relationship between R_c and the probability of an adverse effect on the environment (damage function). Additional work will be done in these areas.

DISCUSSION

The hazard index approach was derived to fill a need for a decision-making tool to be used by toxicology laboratory managers in dealing with their waste disposal problems. Heretofore, no such tool was available for use in this specific application. Until recently, waste disposal from toxicology laboratories was not perceived as an overwhelming burden. The waste was burned (if the laboratory had an incinerator facility) or it was thrown out as ordinary trash. However, federal environmental regulations, the type and quantity of toxic wastes now under safety evaluation, the potential acute and chronic effects of discarded chemicals, an increasingly knowledgeable public sector, and the spiraling costs of hazardous waste treatment and disposal are cause for prudent laboratory managers to review the impact of their operation on the environment and to establish cost-effective waste management programs.

As the toxicologist must evaluate and judge the "safety" of a chemical under test, so must toxicology laboratory managers judge the "safety" of their waste in the context of the various disposal options available. This is not an easy task. Assessment of safety implies that two distinct operations be performed: (1) measuring the level of risk, an objective (and quantifiable) activity and (2) judging the acceptability of that risk (judging safety), an activity that requires both personal and societal value judgments.

The multiparametric risk assessment method discussed here provides the means for measuring item 1 above, the level of risk (hazard index, relative cumulative risk). These parameters, when compared against *acceptable* reference criteria, serve to address the requirements of item 2. Although there are many ways to dispose of hazardous wastes, in reality, for most types of wastes evolving from the toxicology laboratory, incineration or secure landfilling are the only practicable waste disposal modes. The laboratory manager must choose between these two options. A manager's decision to discard laboratory waste considered innocuous in the sanitary landfill (and save the cost of incineration or transportation to a secure chemical landfill) is made with more confidence because it is informed judgment based on scientific data. However, any decision arrived at must have the unanimous concurrence of the hazardous waste management team.

A hazardous waste management committee is an integral part of the risk assessment (hazardous waste management) program. The industrial toxicology laboratory is fortunate in that it has in-house a wealth of expertise from various relevant disciplines. For example, members of such a committee might include a toxicologist, a chemist, a molecular geneticist, a veterinarian, a health and safety professional, a member of management, an employee representative, and a member of the legal staff. The function of this committee would be to recommend to the appropriate laboratory manager the proper and most cost-effective waste disposal option for a particular chemically contaminated waste. The goal would be to match the level of hazard and risk of the waste with the appropriate disposal mode. In this way, the highly toxic, persistent, hazardous residual wastes can be directed to the most stringent, environmentally sound option. Wastes with a lesser degree of potential environmental impact can be directed to less secure (and less expensive) options. Chemically contaminated wastes considered innocuous or not presenting any significant risk could be sent to the least secure (and least expensive) option: the sanitary landfill. The risk assessment methodology discussed here can be used as one of the tools on which the committee can base their recommendation to management. In effect they are performing both items 1 and 2 (discussed above) of an assessment of safety. Professional judgment and the experience of each of the committee members must enter into the recommendation. Only then can management feel confident that the decision made on the committee's recommendation is scientifically and ethically sound.

SUMMARY

Within the laboratory sector, the toxicology laboratory is perhaps the only one that must deal with the handling of such a wide array of chemical substances, ranging from explosives to food additives, in quantities varying from milligrams to hundreds of kilograms. Consequently, the waste generated by these laboratories is potentially contaminated with a variety of environmentally hazardous materials. Because of the impact of federal toxic substances legislation, toxicology laboratories must find cost-effective methods for disposing of this waste. Incineration is judged to be the most effective mode of treatment for laboratory waste, yet the costs of handling all waste by this method can be prohibitive. It thus becomes imperative for toxicology laboratory management to assess the risks associated with the various types of waste and select appropriate alternative disposal modes consistent with safety and cost. A decision-making tool for management in this regard is presented. The methodology uses a dimensionless series of terms in a multiparametric decision logic which considers a chemical's known hazardous properties but also accounts for its concentration in the waste and the total quantity of waste. A hazard index is graphically derived which is an expression of the waste material's intrinsic capacity to do harm or damage. A relative cumulative risk term is defined which extends the risk assessment method to account for periodic and repeated discharge of contaminated wastes. This value can be used by the waste management team to assist managers in making informed and scientifically sound waste disposal decisions.

ACKNOWLEDGMENT

We wish to express our appreciation to the management and staff of Litton Bionetics, Inc., for their support in the development of the concept and preparation of the manuscript.

REFERENCES

1. Toxic Substances Control Act, Public Law 94-469, Enacted September 28, 1976 and 15 USC 2602.
2. Worthy, W. "Hazardous Waste: Treatment Technology Grows," *Chem. Eng. News* 60(10): 10–16, 1982.
3. Metry, A.A. "Comprehensive Hazardous Waste Management," in *The Handbook of Hazardous Waste Management*, A.A. Metry, Ed. (Westport, CT: Technomic Publishing Co., 1980), pp. 45–89.
4. Metry, A.A. "Introduction," in *The Handbook of Hazardous Waste Management*, A.A. Metry, Ed. (Westport, CT: Technomic Publishing Co., 1980).
5. *Laboratory Waste Disposal Manual* (Washington, D.C.: Manufacturing Chemists Association, 1975).
6. Sansone, E.B. *Degradation of Chemical Carcinogens* (New York: Van Nostrand Reinhold, 1980).
7. Lowrance, W.W. *Of Acceptable Risk* (Los Altos, NM: William Kaufmann, 1976).
8. Corbin, M. "General Considerations for Hazardous Waste Management Facilities," in *The Handbook of Hazardous Waste Management*, A.A. Metry, ED. (Westport, CT: Technomic Publishing Co., 1980), pp. 184–185.
9. Walsh, P.J., G.G. Killough, and P.S. Rohwer. "Composite Hazard Index for Assessing Limiting Exposures to Environmental Pollutants: Formulation and Derivation," *Environ. Sci. Technol.* 12(7): 799–802, 1978.
10. Haque, R. "Dynamics, Exposure and Hazard Assessment of Toxic Chemicals in the Environment: An Introduction," in *Dynamics, Exposure and Hazard Assessment of Toxic Chemicals*, R. Haque, Ed. (Ann Arbor, MI: Ann Arbor Science, 1980), pp. 1–3.
11. Johnson, W.G. *MORT Safety Assurance Systems*, National Safety Council Publication (New York: Marcel Dekker, 1980), pp. 90–109.
12. Neely, W.B., D.R. Branson, and G.E. Blau. "Partition Coefficient to Measure Bioconcentration Potential of Organic Chemicals in Fish," *Environ. Sci. Technol.* 8(12):1113–1115, 1974.
13. Veith, G.D., K.J. Macek, S.R. Petrocelli, and J.J. Carroll. *Federal Register* 15926, March 15, 1979.
14. Lu, P. and R.L. Metcalf. "Environmental Fate and Biodegradability of Benzene Derivatives as Studied in a Model Aquatic Ecosystem," *Environ. Health Persp.* 10:269–284, 1975.
15. Banerjee, S., S.H. Yalkowsky, and S.C. Valvani. "Water Solubility and Octanol/Water Partition Coefficient of Organics. Limitations of the Solubility-Partition Coefficient Correlation," *Environ. Sci. Technol.* 14(12):1227–1229, 1980.
16. Chiou, C.T. and D.W. Schmedding. "Partitioning of Organic Compounds in Octanol-Water Systems," *Environ. Sci. Technol.* 16(12):4–10, 1982.
17. Hansch, C. *Biological Activity and Chemical Structure* (Amsterdam: Elsevier, 1977), p. 46.
18. Hallman, T.M. and F.H. Small. "Characterization of Odor Properties of 101 Petrochemicals Using Sensory Methods," *Chem. Eng. Prog.* 69:9–13, 1973.
19. Verschueren, K. *Handbook of Environmental Data on Organic Chemicals* (New York: Van Nostrand Reinhold, 1977).
20. Ott, W.R. *Environmental Indices, Theory and Practices* (Ann Arbor, MI: Ann Arbor Science, 1978).

CHAPTER 18

Chemical-Contaminated Waste Management: Disposal Concerns, Regulations, and Surplus Chemicals

Neil B. Jurinski
NuChemCo, Inc., 9321 Raintree Road, Burke, Virginia 22015

INTRODUCTION

Management of toxic chemicals during their use in industrial processes or in testing procedures has been performed for many generations and is routinely accepted as a normal everyday activity. Unfortunately, in the past these materials were often disposed of as common waste. Thus liquid hazardous and toxic materials have found their way into public sewers, treatment plants, streams, and rivers, and solid materials to public dumps, landfills, and incinerators. Over the past decade environmental investigations have shown the folly of these actions, and much new legislation has been enacted to address these problems. Concurrently, actual and perceived damages have resulted in a marked increase in the frequency and size of lawsuits filed relating to damage due to poor chemical waste management practices. In today's environment chemical waste management is an essential element for all persons handling materials classified as hazardous or toxic.

Development of a chemical waste management program has to be done in a manner consistent with current environmental laws, with an eye to future trends in this area. The future concerns need to be addressed at an early stage in order to avoid embarking upon a capital-intensive path which will be outmoded and useless before its normal lifetime has been reached. Several of the waste treatment options regarding hazardous waste streams are not currently required by law, but it may be anticipated that at some future date there may be need for retrofitting of treatment equipment onto existing utilities. Thus in planning for any new construction it is important to be aware of these potential future demands, and to incorporate their requirements during the design phase of new construction. To illustrate this point one could consider the potential need for pretreatment of sewage discharge to a municipal system. Most current jurisdictions have no such general requirements; however, at some future time they may exist. Thus it would be prudent during the design of sewage line placement to position the lines with a convenient access to facilitate this modification.

Among the current options for waste management, one that has been given only little consideration is the process of recycling of wastes. For chemical materials, either on a large or a small scale, recycling of a waste may be the most economical means of waste management. This is especially true if the material changes ownership during the recycling. When this occurs, the material is never an actual waste, but instead is a useful chemical substance within the commercial sphere. As such, the substance is not regulated as a waste, but is regulated by other laws dealing with common materials of commerce. A chemical waste manager should expend sufficient effort to determine the potential for reuse and recycle of all well-characterized chemical substances prior to classifying them as waste materials for ultimate disposal. Assistance in this area is now becoming more readily available with the advent of "waste brokers," whose business is to match supply with needs, and to facilitate such transfers.

Within a large toxicology testing laboratory there are several different types and sources of chemically contaminated wastes. Chemical waste may appear as gaseous, liquid, or solid phase materials. A mass balance for the distribution of test materials among these three streams (excluding inhalation studies) has been conducted [1] and it has been concluded that approximately 90% of test materials employed for toxicity studies will normally reside in the solid waste stream. This finding implies that air and water pollution sources within a test laboratory are relatively small in quantity. Due to this fact, administrative control of handling procedures for air and liquid wastes may be very effective for achieving compliance with any regulatory requirement, since relatively small amounts of hazardous wastes are generated. This study found it feasible to increase the percentage of test material in the solid stream to 95–98% in several facilities through use of diversion of chemical wastes from the air and liquid streams into the solid stream. This method has been useful in achieving a 50–90% reduction in the load of chemically hazardous materials in the liquid effluents, and similar though smaller reductions in the airborne emissions. Use of these administrative control techniques, rather than engineering controls, made possible achievement of almost the same degree of contaminant control for almost negligible costs. Diversion from one waste stream to another is usually a very cost-effective management option that should be considered during early discussions of any waste handling problem.

DISPOSAL CONCERNS

Air pollution sources are of sufficient levels to present concern when inhalation studies are performed. Sometimes overlooked as a concern is the dosage of chemicals by other routes of administration such as gavage, dosed feed or water, or skin painting.

For materials with a significant vapor pressure these operations may also present a significant hazard. Bulk chemical handling, dosage preparation, and animal handling operations may also be sources of airborne contaminants and should be evaluated for their potential to produce hazardous levels. Most modern toxicology facilities have addressed the problem of chemical control during these work operations and have provided engineering controls and protective equipment for workers assigned to these tasks. The exhaust from fume hoods used for local exhaust may itself be a source of airborne emissions of hazardous chemicals and in need of filter or scrubber controls.

Gavage techniques are frequently used for dose administration to animals when the test materials are volatile. It has been found from measurement of in-room levels of vapors that airborne concentrations in the range of 1–10 mg/ M^3 may be generated even when chemical fume hoods are used for the dosage administration operations [2]. These findings have led to a reliance on respirators for protection of workers during this work. These emissions are eventually exhausted through the air handling and ventilation systems of the building, and are found in the exhaust stream unless filtered in some manner.

Construction of inhalation facilities typically includes the installation of particulate filters in the exhaust streams from the inhalation chambers. In most instances these are high-efficiency particulate air (HEPA) filters with an efficiency rating of 99.9+% for 0.3 μm particles. Unfortunately, many systems do not incorporate charcoal filters for removal of organic vapors that may be on test. The exact design and function of the filtration system should be scrutinized by the waste management program. The same situation applies to noninhalation facilities that may not even be equipped with HEPA filters. By extending the area of concern of a chemical waste management program back to the point of waste generation, a more comprehensive overall program may be established. Use of highly efficient air filters (for both particles and vapors) on fume hood and inhalation chamber exhausts is one of the best means of diversion of air stream contaminants into a solid waste contaminant. The spent filter becomes a part of the solid waste of the facility when replaced and carries with it the contaminant load removed from the exhaust air.

Liquid contaminants may also be a prime concern for control measures. Most liquid wastes of bulk chemical materials are rather easily controlled by use of bulk collection containers. In this manner it is quite common to collect spent solvents or liquid reagents for proper disposal. However, within the toxicology testing laboratory there are several operations associated with sanitation practices which generate the majority of the contaminant load released to the sewage system. These operations concern the cleaning of the soiled cages and racks used for testing, and cleaning the glassware and other equipment used for support operations during conduct of the testing work. In the first instance, cage cleaning, the contaminant concentrations are very low but the hydraulic load is very high. In the second instance, support equipment cleaning, just the reverse situation is true. Due to these opposite situations it is not often cost-effective to apply one treatment concept to both cases. Upon analysis it has been found [3] that administrative controls to accomplish diversion of contaminants on the support equipment from the liquid stream to the solid stream may eliminate much of the need for liquid waste treatment systems, provided that these diversions are applied judiciously at the places with low hydraulic load and high contaminant concentrations.

The levels of contamination of liquid waste streams from toxicology laboratory operations have been examined in an experimental project to study the removal of these contaminants prior to discharge [3,4]. Samples of contaminated waste waters have been treated by use of ultrafiltration, reverse osmosis, cartridge filtration, and carbon absorption processes to determine the economics of applying these treatment processes to typical waste streams from testing laboratories. The results of this study indicated that for some chemical compound classes pretreatment of liquid waste could reduce the contaminant concentrations by 95-99%. At present the only U.S. toxicology laboratory applying these techniques is located at the National Center for Toxicological Research in Arkansas.

Solid wastes generated at a "typical" toxicology laboratory may account for as much as 90-95% of the test compounds used [1]. For this reason considerable attention has been focused on solid waste handling methods in the conduct of long-term bioassay experiments. As mentioned previously, the solid waste stream frequently contains the filtered air contaminants from spent air filters and also a portion of the liquid contaminants from diverted liquid sources. In addition, the solid waste stream contains the "normal" solid wastes such as soiled bedding, animal wastes, spent feed, used support equipment, and discarded protective equipment and clothing items. This diversity of composition creates special handling problems for disposal and may result in more than one standard procedure being necessary to handle properly each type of waste. For example, incineration conditions have been found to vary considerably based upon the ratio of wet bedding to disposable olefinic garments in an incinerator load, and control of the load composition has been found necessary for efficient combustion.

Aside from the bulk test chemical itself, dosed-feed residuals usually represent the highest concentration source of the chemical contaminants in the solid waste stream. Caution in packaging the spent feed is needed to assure safe transport to the disposal site and to minimize the potential for spill contamination.

Caging wastes contain the next highest amount of chemically hazardous material from the test procedures. These materials present a special problem, because it is at this point that a degree of uncertainty in the actual chemical composition of the waste and its chemical hazards may arise if the original material has been metabolized to another substance prior to excretion. The metabolite material may have different and unknown hazardous properties than did the original test material.

Support equipment disposables generally do not contain significant concentrations or amounts of test chemicals. Skilled animal technicians know how to conduct routine procedures in a manner to avoid accidental spill or release of the test compounds. Thus, at the end of a work shift their garments will not be appreciably contaminated with hazardous chemicals except in very rare instances or unusual procedures. Cleaning of support equipment (e.g., blenders and mixers) may generate waste components with significant levels of contamination. Control and containment of these wastes at the point of generation is essential. The most concentrated chemical hazard in the support equipment solid waste stream is usually the spent filter media used for air or liquid purification prior to discharge from the facility. If liquid scrubbing is performed for contaminant control, these sludges will also contain similar hazards. Filter change procedures represent an important part of the chemical waste management program.

REGULATIONS

The handling of chemically hazardous materials falls under the jurisdiction of numerous federal laws. Transport of hazardous chemicals is of concern to both the U.S. Coast Guard and the Department of Transportation, while in transit. If the material is a food or drug the Food and Drug Administration will be involved. If the substance is a workplace chemical the Occupational Safety and Health Administration is concerned. Also involved in this area is the U.S. Environmental Protection Agency (EPA) under the areas of concern of the Toxic Substances Control Act. Prior to a chemically hazardous material being classified as a waste material, all the regulatory requirements of these agencies must be met. However, this discussion shall only deal with these materials after they have achieved the classification of a chemical waste.

The primary law to be dealt with is the EPA's solid waste law, the Resource Conservation and Recovery Act (RCRA) of 1976, PL 94-580 (42 U.S.C. 6921 *et seq.*). Other legislation concerned with air and water pollution emission standards is usually not specifically pertinent to release of chemically hazardous materials as pollutants from a typical toxicology laboratory. For example, the Clean Air Act addresses only a very small number of specific chemicals when specifying control limits. RCRA, however, has as its keystone that hazardous wastes will be "controlled from the cradle to the grave." This approach makes a comprehensive waste management program essential since this legislation has incorporated extensive punitive powers for the enforcement of the supporting regulations.

Hazardous Waste Management Regulations have been published by the EPA [5] and became effective on November 19, 1980. These regulations are very complex and voluminous. They define hazardous wastes (40 CFR Part 261), standards for hazardous waste generators (40 CFR Part 262), standards for hazardous waste transporters (40 CFR Part 263), and standards for owners and operators of hazardous waste treatment facilities (40 CFR Parts 264 and 265). Other sections of these regulations address guidelines for state programs (40 CFR Part 123), and permit requirements (40 CFR Parts 122 and 124).

Identification of a hazardous waste is the first point of concern for a toxicology laboratory. EPA has defined a set of characteristics using standardized tests to enable determination of the applicability of these regulations to a particular waste. Ignitability during routine handling is the first characteristic which will apply to most flammable substances, especially organic solvents. Corrosivity is a concern in relation to whether the waste will corrode standard waste containers. Reactivity is the tendency for the material to explode, to react violently when mixed with water, or to emit toxic gases. Extraction procedure toxicity is the characteristic of the waste emitting toxic materials at levels in excess of specified levels.

A varied waste stream from a typical toxicology laboratory will usually contain one or more individual substances which fall within the boundary of these defining characteristics of EPA; thus these laboratories should consider all the appropriate sections of the regulations. Once a waste stream is identified as included by these definitions, the facility must determine whether it can be considered a small generator, and thereby be exempt from some of the sections of the regulations. In general, generators having less than 1,000 kg per month of the waste are eligible for this consideration. However, certain substances are regulated at levels lower than 1,000 kg per month, and the specific section of the regulation should be studied to determine whether the exemption applies.

A hazardous waste generator must obtain an EPA identification number. If the waste is accumulated and stored more than 90 days on site, a facility permit is needed. Appropriate containers and labeling are required. A manifest of the waste materials must be prepared to accompany the waste in transport. An annual summary of waste activities must be prepared.

Transporters of hazardous wastes must obtain an EPA identification number. During transport the waste materials must be accompanied by a proper manifest describing the materials, and the entire shipment must be delivered to the site designated by the generator of the waste. During transit the transporter must comply with all regulations of the Department of Transportation relative to reporting of spills or discharges, and must clean up any material spilled during transit. A copy of the manifest must be retained for three years after delivery.

Standards applicable to operators of a hazardous waste disposal site pertain to operators of incinerators and chemical landfills. For many toxicology laboratories this will mean the incinerator falls under scrutiny as a hazardous material disposal site. Operation of the incinerator in a manner to assure adequate combustion of the hazardous material is required. Compliance standards from the Clean Air Act, the Clean Water Act, and the Safe Drinking Water Act are used to limit emissions from any facility.

SURPLUS CHEMICALS

In a large-scale chronic toxicity testing program a significant amount of residual chemical material may remain upon completion of the testing protocol. Each compound on test is selected because of its potential ability to cause toxic effects. Therefore, disposal of these materials has to proceed in a manner consistent with the substance potentially being classified as a hazardous waste. The first question to be addressed for each unwanted compound is whether the material can be incinerated. Incineration is chosen as the preferred route of disposal since the substance loses its identity during processing and the possibility of future problems with a material is removed once processing is completed. Certain types of test materials are found to

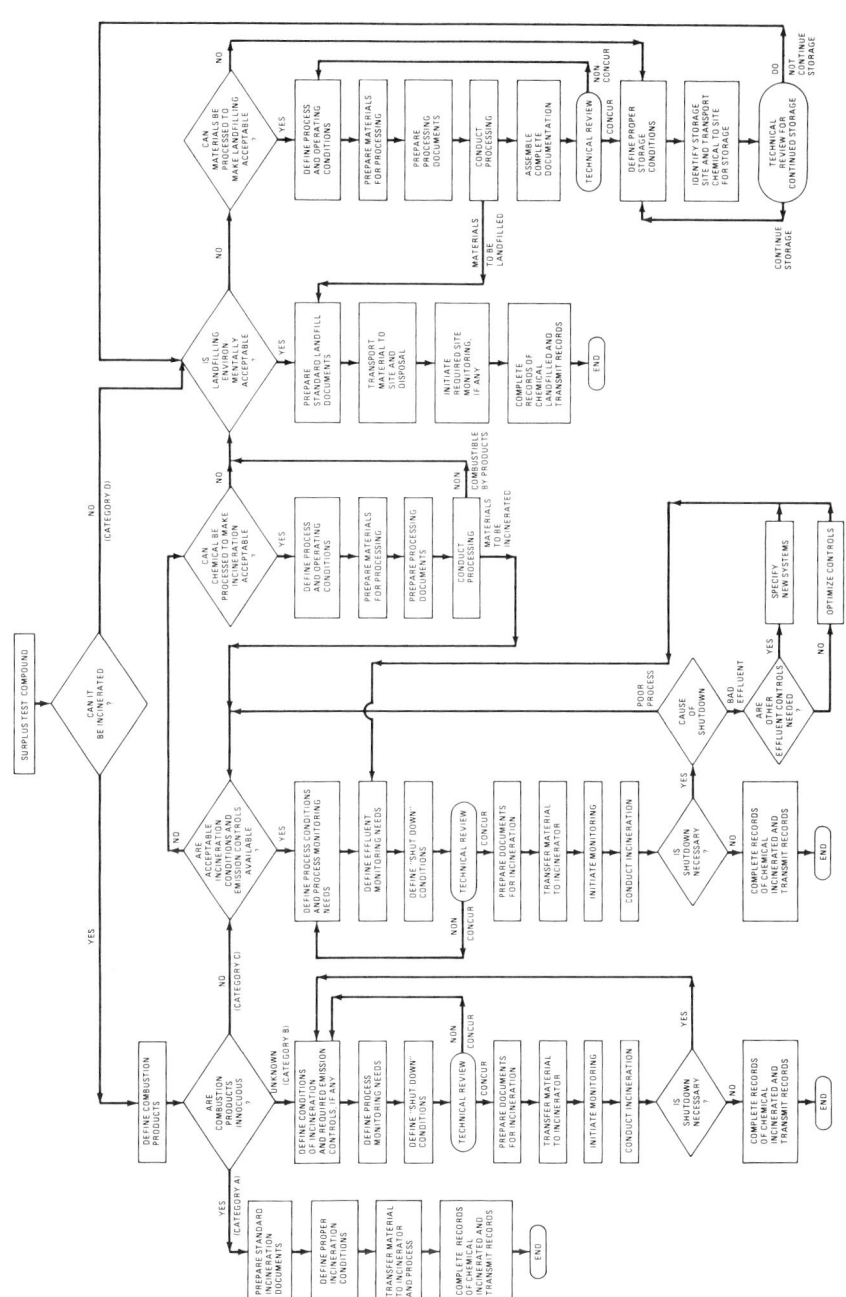

Figure 18-1.   Chemical disposal scheme.

not be disposable through incineration and these are designated for disposal at a secure landfill site.

A more recent approach to control of waste emissions has addressed the problems associated with slow chronic releases of hazardous materials from landfill sites or manufacturing facilities. This type of problem has received considerable publicity and is most vividly characterized by the New York State Love Canal problems. Private insurance carriers are now developing a comprehensive type of insurance to provide coverage for their customers who have potential sites of emission. To protect their interests these companies have developed techniques of an environmental audit for the purpose of premium setting. Knowledge of these findings may help in providing prewarnings of emission problems from such disposal sites. The chemical management program should examine the findings of any environmental audits conducted at the site chosen for landfill.

The general approach to this chemical disposal scheme is represented by a series of decision points that will now be described [6]. As stated, the initial decision concerning incineration selects the options available. For a material that can be incinerated the next question of interest is to define the expected combustion products and their properties. Similarly for a material going to landfill, the acceptability of that choice must be affirmed. If it is found that the combustion products are innocuous, a straightforward incineration may be conducted. In general, this group comprises compounds containing the elements carbon, oxygen, and hydrogen. For materials designated for landfill an uncomplicated process may occur if there is little likelihood of subsequent migration. Highly insoluble inorganic oxides and sulfides are representative of this group.

Materials whose combustion products or whose properties are unknown require further work. Incineration conditions and emission controls must be defined and secured. Environmental monitoring needs must be met. Finally, a trial burn should be made to determine if conditions and controls are adequate. If all these conditions are met then the process may be completed. Materials in this group tend to be organic compounds containing sulfur or nitrogen which produce acidic gases as combustion products.

More difficulty is found when combustion products are not acceptable, but it is felt that acceptable conditions and controls may be used to allow a safe burn. Materials falling in this group are represented by the organophosphates and halogenated organics. Here the process controls, effluent controls, and monitoring needs must be defined to specify the shutdown conditions if the burn does not go smoothly. A trial burn is begun and monitored to determine the need to shut down. If shutdown is required, then a reconsideration of the process and effluents is needed to determine the appropriate changes to be made. It may be that at this stage acceptable controls cannot be found, and that the landfill option has to be reevaluated. Alternatively, it may be feasible to preprocess the material to convert it to a substance more amenable to incineration or landfill.

A similar situation may arise with materials designated for landfill due to lack of the ability to incinerate. Where direct landfill is not an environmentally acceptable choice (for example due to a leachate problem), the substance may be able to be converted into a less hazardous material through chemical processing. If processing for a conversion is not feasible, then the substance may wind up in long-term storage with a periodic review cycle designated. Storage problems may result in the need for an entire review of the material's fate starting right back with the initial decision as to whether the material may be incinerated.

SUMMARY

The problems attendant with handling numerous diverse chemical materials in a toxicology laboratory present many challenges to the chemical waste management program. Many of these problems may be minimized by thorough consideration of handling operations and the reuse and recycle of substances. Several recent government regulations have a great impact on this area that a facility operator cannot ignore. It is important to develop a systematized approach to waste handling to avoid technically inconsistent methods of response to waste disposal choices.

ACKNOWLEDGMENT

I am grateful for support for this work under a subcontract from Tracor Jitco Inc. under prime contract N01-CP-43350 from the National Cancer Institute, Bethesda, MD.

REFERENCES

1. Kemp, D.W. and G.L. Wiegele. "A Pollution Assessment of Chemicals Dispersed to the Environment from Selected Bioassay Research Facilities," Contract No. N01-CP-43350, National Cancer Institute, Bethesda, MD, 1978.
2. Jurinski, N.B., J.J. Beres, and D.B. Walters. "Evaluation of Potential Chemical Exposures in Toxicology Laboratories," in preparation.
3. Light, W.G., K.J. McNulty, and R.L. Goldsmith. "Development of Decontamination Procedures for Aqueous Chemical Carcinogens," Contract No. N01-CP43350, National Cancer Institute, Bethesda, MD, 1978.
4. Light, W.G., K.J. McNulty, and N.B. Jurinski. "Development of Decontamination Procedures for Aqueous Chemical Carcinogens," *Nucl. Chem. Waste Manag.* 1(2): 119-127, 1980.
5. *Federal Register,* 45(98):33066-33588, May 19, 1980.
6. Jurinski, N.B. "Incineration or Landfill—Exploring the Waste Disposal Options," *Haz. Mat. Manag. J.* 2(1):12-16, 1980.

CHAPTER 19

Incinerator Design and Operation for Chemical Waste Disposal

Maurice W. Hunt
Rollins Environmental Services (NJ) Inc.,
P.O. Box 221, Bridgeport, New Jersey 08014

INTRODUCTION

The art of incineration or thermal destruction of combustible material has been practiced for many decades by all types of industries, including municipalities which burned some of their trash. The process was usually not well understood by the operator and often thought about even less. The primary measure of success was, "Did the original combustible material disappear?" ignoring the possibility that substantial amounts of the combustible might be emitted out the stack unchanged or partially changed to some type of material even more dangerous to the environment.

As an example of performance problems resulting from such lack of understanding, consider the following. I was assigned the responsibility of "starting up" the operation of a custom-built, solid ram/liquid injection incinerator for another company as recently as 1970 in which complete successful performance could never be achieved. The consultant designer had apparently never considered, or even understood, the difficulty of retaining a burning piece of trash so it would not be carried out the stack while still aflame. Although the liquid injection part of the system seemed to function satisfactorily, residence time to ensure guaranteed adequacy of destruction efficiency was apparently not considered a major design parameter.

The purpose of this story is to remind us of how far we have come with regard to our expectations and also to stress that the way has not been easy or inexpensive. Each time the design has been improved, analytical methods have been developed almost simultaneously which, instead of measuring in percentages, have inexorably moved to parts per million, parts per billion, and parts per trillion. The fact that the scientist, almost without exception, has been unable to discern the correlation between these minute concentrations of materials and their environmental impact, has not dissuaded the public or the well-intentioned regulation writer from demanding complete disappearance of the material fed to the incinerator.

One other major factor impacting upon the design aspects of an incinerator is that, for a variety of reasons, the waste to be handled is constantly changing, usually becoming more and more difficult due to viscosity, chemical and physical variability, etc. Therefore, although various environmental regulatory agencies have already mandated or are planning to mandate that thermal incineration will be the only acceptable disposal method for certain chemical wastes, the technology requirements for achieving compliance with these regulations is challenging designers of this type of facility.

In contrast, however, subsidiary companies of Rollins Environmental Services, Inc. (RES) have been successfully operating three such facilities for more than 10 years. During that time, the basic incinerator design has not changed significantly except for some performance upgrading of the combustion gas pollution control or purification system to meet the more stringent and constantly changing requirements. Figure 19–1 is a general schematic which shows the incinerator system as presently operated at both the Bridgeport, New Jersey, and the Houston, Texas, facilities. The third unit at Baton Rouge, Louisiana, is similar to the other two except that the combustion gas purification system relies upon a wet wall electrostatic precipitation system. This difference, of course, does not affect the destruction efficiency of the incinerator itself.

The primary purpose of this chapter is to describe what are believed to be key design and administrative control criteria necessary to successfully operate a commercial chemical waste incineration system. Most of the criteria described herein

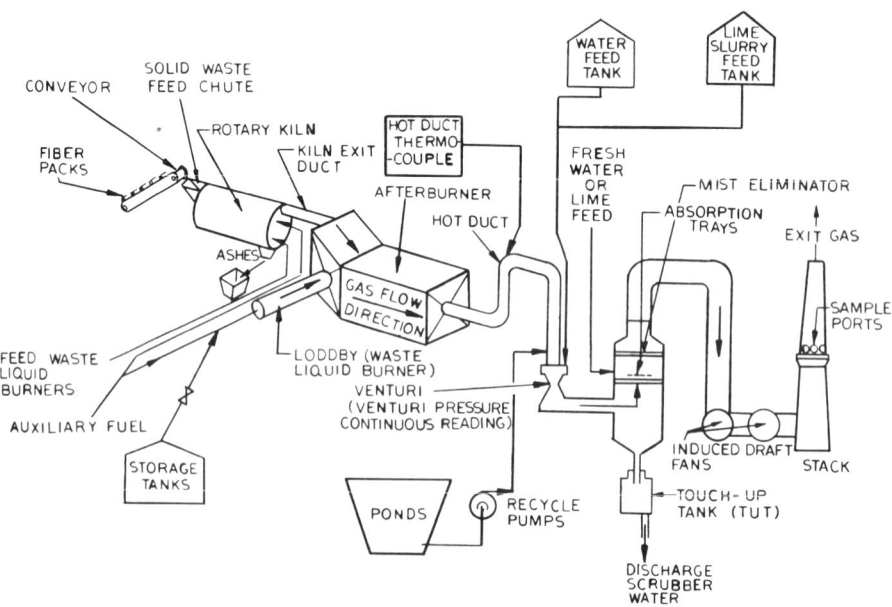

Figure 19–1. Schematic of Rollins Environmental Services incinerator.

have been used or are still in use by at least one of the RES facilities; however, in a few instances, such is not yet in place because of recent innovation. The descriptions follow the normal path of the waste material as it passes through the receiving area to the final reintroduction of the incineration waste residuals into the environment. Equipment design is discussed first, followed by a description of how personnel are to operate the equipment from an administrative control standpoint.

KEY EQUIPMENT DESIGN CRITERIA

Waste Receiving Area

Figure 19-1 does not include this area for the sake of simplicity. However, it is an extremely important aspect of the facility from both a safety and an environmental standpoint. Key points are given below.

Transporter Vehicle Permitting

Obviously, waste transportation equipment comes in a multitude of shapes and sizes; however, the first priority is that the legal requirements be satisfied. Since that subject in itself would take another chapter to describe it, suffice to say that Department of Transportation (DOT) rules must be satisfied. In addition, most states now have their own permitting rules which, in some instances, even require collateral from the transporter. Placarding and manifesting are also important legal requirements, with citations and fines awaiting those who ignore the details. Good starting references for instruction regarding some of these compliance items are: "Transportation," 49 CFR, Parts 100 to 177 and Parts 178 to 199, and "Hazardous Materials: 1980 Emergency Response Guide Book," DOT-P-5800-2.

Transporter Vehicle Design

With the paperwork of transportation behind us, the next important step is to match the equipment design to the waste characteristics. Materials of construction are of major importance to ensure avoidance of catastrophic failure. A good source for corrosion information is the waste generator.

If the material is to be shipped in some type of small container rather than a bulk tanker, box trailers or vans are most frequently used. Open flat bed trailers were often used in the past and are still permissible; however, closed trailers offer more spill protection in case of container failure or vehicle accident. Many of the closed vans now in use even offer sealed floors to enhance emergency containment capability. Frequently, absorbent materials and safety gear are also carried in order to enhance spill clean-up response. Obviously, all trailers must be well maintained so as to avoid waste container damage or potential spills.

If the material is to be shipped in bulk liquid quantities, standard tankers or vacuum trailers are used. Assuming that the DOT requirements have already been fulfilled, some of the important trailer ancillaries that must be available for delivery to RES incinerator facilities include sample points, relief valves, vent lines, vapor line for nitrogen gas blanketing and electrical grounding connectors.

The RES liquid waste bulk delivery system requires that an electrical grounding permissive interlock and gaseous nitrogen feed permissive interlock be satisfied prior to any actual waste liquid flow. By so doing, the risks associated with potential fires or explosions are essentially eliminated. The grounding connector safely removes any static electricity and the presence of a nitrogen atmosphere instead of air prevents any volatile wastes from reaching their explosive limits because nitrogen is an inert gas.

Vent lines and relief valves are needed as the final protection against pressure build-up in the trailer to avoid an uncontrollable rupture and its attendant hazards. As an alternate procedure, sometimes during unloading, vent lines can be connected between the trailer and the receiving tank. Such practices can reduce nitrogen consumption. However, some additional unloading risk may be experienced because of potential incompatible chemical mixtures.

Sometimes waste solids are shipped in bulk, but possible system designs for their incineration are not described here. Such systems are available and would be installed if the need developed. Most waste solids bulk shipments are made to landfills.

The other major option for bulk waste shipments is the rail car. Thus far, most waste shipments are in smaller than rail car quantities, since waste generators usually prefer to maintain a minimum inventory for control and liability purposes. No further description of rail car transportation options will be given here except to state that they can be made available when economic justification exists.

Sampling/Unloading

In order to minimize safety hazards, particularly during inclement weather, platforms with stairways and drop gates must be provided. Since waste deliveries must be sampled prior to acceptance for unloading, and many wastes could cause injury, either chronic or acute if direct exposure occurred, it is absolutely imperative that the personnel doing such tasks have easy access to the dome of the trailer. A person in fully enclosed safety gear with self-contained breathing apparatus is significantly hampered in mobility and agility.

At one major chemical manufacturing facility, I reviewed records which showed that almost 50% of all injuries that occurred over a 30-year period happened while the worker climbed around on tank cars or trailers. It is a commonly underemphasized risk in many safety programs. Also of importance is the need to use closed sample containers, preferably not glass, with a sample carrier equipped with a handle for ease of control. Sampling techniques for each type of container and waste must be specifically developed. In all cases, the sample takers have not finished their job until the container exterior is completely clean and properly labeled.

Secondary Containment

Although not necessarily mandated by regulations, it is recommended that all sampling activities be carried out within a secondary containment area. By so doing, any spillage can be washed immediately from the equipment, collected and removed for proper treatment. The containment area should include a sump system with enough capacity to hold well in excess of the largest container (trailer) to be handled in case of a complete rupture of the unit. Easy access for removal of the accumulated liquid or solids buildup is a must. It is important that the material collected in the sumps be carefully sampled and analyzed prior to mixing with other materials in order to avoid compatibility problems.

Waste Storage Systems

Satisfactory storage of steel or fiber drums is quite easily accomplished. It is acceptable in many instances to leave the fiber drums in the box trailer until they are fed to a rotary kiln. However, the trailers must be kept in a secure area and, of course, be accessible for necessary sampling. If unloaded, storage must be equipped with a cover at minimum to ensure necessary protection against weather. Damage to the drum or label must be avoided.

Steel drums containing liquids must be handled somewhat similarly. Additional safety factors such as secondary containment and segregation according to characteristics must also be addressed. Often, local fire codes must be observed.

Although small container storage and handling is important, bulk liquid waste storage offers even greater complexities. A typical example of such a system is shown in Figure 19–2.

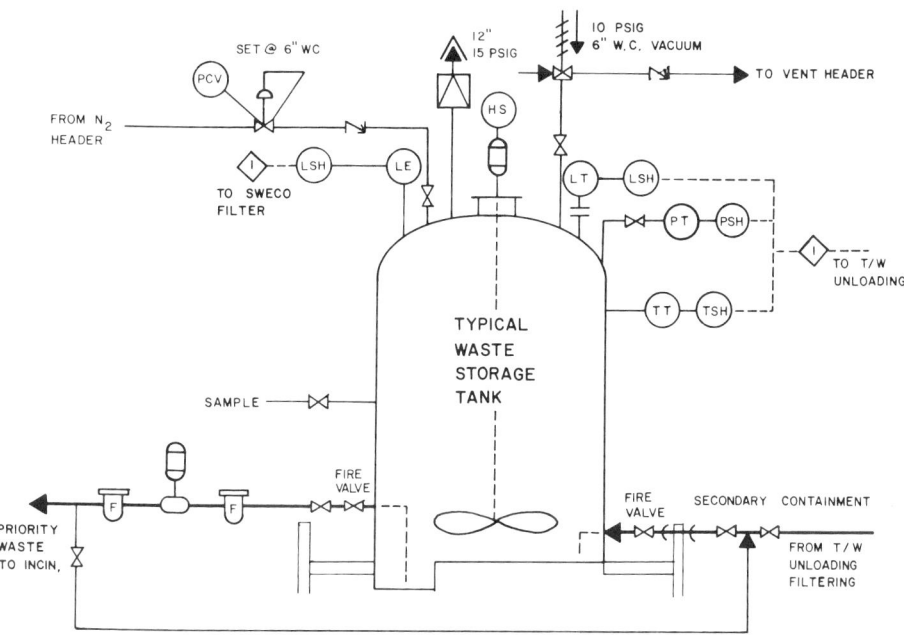

Figure 19–2. Waste storage tank.

Since commercial liquid incineration systems must rely upon a multitude of different suppliers of waste and must maintain the capability of handling those wastes without being solely dependent upon commercial fuel for its heat source, a substantial amount of waste blending must be done in order to provide a liquid waste feed of adequate consistent heat content. Other reasons for blending include ash content, heavy metal content, chlorination levels, viscosity, etc. Administrative control, based upon accurate laboratory data, is the single primary control point which must be rigorously executed in order to avoid problems during waste blending. Even with perfect execution of those systems, equipment design is also very important.

Good control of a liquid waste system is achieved only if unexpected pluggages and/or leakages can be avoided and some level of waste homogeneity can be provided. A starting point for that objective is to carefully evaluate materials of construction just as was done during selection of the shipping container. All lines, pumps, and tanks must be considered from a worst-case exposure potential. Corrosion tables from vendors are of great value, but due to the nature of waste mixture, actual testing must sometimes be done. Of course, a key source of information is the waste generator. However, the incinerator operator must blend many wastes together, which means that, in most cases, he or she is the sole authority on probable corrosion potential. Allowances must be made for velocity variation and type of exposure, whether wetted, interface, or vapor. Ultimately, the operator must use good judgment for the best economically available construction material, overdesign to allow for sacrificial wear, and monitor routinely with good documentation so as to anticipate need for replacement. The final measure of success of this overall program will be the number of unexpected leaks or major equipment failures experienced.

Since liquid injection incineration generally relies upon some type of waste atomization or fine droplet formation at the burner entry port, an important design parameter is to ensure that the suspended solids content in the waste can be successfully handled with the equipment provided. Orifice or nozzle size must be protected by adequate filtration. Even more important, wastes cannot be mixed which might polymerize unless the system is so designed to handle this factor.

The starting point for this control is at the laboratory, as far as determining proper or safe waste mixtures, followed by some type of filtration or suspended solids removal system at the trailer unloading point. Additional filtration is typically done after unloading, because even if a waste mixture does not polymerize, solubilities can be adversely affected which might generate more suspended solids after unloading and blending. In order to provide continuity of operation, dual filters or strainers are needed to allow one to be cleaned while the other is in use.

Each storage tank, even though constructed according to the best engineering design, must be diked so as to provide secondary containment in case of overfilling, leaks, complete tank failure, etc. Some states allow more than one tank to share the same secondary containment. In any case, the dike must have enough capacity to contain at least 100% of the volume of the largest storage tank within the diked area with necessary allowances for any volume displaced by other equipment or tanks within the dike. In addition, good engineering practice should be followed to allow enough distance between tanks for proper maintenance, including replacement, fire protection, cleaning, etc. Space is needed to permit easy access for internal inspections as well. Some states and/or cities have very specific requirements as to distance between tanks and even dike height.

Other key requirements for proper liquid storage include remote readout of level, temperature, and pressure with audio alarms to indicate outer limits of proper range. Tank design should permit essentially complete emptying so as to avoid waste heel problems and/or sludge buildup.

Special designs for difficult-to-handle wastes should include at least one piping, pump, and tank system equipped with heat tracing or jacketing and insulation. This type of system is required to permit handling viscous wastes susceptible to elevated temperature thinning. Similarly, at least one system solely dependent upon gaseous nitrogen to provide motive force from the delivery trailer into a special pressure waste storage tank and hence into the incinerator, is very helpful and even mandatory for certain reactive or particularly odiferous wastes. Nitrogen blanketing on all tanks is a very important safety factor. It also helps to minimize odors because when used in conjunction with pressure tanks it suppresses the waste volatility somewhat.

The system in Figure 19–2 depicts a typical storage tank used at the Bridgeport, New Jersey, facility. It includes the standard diking for secondary containment, filtration, level, pressure, and temperature remote monitors. In addition, the level, pressure, and temperature instruments are all part of a safety interlock system which will automatically stop the waste transfer into any given tank if preset outer control limits are reached.

All are pressure tanks and have an automatic gaseous nitrogen feed system and double-stage vent relief system. Thus, if liquid is being pumped from the tank, a vacuum would be avoided by automatic inlet gaseous nitrogen flow. Conversely, if a tank is being filled, the feed nitrogen automatically shuts off, and when the pressure reaches about 10 psig, gas is released from the tank vapor space to a vent header. This vent gas is injected through a flash-back system into the incinerator for destruction. If the incinerator is shut down, the vent gas is automatically fed to an activated carbon absorber before exiting to the atmosphere. Should this vent system fail or have its capacity overloaded, a backup relief valve system would allow escape of gases directly to the atmosphere to avoid tank overpressurization. Agitation is provided on most of the tanks so as to maintain some semblance of homogeneity and sample points are provided to allow for follow-up analyses, if necessary. Finally, fire valves are provided to prevent escape of the tanks' contents if an external line fails and a fire starts.

Combustion System

Many different incinerator designs have been used in the past and some, of course, have been designed specifically for only one or a few specific captive wastes to be burned on site by the waste generator facility.

The commercial waste incinerator operator has a substantially more difficult task, however, because of the multiplicity of wastes to be handled. Rather than provide a liturgy describing systems that have been used both successfully and unsuccessfully by others, the following describes the basic parts of the incinerator presently operated by all three of the RES subsidiary facilities.

Figure 19–3 shows the vortimetric burner system, equipped with a Loddby design burner, where most of the liquid waste and all the gaseous waste is fed to the incinerator system. Figure 19–4 shows the rotary kiln system where all the solids and sludges are fed, contained in fiber or plastic drums or boxes. Figure 19–5 shows the afterburner system where the combustion gases from the kiln and vortimetric systems mix and are retained long enough at the required temperature to achieve the desired destruction efficiency. Slightly contaminated aqueous wastes are also injected directly into the afterburner, where they mix with the other combustion gases and are thermally oxidized themselves.

As can be seen from these figures, all the combustion units are refractory-lined to allow operation at the high temperature required for the thermal oxidation process. The refractory used in the RES incinerators is available from several different companies. However, no attempt will be made to describe the design in detail because of the complexity of the topic. Suffice to say that choices are usually based upon experience and usually are somewhat subjective as well as design limited.

Destruction efficiency of the chemical waste is controlled by three variables in the combustion zone, i.e., excess oxygen, residence time, and temperature. It is defined as 100 times the ratio of the input less the output to the input. Present regulations now require that the chemical destruction efficiency for incineration exceed 99.99%. Actual performance of the RES incinerator during a recent test burn

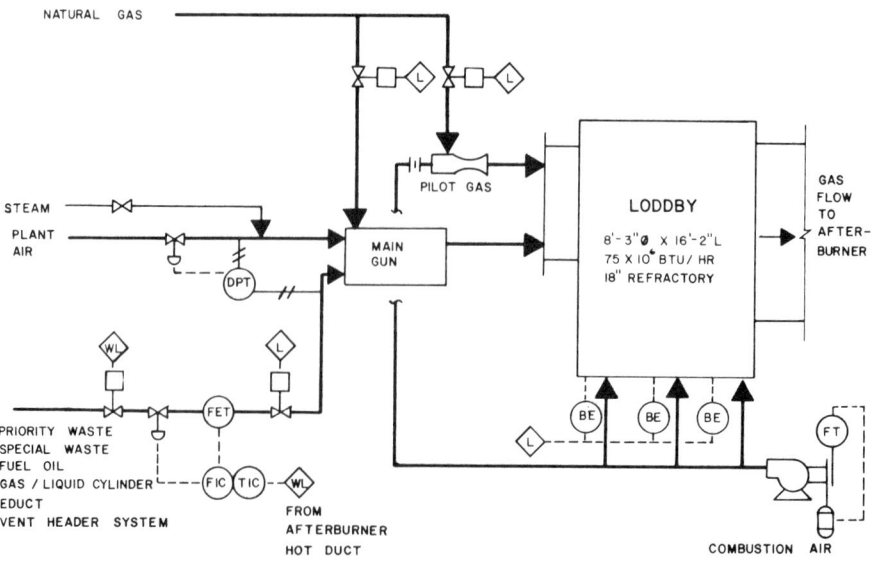

Figure 19–3.   Loddby burner.

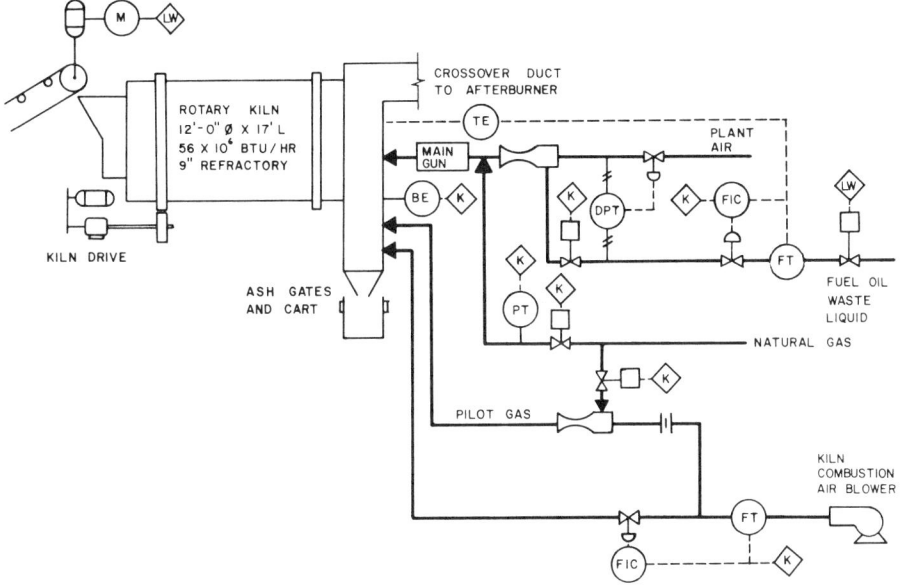

Figure 19–5.   Afterburner.

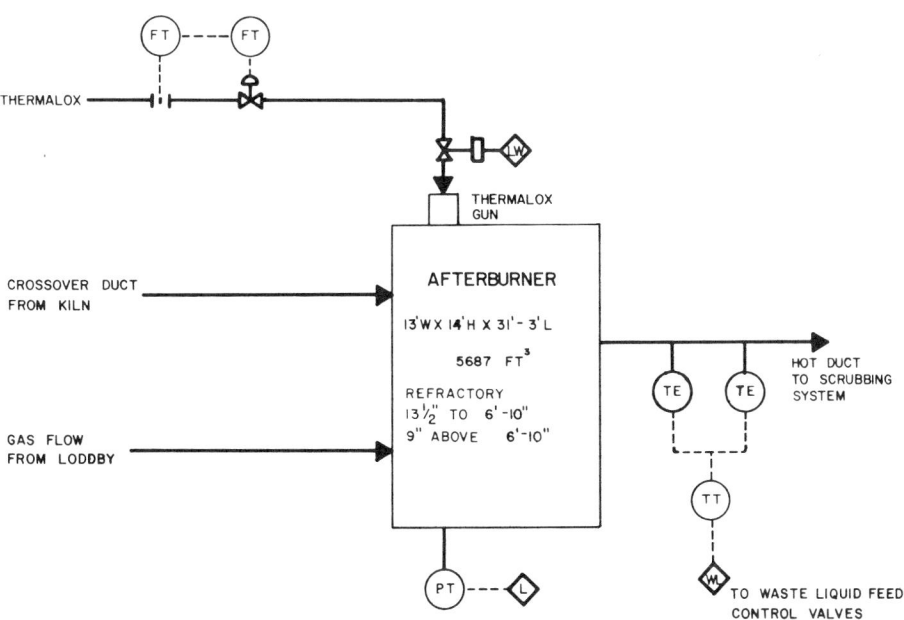

Figure 19–4.   Rotary kiln.

on polychlorinated biphenyls (PCBs) consistently demonstrated destructive efficiencies >99.9999%. In order to achieve these high-level efficiencies, the following conditions for the three key variables are typically maintained.

- *Residence time.* This is basically controlled by the dimensions of the combustion zone of the incinerator internals and the volume of combustion gases generated. The RES design always provides >2 seconds and ranges up to 3 seconds, depending upon the waste type and feed rate.
- *Excess oxygen.* This is controlled by the ratio of waste feed to the amount of combustion air fed to the vortimetric burner and the rotary kiln. The RES design typically provides from 50% to 100% in excess of stoichiometric oxygen requirements.
- *Operating temperature.* The required operating temperature to achieve the destruction efficiency objective is almost directly related to the chemical bonding (sometimes considered to be heat of formation) of the specific waste, assuming uniformity of the other variables. Many wastes can be adequately destroyed at temperatures as low as 1,600° F to 1,800° F. However, the New Jersey incinerator maintains a minimum of 2,000° F at the hot duct control point (temperature sensor located at a prespecified position in the hot duct or flue exit from the afterburner chamber prior to entry to the scrubber system). The Texas unit maintains at least 2,102° when burning PCB wastes.

Even if the three key variables are properly maintained within the desired operating ranges, there is need to include a number of interlock systems so as to minimize the possibility of inadequate destruction efficiency or equipment damage. The RES incinerators operate with some or all of the following interlock systems:

- *Waste Feed Shut-Off No. 1.* If the hot duct control point temperature falls below the desired preset temperature, all waste feeds, including the rotary kiln belt conveyor, automatically shut off. This system cannot be bypassed. Therefore, no waste can be fed until the proper incinerator operating temperature is regained by the combustion of nonhazardous fuel.
- *Waste Feed Shut-Off No. 2.* Although not presently required except for PCB wastes, a system has been developed which will shut off all waste feeds if the excess oxygen decreases below 3% or if the carbon monoxide concentration increases above 100 ppm in the combustion gas in the hot duct.
- *Exit gas opacity.* The RES incinerators do not use in-line opacity meters because the other controls are far more sensitive. It is also questionable whether or not such a meter would function due to the water-saturated nature of the exit plume. Visual readings are made by certified opacity readers during daylight hours.
- *Equipment protection.* Several interlock systems are used, such as automatic induced draft fan shutdown. If the fans become unbalanced, scrubber cooling water flow is lost, or if certain scrubber control temperatures are exceeded the system is automatically shut down.

Emission Control System

Fugitive emission control around the incinerator is accomplished by maintaining a slight draft throughout the incinerator from the induced draft fans backward to the feed entry point. It is imperative to maintain the entire incinerator system leak free to minimize air in-leakage to ensure accurate excess oxygen measurements. Ideally, the only air inlet should be from the controlled addition of the combustion air supplied to the vortimetric burner and rotary kiln by their forced draft fans plus that which enters during the kiln charge or ash discharge cycle.

Aside from fugitive emission control is the basic process need to purify the combustion gas prior to discharge to the atmosphere from the 100-foot-high stack. Purification or combustion gas scrubbing is necessary because the chemical wastes fed to the incinerator usually contain varying amounts of heavy metals which fluidize to some extent in the combustion process. Also, much of the waste material is chlorinated or contains sulfur, both of which are converted to acid gases upon combustion.

This purification process can be accomplished in several different ways with or without energy recovery. The New Jersey and Texas plants use a wet scrubbing system, as shown in Figure 19-6. Fresh creek water or a lime slurry are injected at the high-energy Venturi scrubber and scrubber tower. The gas/liquid mixing and reaction which occurs cools the combustion gas from $>2,000°$ F down to $150°$ F at the

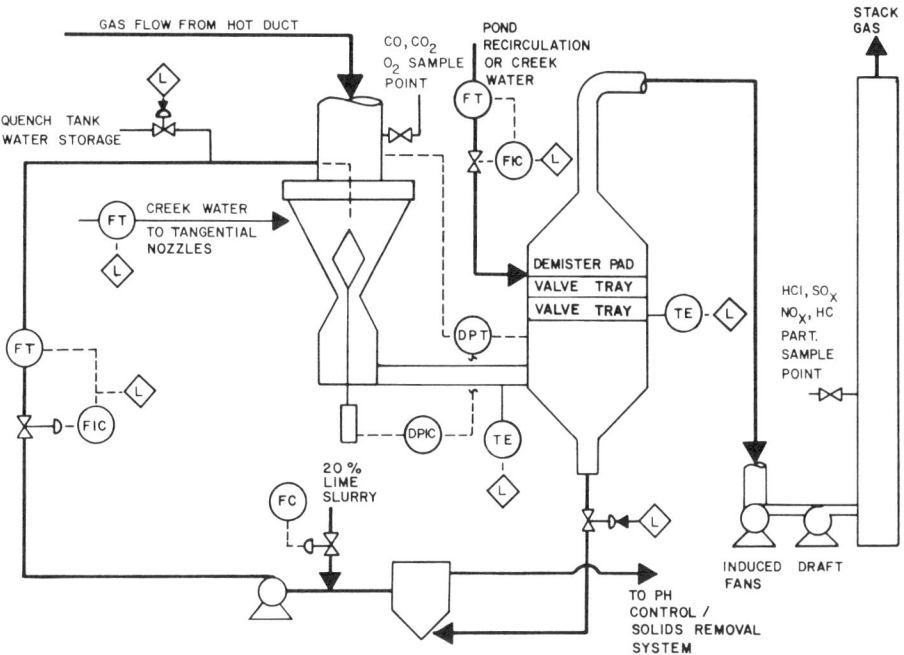

Figure 19-6.   Scrubbing system.

stack discharge. In addition, the fine heavy metal or inorganic particulates are agglomerated and removed as a slurry with the unreacted lime which is discharged from the bottom of the scrubber tower. Concurrently, the lime solution reacts with the acid gases such as hydrochloric acid, and the resultant neutralization products also exit the bottom of the scrubber tower.

The purification system is operated to ensure compliance with current regulations on emission limits which in New Jersey are:

Chemical	lbs./hr.
sulfur oxides (SO_x)	<120
hydrochloric acid (HCl)	<50
oxides of nitrogen (N_xO_x)	<75
particulates	<0.1 grains/DSCF corrected to 12% CO_2
hydrocarbons as methane	<1.5

As was mentioned earlier in the combustion control instrumentation section, this system includes a number of safety interlocks. These function to protect the fiberglass equipment from being damaged due to overheating as well as to protect the environment by ensuring that proper gas scrubbing is taking place.

In addition, sample points are provided in the hot duct and the exit stack for in-line or static grab sample testing. No specific testing frequency is presently mandated except when burning PCBs. Capability exists to measure all of the permit parameters. Typical in-line instrumentation can measure excess oxygen, carbon monoxide, and hydrocarbons.

Construction is presently under way at the New Jersey plant to install an improved wet scrubber design in order to meet more stringent emission standards recently promulgated. Engineering studies have been completed and consideration is being given to installation of energy recovery systems in the New Jersey and Texas plants.

Wastewater Control System

Although some amount of lime water recycling is done, both from the scrubber tower and from the cooling lagoons, most of the wastewater discharged from the bottom of the scrubber tower must be treated to allow discharge into a nearby waterway under state and federal permits (NPDES, or National Pollutant Discharge Elimination System). Figure 19–7 is shown which depicts a system presently being designed for the New Jersey plant.

The basic processes included in the new design are multi-stage lime neutralization tanks, polymer addition, clarification and dewatering prior to discharging into cooling lagoons. Discharge into the local waterway is batchwise or continuous depending on the permit. The existing system relies upon one tank and a series of lagoons to accomplish the same objective. An example of typical wastewater quality as discharged is shown in Table 19–1.

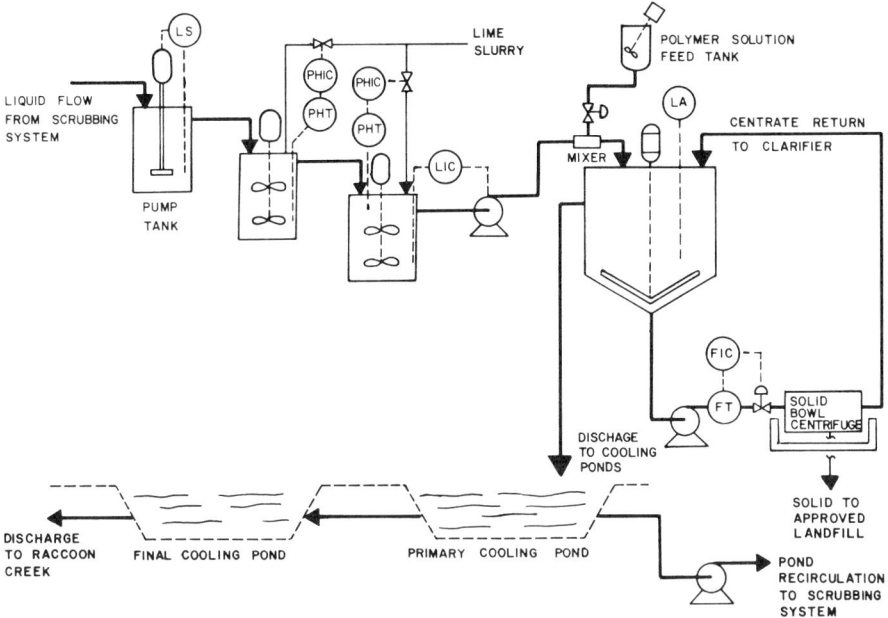

Figure 19-7.   pH control/solids removal.

RESIDUAL DISPOSAL

In addition to the stack emission, waste incineration produces two types of residuals that must be disposed of in an environmentally sound manner.

Kiln Ash

This material has been water quenched and consists of inorganic ash from the discharge end of the kiln as well as the metal rings and lids from the fiber drums. Although EP leachate tests indicate that this material is not hazardous by definition (test leachate must contain <100 times parameters specified in drinking water standards), a petition for delisting has not been submitted yet, so all such materials must be disposed of in a secure chemical landfill.

Emission Scrubber Sludge

The combustion gas scrubber system generates a lime sludge which flows continuously to a series of settling lagoons where clarification occurs. The sludge is periodically dewatered and removed for disposal in a secure chemical landfill. This material also appears to pass the EP leachate tests regarding toxicity, but a delisting petition has not yet been submitted.

Table 19-1. Incinerator Effluent Discharge

Parameter	Average Concentration (mg/l)
BOD_5	<15
COD	<50
Oil and grease	<9
Suspended solids (total)	<30
Dissolved solids (total)	<5,400
Ammonia (as nitrogen)	<20
Aluminum	<1
Arsenic	<0.05
Barium (soluble)	<1
Beryllium	<0.05
Cadmium (total)	<0.02
Chromium (hexavalent)	<0.05
Copper	<0.1
Lead	<0.15
Mercury	<0.005
Molybdenum	<1
Titanium	<2
Zinc (total)	<0.3
pH	6–9
Flow (maximum)	1,120,000 (gal/day)

*These data are based upon actual discharge data; however, they have been corrected to adjust for contribution from other sources such as the biological treatment process.

EMERGENCY SYSTEMS

Because all the wastes fed to the incinerator are either combustible or ignitable, an on-site emergency diesel-powered fire protection system using both water and foam is considered to be a necessity. A guaranteed source of water, adequate in volume to supply the fire protection system for several hours, is also a requisite. Distribution should be by both standard hydrant/hose systems and fixed fire monitors. A diesel-powered electric generator is also needed in order to ensure a continuous power supply to critical control instrumentation. These systems must be regularly maintained and tested and drills executed. Drills should involve the local fire departments and police as often as possible in order to minimize risks to everyone involved.

ADMINISTRATIVE CONTROLS

Successful operation of a hazardous waste treatment and/or disposal facility, particularly a commercial incinerator, is dependent upon a number of important administrative controls. Many of these controls are similar to those followed by any chemical manufacturing operation; however, many are unique to the waste disposal business. In order to adequately describe these differences, a step-wise explanation of the procedures used by the RES New Jersey facility follows.

Pre-Acceptance Qualification of the Waste

Once the waste generator has determined that they have material that is of no commercial value to them as a processor, such material is classified as a waste. The term hazardous is added if it meets certain criteria specified by the federal government's Resource Conservation and Recovery Act of 1976. Generally, the definition either identifies the waste by chemical name, generating process, or by one of four characteristics—ignitability, corrosivity, reactivity, or toxicity. The Rollins' facility is accessible for any waste that is compatible with our system and whose generator wishes to contract it. All wastes, however, are subjected to the hazardous waste control system, whether they are so defined or not.

The first action required by the generator, therefore, is to establish the key characteristics of their waste. If they contract Rollins, such information is documented by use of a Waste Data Sheet (Figure 19–8) and submitted to our Technical Department, so it can be determined if and how the waste can be treated. There are several key pieces of data to be included on this form, some of which are mandated by law, such as the EPA identification number, concentration of mercury, lead, sulfur, chlorinated compounds, and Btu value. Other information is needed to ensure compliance with state regulations or ensure operation with process limitations.

Once the treatability decision is made and concurred with by the operating department, a treatment price is calculated by the Technical Department. This price is unique for that particular waste and includes limitations on the variability of key parameters such as heat content, ash content, and halogenated content. The price must then be approved by Operations, Sales, and the vice president.

The sales representative then presents a proposal to the prospective customer based upon the above information. Normally, this proposal specifies a check burn volume that must be evaluated prior to a final proposal.

No wastes are priced nor are any wastes accepted at any Rollins plant until information is submitted to Rollins as specified on the Waste Data Sheet. If the generator cannot provide such information or chooses not to, Rollins will agree to provide the necessary analytical service at a preestablished price.

Prices for disposal by incineration vary significantly, as a function of the wastes' key characteristics. This variation is far more pronounced than for secure landfill, as an example, because variable costs are directly related to heat incineration content, halogen content, ash content, and throughput rate. In addition, fixed costs have steadily increased as a result of regulatory mandated capital requirements such as secondary containment, more stringent emission standards, continuous monitoring, and instrumentation. Generally, current incineration prices at the RES New Jersey facility range as follows:

Container Type	Price Range
bulk liquid (40,000 lbs.)	$0.05 to $0.40 per pound
drums (55-gallon steel drums)	$60 to $400 each
drums (20-gallon to 40-gallon fiber drums)	$40 to $300 each
pharmaceuticals (misc. package size)	$0.30 to $0.40 per pound

Rollins ®
Environmental Services

CUSTOMER INFORMATION:

Company Name	RES Stream No.
Plant Address	Mailing Address
State	State Zip
Company Contact, Technical	Phone
Company Contact, Business	Phone
USEPA Generator I.D. No.	State Generator I.D. No.

GENERAL WASTE DESCRIPTION:

Type of Process Generating Waste: ————————————————

Quantity Generated (per mo.)	Frequency (of removal)

TRANSPORTATION INFORMATION:

Hazardous Material:

Hazardous Substances:	Concentration	Hazardous Substances	Concentration

Hazardous Characteristics: ————————————————————

Transporter: _____   Placarding _____

TRANSPORTATION EQUIPMENT:

Tank Truck ☐	Vacuum Truck ☐	Flatbed ☐	Dump Truck ☐
Bin ☐	Barge ☐	Tank Car ☐	Other ☐ _____

Method of Collection:

Fiberpaks ☐   Drums ☐   Tanks ☐   Sumps ☐   Other ☐ _____

Other available transportation information: _____

RES 419 7/82

RNB:vjd
9/30/80

Figure 19–8.   Waste data sheet.

DETAILED WASTE DESCRIPTION AND REGULATORY COMPLIANCE:

RCRA Characterization Codes _____ _____ _____

Reason for above characterization: _____

_____

State Characterization Codes _____ _____ _____

OSHA: Contain listed compounds? _____   EPA : PCB conc > 50 ppm? _____

NRC: Radioactive? _____   PHS: Infectious Wastes? _____

FIFRA: Does this waste contain a pesticide for which the EPA
       has issued specific disposal requirements? _____

CHEMICAL COMPOSITION:

Compound Name	Norm. Conc. Range % W	Chemical Formula

LABORATORY ANALYSIS

Metals		CN	___ Mg/L
Pb	___ Mg/L	TOC	___ Mg/L
Hg	___ Mg/L	COD	___ Mg/L
Cd	___ Mg/L	BOD	___ Mg/L
Be	___ Mg/L	SS	___ Mg/L
As	___ Mg/L	TDS	___ Mg/L
Na/K	___ Mg/L	Br	___ % Wt
Other	___ Mg/L	Cl	___ % Wt
	___ Mg/L	F	___ % Wt
	___ Mg/L	I	___ % Wt
	___ Mg/L	S	___ % Wt

PHYSICAL PROPERTIES

PHYSICAL STATE @ $25^{\circ}C$
GAS ___ LIQUID ___
SOLID ___ SLUDGE ___
SLURRY ___ PASTE ___
GRANULAR ___ CRYSTAL ___
POLYMERIC ___ AMORPHOUS ___

SINGLE PHASE ___
MULTI PHASE ___
OIL/WATER ___
VISCOSITY ___

BTU _____ /lb
ASH _____ %
VAPOR PRESS _____
                @ _____
SPEC. GRAVITY _____

MELTING PT _____
BOILING PT _____
pH _____
FLASH PT _____

Is the waste reactive with water? _____   with air? _____

Is a representative sample provided? _____

Give any other additional information on the hazards of the waste: _____

_____

I hereby certify that the above information is complete and accurate.

_____   _____   _____
   Customer Signature   Title   Date

Figure 19–8. *(continued)*

CONTRACTUAL AGREEMENTS

The treatment proposal is accomplished by a standard contract form. If the customer accepts the treatment price, Rollins prefers that this acceptance be documented by returning a signed contract along with a purchase order. In some cases, more involved contracts are negotiated in order to meet special customer needs.

Key portions of the standard contract are:

- *Indemnification*. Specifies when transfer of waste ownership occurs (Rollins, by preference, transports most of the wastes between the generator and the treatment site, and therefore, as owner of the waste upon pickup accepts the transportation liability).
- *Warranties*. Addresses needs for proper regulatory compliance by Rollins and proper waste identification by generator.
- *Force majeure*. Protects either party against uncontrollable situations.
- *Payment terms*. Requires timely payment.
- *Safety and health conditions*. Requires that both parties must have specific knowledge regarding known carcinogens as required by the Federal Occupational Safety and Health Act.

In summary, use of such a contract minimizes potential liability difficulties by clearly defining the limits of the business relationship.

The specifics of each waste stream are handled by an appendix so that detail modifications can be readily handled without disturbing the nature of the basic relationship.

WASTE DELIVERY QUALITY CONTROL

If the customer agrees to this proposed business relationship, each of the individual wastes are assigned a unique, four-digit number, consecutive in nature from the first day of operation, with a prefix which initiates the creation of a unique set of documentation and thereafter controls all future handling of that specific waste stream.

A waste safety sheet (Figure 19-9) is jointly prepared by the Safety and Technical Departments. Prior to any acceptance of such waste, a copy of that specific waste safety sheet must be provided to the following:

- *Truck driver*. Must have a copy of such for whatever waste is being transported.
- *Security*. Must have a safety sheet for every waste on site and identified by waste location. This is important in case of an emergency. A copy for the waste involved would accompany an injured person in case of chemical exposure which required off-site medical treatment. This same information would be made immediately available to community emergency response personnel, such as a fire department.

Rollins ®
Environmental Services

Waste Designation: _____

Rollins # _____   EPA # _____   STATE # _____

CHEMICAL COMPOSITION:

Component Name	Formula	Range W %	Flash Pt. °F

PHYSICAL PROPERTIES:

Physical Character: _____

Color: _____   Odor: _____

Flash Point ☐ <100°F   ☐ <140°F   ☐ >140°F

INSPECTION FOR RECEIPT APPROVAL:

Parameter	Min. - Limits - Max.	

TREATMENT METHOD/PROCESS NOTES:

_____
_____
_____

☐ There is a special procedure for this waste.

HAZARD CODE INFORMATION

4=Red-Severe   3=Orange-High

2=Yellow-Moderate   1=Blue-Low

CHEMICAL COMPATIBILITY:

_____
_____
_____
_____
_____

REQUIRED PERSONAL PROTECTIVE EQUIPMENT:

☒ Hard Hat   ☐ Safety Glasses   ☐ Air-Supplying   ☐ Protective Suit
☒ Rubber Gloves   ☐ Splash Goggles   Respirator   ☐ Other _____
☐ Rubber Boots   or Face Shield   ☐ Air-Purifying
                                              Respirator

                                           Type: _____

RPE:v
8/7/80

_____   _____
Date Completed   Author's Name

Figure 19-9.   Waste safety sheet.

Waste Designation: _____ Rollins # _____

HEALTH PROTECTION:
  Effects of Exposure: _____
_____
_____

  First Aid: ' Eyes _____
_____

           Skin _____
_____

           Inhalation _____
_____

           Ingestion _____
_____

  Notes for Physician: _____
_____
_____

FIRE PROTECTION:
  Explosion or Fire Hazard _____
_____

  Fire Fighting Procedures _____
_____

REACTIVITY
  Conditions to Avoid _____
_____

  Incompatibles _____
_____
_____

  Hazardous Products _____
_____
_____

SPILL RESPONSE PROCEDURES _____
_____
_____
_____

TRANSPORTATION INFORMATION:
Hazardous Material:

Hazardous Substances	Concentration	Hazardous Substances	Concentration

Hazardous Characteristics: _____

Placarding: _____

Figure 19–9.   *(continued)*

- *Laboratory*. Must have a complete set of safety sheets for all wastes handled.
- *Safety supervisor*. Must have a complete set for emergency reference.
- *Unloading/storage control room*. Must have a complete set of safety sheets. However, only those for wastes which are presently in storage or being unloaded must be visibly displayed and identified as to waste location.
- *Incinerator control room*. Must have a complete set of safety sheets. However, only those for wastes presently being fed to the incinerator must visibly be displayed and identified as to waste location.

WASTE TRANSPORTATION MANIFEST

When the waste leaves the generator, a hazardous waste manifest must be initiated by the generator and must accompany the transporter. Figure 19-10 gives an example of such a manifest as required by New Jersey and subsequently revised to meet RCRA requirements. It now consists of a two-part, six-copy form. This type of manifest is intended to provide "cradle-to-grave" documentation for every hazardous waste shipment throughout the United States. It permits tracking of each hazardous waste from the generator through every step of handling and requires reporting of any deviation from the norm up to and including the final disposal.

Three copies of Part A are left at generator's site after waste pickup. Upon delivery of the waste to Rollins and laboratory acceptance of same, remaining copies are distributed as follows: one copy of Part B to the New Jersey Department of Environmental Protection (site of the disposal facility); one copy of Part B to the generator's state; one copy of Part B to the generator. If the waste was transported by someone other then Rollins, that company would receive a transporter's copy of the manifest. All other copies of both parts are retained by Rollins for at least three years.

Upon arrival at the treatment facility, each waste must be sampled and analyzed for key parameters to verify that it is definitely the same waste as was originally characterized by the waste data sheet, waste safety sheet, and manifest. If the laboratory confirms the shipment, the manifest is signed and the waste unloading personnel are instructed, in writing, as to the required disposition of that waste. This includes unloading instructions (specific receiving tank) and type of treatment to be done.

If the waste delivery does not conform to specifications, the laboratory immediately determines if the out-of-specification waste can be properly treated at the Rollins plant. If it can be treated, but at a higher cost, or if it cannot be treated due to process limitations, the sales representative advises the generator of the new situation. The generator then specifies its disposition. If the price revision is acceptable, the material is unloaded for treatment. If the price revision is rejected or if treatment is not possible, the generator specifies the return delivery location and absorbs all resultant costs under previously specified contractual conditions. Rejections must be noted on the manifest. In all cases, Rollins is responsible for distribution of the manifest copies as described earlier.

This entire quality control procedure is extremely critical in order to ensure proper compliance with safety and environmental requirements as well as to fulfill all mutual contractual obligations.

PART A: SEND TO DISPOSER'S STATE   DOCUMENT NO. NJ 0106256

Generator Name	Phone (inc. area code)	EPA I.D. NO.

Address (Street-City-State-Zip Code)

Transporter No. 1	Phone (inc. area code)	EPA I.D. NO.
Transporter No. 2	Phone (inc. area code)	EPA I.D. NO.

Address (Street-City-State-Zip Code)

Treatment, Storage or Disposal (TSD Facility)   Phone   EPA I.D. NO.

IF MORE THAN TWO TRANSPORTERS ARE TO BE UTILIZED, FILL OUT THE FOLLOWING, AS APPROPRIATE:
THIS FORM IS NO._____ OF A TOTAL OF _____. THE FIRST MANIFEST DOCUMENT NO. IS NJ_____

PROPER US DOT SHIPPING NAME	US DOT HAZ-ARD CLASS	UN NO.	FORM	NET QTY.	UNITS	CONTAINERS NO.	TYPE	EPA HAZ. CODE	EPA WASTE TYPE
1.									
2.									
3.									
4.									
5.									

Special Handling Instructions Including Container Excemption (i.e. Identification of Additional Wastes Included in Shipment of a Non-Hazardous Nature which do not have to be manifested)

GENERATOR'S CERTIFICATION: This is to certify that the above-named materials are properly classified, described, packaged, marked and labeled and are in proper condition for transportation according to the applicable regulations of the Department of Transportation, USEPA and the State. The wastes described above were consigned to the Transporter named. The treatment, storage or disposal facility can and will accept the shipment of hazardous waste and has a valid permit to do so. I certify that the foregoing is true and correct to the best of my knowledge.

GENERATOR'S SIGNATURE	TITLE	DATE SHIPPED	EXPECTED ARRIVAL DATE
Treatment stroage signature & certification of receipt of shipment	TITLE	DATE RECEIVED	

Figure 19–10. State of New Jersey Department of Environmental Protection hazardous waste manifest.

PART B: SEND TO DISPOSER'S STATE   GENERATOR'S EPA I.D. NO.

Transporter No. 1 Signature and Certification of Delivery and Non-Tampering with Shipment. Also Print Signature	Date Delivered
Transporter No. 2 Signature and Certification of Receipt of Shipment - Also Print Signature	Date Received
Transporter No. 2 SWA Registration No.	
Transporter No. 2 Signature and Certification of Delivery and Non-Tempering with Shipment. Also Print Signature	Date Delivered
Treatment, Storage or Disposal Facility of any differences between Manifest and Shipment or listing of reasons for and disposition of Rejected Materials. TSD FACILITY EPA I.D. NO.	Handling Method 1._____ 4._____ 2._____ 5._____ 3._____ 6._____
Treatment, Storage or Disposal Facility Signature & Certification of Receipt of Shipment. Also Print Signature	Title	Date Received

In case of emergency or spill, immediately call the State the emergency occurred in and the New Jersey Department of Environmental Protection:
        609-292-5560 (day)   (609)292-7172 (night)

                                        DOCUMENT NO. NJ 0106256

Figure 19-10.   *(continued)*

PREINCINERATION TREATMENT PROCEDURES

Additional standard operating procedures (SOPs) must be rigidly followed once the waste has been accepted by Rollins for disposal. Part of these are mechanical type safety/environmental procedures such as:

- Determination of the receiving vessel or location.
- If bulk liquid delivery, a fail-safe electrical ground and nitrogen vapor space must be established on the delivery trailer.
- Proper prespecified safety gear must be worn.
- Determination of compatibility of new waste with wastes already in storage.

Assuming that the earlier procedures have been followed, the next critical step is to make a check burn with any new waste so as to evaluate its treatability from a control and throughput standpoint. This is *not* the test burn procedure mandated by RCRA, however, but instead consists of carefully monitored incineration of limited quantities of a single waste (i.e., six-fiber pack drums to the kiln). Upon completion of the check burn, the other controls reviewed earlier are normally adequate to achieve proper incineration.

PERSONNEL QUALIFICATIONS

Due to the rather limited opportunities for people to gain experience in hazardous waste management because of the small number of such operations in existence for only the past few years, staffing is somewhat challenging. The New Jersey facility census consists of about 90 people (including sales personnel), approximately half of whom are supervisory and clerical. About 35% of the total are degreed professionals, specializing in engineering, chemistry, or industrial safety and health.

Management must then ensure that all personnel are adequately trained so that each person will instinctively and effectively perform according to the following priorities:

- facility personnel and community safety
- environmental compliance
- process security
- profitability improvement

In order to accomplish this objective, it is necessary to rely heavily upon written standard operating and emergency response procedures as well as effective inspection and preventive maintenance programs, supported by a cadre of experienced personnel.

Examples of the types of plans and procedures in effect at the RES New Jersey facility are listed below:

- safety/health program
- environmental program
- standard operating procedures
- best management practices program
- contingency plan
- waste analysis plan
- quality assurance plan
- spill/discharge prevention control and countermeasures
- discharge cleanup and response
- rainwater management and flood control plan
- facility closure program

SUMMARY

In summary, keys to successful operation of a chemical waste incinerator are:

- Good process and equipment design with a reasonable safety factor for all parameters.
- Full knowledge of the waste prior to any action, particularly with regard to reactivity, ignitability, corrosivity, and toxicity.
- Thorough quality control procedures from waste characterization, operation, effluent/emission control, and quality assurance programs.
- Sound management practices such as qualified personnel, training, preventive maintenance, and compliance with regulations.

INDEX

Barrier laboratory, 91. See also Toxicity Testing Laboratory, Hazardous Materials Laboratory and Chemical Containment
barrier concept, 92–93
corridor design, 99
double-corridor concept, 97–98
exit signals, 99
fire control, 91–92
fire control center, 100
fire detection, 99–100
fire propagation, 94–96
fire safety, 93–94
ignition sources, 94–96
site selection factors, 107–108
smoke, fire, and heat movement, 96–97
structural integrity, 106–107
Barrier systems, 23. See also Barrier Laboratory
Biological monitoring. See Medical surveillance
Bulk chemical management, 221–222
chemical handling, 225
cleanup, 238
facility requirements, 230–231
homogenization, 236–237
operations, 233–234
particle size reduction, 234–236
protective clothing, 231–233
random sampling, 237
repackaging, 237–238
documentation, 224–225, 226–229
procurement
experimental design, 222–223
purchase, 224
source identification, 223–224
shipment, 238. See also Packaging and Shipping

Chemical containment
design criteria, 33–34
principles, 33
source, path, receivor concept, 16, 36–37, 130–131
Chemical handling. See Bulk Chemical Management
Chemical health and safety program
discipline areas, 4
Chemical monitoring. See Monitoring
Chemical repository, 8. See also Hazardous Materials Laboratory
Chemical Safety Data Sheets. See Health and Safety Documents
Chemical storage. See also Chemical containment
macro containment, 39
micro containment, 38–39
Containment laboratory. See Barrier Laboratory or Toxicity testing laboratory
Contractor monitoring
annual program review, 13–14
chemical monitoring, 14, 16
concerns, 16
follow-up site visit, 15–16
health and safety baseline survey, 14
monthly reports, 15
site visit, 13–14

Data Sheets. See Health and safety documents
Disposal. See Incinerator and Waste
DOT regulations. See Packaging and shipping.

Engineering controls, 24–25
Epidemiological studies, 159

Ergonomics. See Human factors
Exposure, chemical
    cage dumping, 276–277
    control measures, 247
        administrative controls, 247–249
        engineering controls, 249–251
        operational practices, 247–249
        personal protective equipment, 251–
            252
    determinants, 243
    dosage preparation and administration,
        244–245, 276
    material handling, 244
    posttreatment animal holding, 245
    routes, 242, 275–277
    sampling, 26
    servicing and maintenance of equip-
        ment, 246–247
    waste handling and disposal, 246

Firefighting operations, 101–102. See also
    Barrier laboratory
    access, 102
    exposures, 104
    locating, confinement and extinguish-
        ment, 103–104
    overhaul, 105
    rescue, 102–103
    salvage, 105
    ventilation, 104–105
Fire suppression systems
    automatic sprinklers, 100–101
    halons, 101
    manual systems, 100
Flash points, 18
Formaldehyde control, 26. See also Monitor-
    ing, biological, formaldehyde

Glove boxes. See Ventilation

Hazardous Materials Laboratory, 45–46
    atmospheric control, 56–57
    chemical storage, 67, 69
    chemical traffic flows, 53–55
    communication, 70
    critical systems control, 63–64
    design components, 47
        mechanical, 55
    effluent control, 58–62

equipment design component, 66–69
    equipment placement, 65–66
    exhaust air, 58–59, 61
    fire control, 70
    fume hoods, 66–67
    glove boxes, 67, 68
    interior surfaces treatment, 66
    laboratory furniture, 67
    location, 48
    personnel traffic flow, 53–55
    safety design component, 69–70
    safety equipment, 69
    security, 70
    spatial design components, 47–48
    spatial elements, 49–53
    structural design component, 64–66
    utilities, 62–63
        access, 64–65
    visibility, 69–70
    wastewater, 60–62
    workspaces, 48–53
Health and safety
    duties, 17
    functions, 7, 8
    handbook, 11
    minimum requirements, 9–11
        bioassay laboratories, 21–26
        cellular and genetic toxicology labora-
            tories, 28–30
        inhalation studies, 27
        pathology laboratories, 31–32
    plans, 12, 23–24
    research areas, 17
    standard operating procedures (SOPs),
        12–13, 25, 37
Health and safety documents, 137–138
    chemical data sources, 148–153
    chemical safety data sheets, 219
    chemical-specific health and safety guide-
        lines, 6, 13, 138–142
    databases and databanks useful for docu-
        ment preparation, 154–158
    emergency procedures document (EPD),
        12, 17, 143, 219
    literature search scheme, 145–146
    preparation, 144
    protocol for hazardous use, 13
    safety and handling document (SHD), 12,
        142–143, 219

Health and safety officer
    minimum requirements, 21–22
High hazard laboratory. See Hazardous
    mateials laboratory
Hood monitoring and evaluation, 258–259
    daily visual inspection, 259–261
    face or capture velocity measurement,
        265–271
    quarterly inspection, 261–271
    routine maintenance, 272–273
    smoke candles, proper use of, 263
    smoke tube, proper use of, 261, 263
    training, 271–272
Hoods. See Ventilation
Human factors, 40–41, 121
    anthropometry, 123–125
    biomechanics, 127
    coding, 129
    design
        objectives, 121–122, 131–132
        procedures, 133
    environmental factors
        lighting, 127–128
        noise, 128
    human variables, 122–123
    negative transfer, 129
    population stereotypes, 128
    protective clothing, 132–133
    reach envelope, 123, 126
    work practices, 132

IATA regulations. See Packaging and
    shipping
Incineration, 309–311
    pretreatment, 331–332
Incinerator. See also Waste
    administrative controls, 322
        pre-acceptance qualifications, 323
    design criteria
        afterburner, 317
        combustion system, 315–318
        destruction efficiency, 316, 318
        emergency systems, 322
        emission control system, 319–320
        interlock system, 318
        pH control/solids removal, 321
        purification process, 319–320
        rotary kiln, example, 317
        sampling/unloading, 312

    secondary containment, 312–313
    transporter vehicle design, 311–312
    transporter vehicle permitting, 311
    waste receiving area, 311
    waste storage systems, 313–315
    waste water control system, 320
    efficacy for PBB, 18
    keys to successful operation, 333
    residual disposal
        effluent discharge, 322
        emission scrubber sludge, 321
        kiln ash, 321
    schematic, 310
Industrial hygiene monitoring. See
    Monitoring
Inhalation toxicology laboratory, 111–112
    chamber exhaust, 116
    chamber pressure control, 115–117
    exposure chamber ventilation, 113–115
    hazard containment, 112
    laboratory ventilation, 112–113
    safety equipment, 118
    waste control and decontamination, 116

Laboratory design, 40. See also Hazardous
    Materials Laboratory
    design phases, 41–42
    Laboratory hoods. See also Ventilation
    poor exhaust duct, example, 260
    typical clutter problems, examples, 264

Material Safety Data Sheets. See Health and
    Safety documents
Medical surveillance. See Monitoring,
    medical
Monitoring
    biological, 161–164, 165
        formaldehyde, 177–178
        future development, 172
        industry programs, 175
        interpretation, 166–167
        NTP contract laboratories, 172–
            173, 176
        NTP test compounds, 176–177
        OSHA requirements, 167–168
        pitfalls, 164, 166
        program development, 168–169
        program implementation, 170–171
        US government laboratories, 173–175

environmental (chemical), 162, 277–278
  interpretation, 278–279
  techniques, 278
genetic, 167
medical, 22–23, 162–163

National Cancer Institute
  guidelines for research, 160
National Institute of Environmental Health
  Sciences
  guidelines for research, 160
National Toxicology Program, 161
  Board of scientific counselors, 5
  carcinogenesis and toxicological bio-
    assays, 7, 10
  cellular and genetic toxicology, 7, 10, 12
  chemical manager, 6
  chemical pathology, 7, 10
  in-house studies, 7
  program resources branch, 6
  systemic toxicology, 7
  toxicology design committee, 6

Occupational Safety and Health Administration
  carcinogen regulations, 160

Packaging and shipping, test chemicals, 213–
  214. See also Bulk chemical management,
  shipping.
  chemical stabilization, 218–219
  cover letter, advance notification, 220
  decontamination procedures, 214
  DOT exemption, 217
  DOT hazard classes, 216
  DOT regulations, 215
  durability tests, 214
  IATA regulations, 217–218
  inert atmosphere packaging, 218
  receipt acknowledgement card, 219–220
  refrigeration, 218
  shipment inventory list, 220
  shippers, types of, 216–218
  solids and liquids, 214
Protective Equipment
  minimum requirements, 22

Resource Conservation and Recovery Act,
  284, 287, 303

Respirator protection program
  air-purifying respirators, 195–197
  equipment (general), 194–195
  fit-test procedures, 202–204
  issuance and training, 204–205
  medical assessment, 200–202
  minimum requirements, 22
  need and selection, 199–200
  OSHA regulations, 193, 199
  program administration, 205–206
  supplied-air respirators, 197–199
Risk assessment, 285, 296
  hazard index, 290–293
  hazard value, 288–290
  hazardous waste management committee,
    295–296
  multiparametric method, 286–288, 295
  relative cumulative risk, 293–294
  waste classification systems, 286

Shipping, Chemicals. See Packaging and
  Shipping

Thermal destruction. See Incineration,
  Incinerator
Toxicity testing laboratory, 34. See also
  Barrier laboratory
  chemical storage, 74–75
  chemistry laboratory, 83–84, 130
  chemistry support, 35–36
  design, 73
  dose preparation and administration,
    75–81
  exhaust, 87–90
  incinerator, 85
  in vitro, 35, 130
  in vivo, 34–35, 130
  necropsy and histology, 81–83
  receiving, 73, 75
  utilities support, 85, 87
  waste disposal problems, 283–284
Toxicology testing laboratory. See Toxicity
  testing laboratory
Tracer studies, 159
Training
  laboratory safety, 183–184
    custom-made training modules, 189
    implementation, 185–186
    measures of effectiveness, 188–189

modular approach, 187–188
objectives, 184–185
requirements and needs, 183–184
resource material, 186–187
Transportation. See Packaging and shipping

Ventilation
chemical fume hoods, 39
dilution, 39
glove box, 39
local exhaust, 39, 256, 260
design criteria, 256–258, 260
exhaust stacks, proper placement,
example, 263
reentrainment, example, 262
tissue trimming stations, 39–40

Waste. See also Incineration
data sheet, 324–325
delivery quality control, 326, 329

disposal, 25. See also Toxicity testing
laboratory, Waste disposal problems
disposal scheme, 305–306
management, 299
caging wastes, 302
contractural agreements, 326
disposal concerns, 300–303
exhaust stream concerns, 301
liquid waste streams, 301–302
personnel qualifications, 332
recycling, 300
solid wastes, 302
support equipment disposables,
302–303
regulations, 303–304. See also Resource
Conservation and Recovery Act
safety sheets, 327–328
surplus chemicals, 304, 306
transportation manifest, 329–331